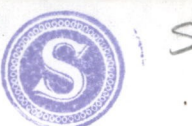

CAROL TURKINGTON

THE
BRAIN
ENCYCLOPEDIA

Checkmark Books™

An imprint of Facts On File, Inc.

THE BRAIN ENCYCLOPEDIA

First paperback printing 1999

Checkmark Books
An imprint of Facts On File, Inc.
11 Penn Plaza
New York NY 10001

Library of Congress Cataloging-in-Publication Data

Turkington, Carol.
  The brain encyclopedia / Carol Turkington.
    p. cm.
  Includes bibliographical references.
  ISBN 0-8160-3169-X (hc)   ISBN 0-8160-3170-3 (pbk)
  1. Brain—Encyclopedia. 2. Neurology—Encyclopedias. I. Title.
  QP376.T87 1996
  612.8′2′03—dc20   95-49503

INTRODUCTION

Swiftly the brain becomes an enchanted loom, where millions of flashing shuttles weave a dissolving pattern—always a meaningful pattern—though never an abiding one.
> —Sir Charles Sherrington (1906),
> (British physiologist)

The body can get along without an appendix or a tonsil and barely notices a missing kidney or gall bladder, but even a momentary bobble can be devastating to the brain, the guardian of the self. Tucked away in its loops and folds is the scent of the sea wind, the taste of grandma's molasses cakes, the image of the beloved.

Up until the last few years, progress in understanding our "enchanted loom" had been agonizingly slow, but scientists are now beginning to understand some of the brain's knottiest puzzles: How does the brain actually *work*? Where does memory reside within the brain? Is our brain separate from, or completely intertwined with, our body? From *acetylcholine* to *white matter*, *The Brain Encyclopedia* takes the reader on a guided tour through the brain, looking at brain diseases and disorders, structure, and function. An extensive glossary explains all terms related to neurology, and there is also a detailed index. Appendixes include extensive listings of self-help organizations related to neurological problems, professional organizations, and governmental groups.

A

abducent nerve Also known as the sixth cranial nerve, this nerve (together with the third and fourth cranial nerves) is responsible for eye movements. It supplies just one muscle of each eye, which is responsible for moving the eye outward. This nerve originates from the abducens nucleus in the PONS (part of the BRAINSTEM) and emerges from the brain right below it. It then extends through the skull, entering the back of the eye socket through a gap between the skull bones.

Because it has such a long way to travel through the skull, this nerve is often injured in fractures along the base of the skull or by a disorder (such as a tumor) that distorts the brain. Damage to this nerve can cause double vision or an eye disorder called *strabismus.*

abscess, brain A collection of pus surrounded and caused by inflamed tissue in or on the brain. Abscesses cause symptoms because of the increase in local pressure and/or local nerve-tract damage. They are most often found on the frontal and temporal lobes of the CEREBRUM in the forebrain.

Brain abscesses are relatively rare today because the widespread use of antibiotics controls many inflections in the early stages. They are fatal in about 10 percent of cases; many of the remaining 90 percent suffer brain dysfunction (such as EPILEPSY).

Causes Except for head injuries, brain abscesses are almost always caused by infection from other areas of the body. About 40 percent of these abscesses are caused by sinus or middle-ear infections; the rest are caused by infection following penetrating brain injury or blood-borne infection. There may be multiple abscesses from blood-borne infections such as endocarditis and some of the immunodeficiency disorders.

Symptoms The most common symptoms are headache, memory problems, drowsiness and vomiting, visual problems, fever, epileptic seizures due to raised local pressure, and local damage to nerve tracts.

Treatment Abscesses are treated with high doses of intravenous antibiotics, but because antibiotics alone may not cure the problem, surgery may be needed to drain or remove the abscess. After the operation, antibiotics are usually given for up to two months. During surgery, a section of the skull is opened to provide access to the abscess and to facilitate drainage. If the abscess has penetrated any area of the skull, some of the affected area may be removed. It is sometimes difficult to locate and remove all traces of the infection, and recovery may be complicated by reinfection. Because many patients experience epilepsy after brain abscesses, anticonvulsant drugs are often administered after removal or drainage of the abscess. (See also CRANIOTOMY.)

Academy of Aphasia A professional organization of neurologists, psychologists, linguists, speech pathologists, and others who specialize in APHASIA (the impairment of language caused by local BRAIN DAMAGE). The academy encourages research and promotes communication among the scientific disciplines that contribute to the understanding of aphasia. Founded in 1962, the group has 189 members and holds an annual convention in October.

acalculia Generalized difficulty in dealing with mathematical concepts.

acetylcholine A common NEUROTRANSMITTER (a chemical messenger) found in the central and peripheral nervous systems. Acetylcholine was the first neurotransmitter discovered by scientists; it was isolated in the 1920s from one of the nerves that regulate heart function.

Acetylcholine is found at all nerve-muscle junctions, as well as many sites in the central nervous system. The actions of acetylcholine are called *cholinergic actions;* those actions are blocked by *anticholinergic* drugs. Acetylcholine is stored in tiny vessels (synaptic vesicles) at the tips of cholinergic axon terminals. After acetylcholine is released and acts on nerve or muscle fibers, it is broken down into choline and acetate by an enzyme called *acetylcholinesterase.* This breakdown of acetylcholine by acetylcholinesterase helps reabsorb choline and acetate back into the releasing neuron.

Acetylcholine is a common neurotransmitter in humans and also in other animals (including insects). Because of this, many insecticides contain substances that interfere with the activity of acetylcholinesterase (the enzyme that destroys acetylcholine). While these insecticides kill pests, they can also poison humans.

Acetylcholine operates as a primary neurotransmitter in brain areas that handle processing of learning and memory, of states of vigilance and awareness. As such, it was no surprise that Alzheimer's disease would be related to acetylcholine dysfunction. In this disease, the region of the brain chiefly responsible for the synthesis of acetylcholine undergoes degeneration.

acoustic nerve   Also known as the auditory nerve, this is part of the VESTIBULOCOCHLEAR NERVE (eighth cranial nerve), the nerve that carries sensory impulses from the cochlea (the part of the inner ear that detects sounds) to the hearing center in the brain, where the impulses are translated as sounds.

acoustic neuroma   A tumor of the cells that surround the auditory nerve, a branch of the VESTIBULOCOCHLEAR NERVE (eighth cranial nerve), which is responsible for balance and hearing. This type of tumor is also known as an eighth-nerve tumor, a neurinoma, or an auditory nerve tumor.

Acoustic neuromas can cause hearing loss on the affected side and are usually slow growing and benign. Although several types of tumors can grow on the auditory nerve, the most common is an acoustic neuroma.

Untreated, the tumor first distorts the eighth cranial nerve and then, as it grows larger, can press on the seventh, fifth, and ninth cranial nerves. Eventually it can grow so large that it protrudes from the canal into the brain behind the mastoid bone and, if untreated, can eventually lead to death. See also Appendix A (Acoustic Neuroma Association).

Cause   The cause is unknown, except for the few associated with NEUROFIBROMATOSIS (hereditary neurologic disorder).

Symptoms   There are no typical symptoms, but people who have inner-ear problems should be evaluated to eliminate the possibility of an acoustic neuroma. Most people with this type of tumor have balance problems, headache, tinnitus (ringing in the ears), facial numbness, and hearing loss in one or both ears.

Diagnosis   Auditory, balance, and hearing tests (including a brainstem auditory-evoked response test and a CAT SCAN).

Treatment   If diagnosed early, the tumor can be removed without damaging the person's hearing, but if detected too late these tumors, while not malignant, can be life threatening. Although the surgical removal of such tumors is complex and delicate, few patients die from the surgery because of modern technology and early detection. Long-term eye problems affect at least half of those who have had an acoustic neuroma removed, in addition to possible taste disturbances, problems with voice or swallowing, and (if the facial nerve has been injured or removed during surgery) some degree of facial paralysis.

With small tumors, it may be possible to save what is left of the patient's hearing, but medium or large tumors have usually destroyed enough of the nerve that the ability to hear cannot be restored through surgery. The particular hearing problems common to people who have had acoustic neuromas include locating the direction of sound, hearing persons who are speaking softly, and understanding speech in a noisy environment.

Acoustic Neuroma Association A support group for those who have had ACOUSTIC NEUROMA (a tumor growing in the inner ear) and those who have had tumors that affect the cranial nerves and nearby brain tissue. The group provides support and encouragement to overcome the effects of these tumors and furnishes information on rehabilitation and the formation of mutual-support self-help groups. The association promotes research, disseminates information, and publishes quarterly newsletters as well as numerous brochures. For address, see Appendix A.

acoustic reflex An important reflex that serves a protective role in the brain. Because of links between the cochlear nerve and the RETICULAR FORMATION (the network of cells in the BRAINSTEM that plays an important role in sleep and arousal), a person will wake up when hearing a loud, unexpected noise.

ACTH See ADRENOCORTICOTROPIC HORMONE.

acute idiopathic polyneuritis The medical name for GUILLAIN-BARRE SYNDROME.

addiction The physiological and psychological dependence on a particular chemical substance produced by the habitual use of a certain drug. Addiction is typically an interaction among personality, environment, biology, and social acceptability. Denied the required dose (or "fix"), a user goes through a period of agonizing withdrawal. Experts are still debating whether the motivation for continual drug abuse springs from a wish to avoid withdrawal or to achieve the drug-related pleasure.

Many types of drugs are abused, including MARIJUANA, AMPHETAMINES, HALLUCINOGENS (such as LSD), TRANQUILIZERS, and ANTIDEPRESSANTS. ALCOHOL and tobacco are probably the substances that have addicted the largest number of people. Most drugs, when abused, carry the risk of dependency.

Currently, the most rapidly addictive substance is COCAINE, especially when it is smoked in the form of crack; the cocaine high is swift, a sudden euphoria that explodes in a rush within 15 seconds of the first puff. Unfortunately, this euphoria is short lived, evaporating within 5 to 15 minutes. The sensation of confidence and clarity can suddenly vanish, leaving the user with an overpowering urge to retain that state again with another "hit."

Not all drugs are *physically* addicting; marijuana and hashish seem to be psychologically addictive. In addition, the psychedelic drugs LSD and mescaline, which interfere with transmitters like SEROTONIN and NORADRENALINE, appear to set off neither a physical nor psychological dependency. Even cocaine, which may create a strong psychological dependency, seems to create only a mild physical dependency.

Surprisingly, even the "hard" drugs such as heroin and cocaine (the OPIATES) don't always result in addiction. On average, only about 10 percent of the people who snort cocaine or shoot heroin will go on to become full-fledged addicts, but the reason why some people become addicted and others don't has never been fully understood. Experts believe that environment and heredity play a part. Because human beings appear to crave stimulation, satisfaction, and pleasure, they are capable of turning to chemicals if a healthy path to these goals is not found.

There is a wide range of addictive drugs. Rapid-acting opiates (including HEROIN, MORPHINE, and meperidine) provide pain relief, contentment, and emotional detachment; long-term effects include weight loss, reduced sex-hormone levels, and physical and psychological dependence. Withdrawal can cause cramps, gooseflesh, and diarrhea.

The NICOTINE in tobacco increases the pulse rate and blood pressure, reduces appetite, and relaxes regular users; long-term use can cause physical and psychological dependence, respiratory disease, and certain cancer risks.

Minor tranquilizers such as the BENZODIAZEPINES reduce emotional responses and alertness and relax muscles; long-term use causes physical and psychological dependence. Withdrawal may cause anxiety and sleep problems.

Amphetamines can cause appetite and sleep loss and increase heart rate and blood pressure; long-term use can lead to malnutrition and psychological dependence. Withdrawal can cause protracted sleep, depression, and increased appetite.

BARBITURATES can reduce tension, enhance sleep, and cause intoxication in high doses; long-term use can cause physical and psychological dependence and lead to sleep disturbances. Withdrawal can cause anxiety, possible DELIRIUM TREMENS, and convulsions.

Alcohol can cause poor coordination, suppressed inhibitions, and slow mental processes. It can produce physical and psychological dependence, the risk of brain, nerve and heart damage, cirrhosis, and certain cancers. Withdrawal can lead to delirium tremens and convulsions.

Marijuana and hashish can cause euphoria and, after long-term use, can lead to loss of drive and impaired learning ability. There are no withdrawal symptoms.

Hallucinogens (LSD, mescaline, and MDMA) causes perceptual distortions and arousal; long-term use can lead to flashbacks and possible brain damage.

adenosine triphosphate (ATP) Called the "universal energy molecule," ATP is created in the mitochondria of the cell with the energy from dietary food. All non-passive cellular activities in the body use the energy released by splitting ATP.

adrenaline Secreted by the adrenal glands, this is both a neurotransmitter and a hormone that readies the body for action. Adrenaline is also known as EPINEPHRINE. The release of adrenaline increases heart rate and blood pressure, and diverts blood flow from the skin and gastrointestinal area to parts of the body where it is needed in times of survival-oriented action.

adrenocorticotropic hormone (ACTH) Also called *corticotropin*, this hormone is produced by the pituitary gland and stimulates the outer layer of the adrenal gland to release various corticosteroid hormones. ACTH is also needed to maintain the adrenal cortex cells. ACTH production is partly controlled by the HYPOTHALAMUS (an area in the center of the brain) and partly by the level of hydrocortisone in the blood. When ACTH levels rise too high, hydrocortisone production is increased, which suppresses the release of ACTH from the pituitary gland. If ACTH levels are too low, the hypothalamus releases its hormones, stimulating the pituitary gland to increase ACTH production.

ACTH levels increase in response to stress, emotion, injury, infection, burns, surgery, and low blood pressure.

Disorders of ACTH include Cushing's syndrome, a pituitary-gland tumor that causes excess ACTH production, which in turn results in an excess of hydrocortisone produced by the adrenal cortex.

aging and the brain Today scientists realize that aging does not necessarily cause an irreversible loss of cells in the cerebral cortex; major cell loss appears to be in the basal forebrain, in the HIPPOCAMPUS and AMYGDALA (site of memory and learning). The loss of these cells, in turn, causes a drop in the production of the neurotransmitter ACETYLCHOLINE, a chemical that is vital to memory and learning. Not surprisingly, ALZHEIMER'S DISEASE patients have markedly low levels of this vital neurotransmitter.

Unfortunately, the hippocampus—probably one of the most important brain structures involved in memory and learning—is highly vulnerable to aging, and up to 5 percent of the nerve cells in the hippocampus evaporate with each decade past middle age. This could add up to a loss of up to 20 percent of total hippocampal nerve cells by the time a person enters the eighth decade of life.

Damage to this area of the brain may be caused by stress hormones such as cortisol, according to researchers at Stanford University and the University of Kentucky. Their rat studies have found that stress-induced increases in cortisol prematurely age the hippocampus. In addition, excessive amounts of FREE RADICALS (toxic form of an element) can also build up as a person ages, damaging the hippocampus.

However, the aging brain can also be negatively affected by a whole host of other factors, such as MALNUTRITION, ALCOHOL, DEPRESSION, and medications (especially the BENZODIAZEPINES used to treat anxiety). In addition, there are a range of organic problems that can occur in the brain itself. Functional brain problems may also be caused by dying neurons or decreased production of neurotransmitters (chemicals like ACETYLCHOLINE that allow brain cells to communicate with each other).

In addition, there are *physical* changes in the aging brain—tissue actually shrinks and the cells become less efficient, according to researchers at the Neuroscience Laboratory of the National Institute of Aging in Bethesda, Maryland. In addition, hereditary problems, environmental toxins, or poor lifestyle choices (smoking, substance abuse, etc.) can accelerate the decline in brain function.

About half of the elderly men and women with severe intellectual impairment have ALZHEIMER'S DISEASE; another fourth suffer from vascular disorders (especially multiple STROKES), and the rest have a variety of problems, including BRAIN TUMORS, abnormal thyroid function, infections, pernicious anemia, adverse drug reactions, and abnormalities in the cerebrospinal fluid (HYDROCEPHALUS). A good diagnosis is important because most of these other disorders can be treated.

Symptoms The chief problem among healthy older people is a decline in their ability to perform several tasks at once or to switch back and forth rapidly between them. While general vocabulary and knowledge about the world often stays sharp through the 70s, memory for names begins to decline as early as age 35. Moreover, the ability to recognize faces and find one's car (spatial ability) has already begun to wane by the time a person enters the 20s. While short-term memory does not usually decline as a person ages, long-term and episodic memory (remembering the time and place something occurred) does deteriorate with age.

While some specific abilities do decline with age, overall brain function remains good through the 70s. In fact, many people in their 60s and 70s score significantly better in verbal skills than young people.

However, brain deterioration may not be inevitable, according to experts at Harvard University. Studies of nursing-home populations controlled for age bias and excess anxiety showed that patients were able to make significant improvements in cognitive ability when given rewards and challenges. Furthermore, physical exercise and mental stimulation can even *improve* mental function in some people as they age. With age, scientists found that a stimulating environment encourages the growth of these dendrites, and a dull environment lowers their number.

The brain often becomes less *effective* as a person ages because of disuse rather than disease, and just as it's possible to strengthen a muscle by lifting weights, it's also possible to challenge the brain to become more efficient. Some scientists believe that by mentally challenging the brain, such as practicing daily mental drills and problem-solving challenges, a person can prevent intellectual breakdown and reverse a decline. Furthermore, engaging in mental activity in early years is related to a lower incidence of Alzheimer's disease.

Researchers believe that after about age 30, most people reach an intellectual plateau which is usually maintained until about age 60; after that, there are small declines, depending on ability and sex. It's not until the 80s that any sort of serious mental slowdown occurs. The capacity to focus on a task or follow an argument remains strong throughout life.

Evidence from animal research suggests that brain stimulation cannot only stop cells from shrinking, but it can also actually *increase* brain cell and dendrite branching. Studies show that rats living in an enriched environment had larger outer brain layers with healthier neurons and more cells responsible for providing food for the neurons, according to scientists at the University of California. Rats kept in a barren cage had smaller brains and apathetic behavior. Some scientists now believe that humans can also improve their brain function or reverse a decline by challenging themselves with active learning or by living in an "enriched" environment. Maybe a person's socioeconomic status can predict mental decline because poverty may go hand-in-hand with an unstimulating environment. Fewer, smaller brain cells is the price a person pays for failing to stimulate the brain.

agnosia A neurological condition, meaning "state of not knowing," in which patients with no sign of sensory problems can't recognize objects, people, or occurrences by using the senses. While the senses are normal, the brain somehow short-circuits the information it receives from the sense organs.

If only one sense is affected, the agnosia may be labeled according to the problem sensory mode, such as "auditory (hearing) agnosia" or "visual (sight) agnosia."

Children with learning disabilities often have partial agnosia that involves visual or auditory skills.

Cause Agnosia is caused by damage to those parts of the brain responsible for the interpretation of the specific sensory information. The most common causes of this type of brain damage are STROKE, HEAD INJURY, or TUMORS in the parietal lobe of the cerebral hemispheres.

Symptoms Agnosia is often restricted to certain types of stimuli. For example, in "facial agnosia," patients *can* recognize a person's voice but not the face. (Some facial agnosics can't even recognize their own faces in a mirror.) *Autopagnosics* can't recognize or localize parts of their own body. There are other types: *visual agnosics* can't identify visual material, even though the person may be able to indicate recognition of it by other means (such as gestures). *Color agnosics* can't recognize colors, despite having normal eyesight—the person is not color blind; it is just that colors have no meaning to him or her.

There are many types of auditory agnosias, including *pure word deafness* (inability to recognize spoken words although the patient can read, write, speak, and react to sounds), and *cortical deafness* (problems in sound discrimination).

Somatosensory agnosics can't recognize objects by shape or size by touching them. Reduplicative paramnesics can't recognize other people and places they know well. A person with this disorder will see a picture and a few minutes later, when seeing the picture again, will say that he or she has seen a similar picture but that it is definitely not the one he or she is now looking at.

agraphia A form of APHASIA, this is the loss or lessened ability to write, although the patient has normal hand- and arm-muscle function. Agraphia is caused by brain damage (usually within the parietal-temporal-occipital association cortex), such as from a brain tumor (see TUMORS, BRAIN) or HEAD INJURY.

Writing requires a complex sequence of mental processes, including word selection, spelling recall, execution of hand movements, and visual agreement that written words match their mental representation. These varied processes apparently take place in a number of connected brain areas; damage to any of them can cause different types and severity of agraphia. Agraphia rarely occurs alone; it often appears with loss of the ability to read (alexia) or a general disturbance in speaking. While there is no specific treatment for agraphia, some of the lost writing skills may eventually return.

See also ALEXIA; APRAXIA; DYSPHASIA.

AIDS and the brain Neurological complications occur in at least 70 percent of patients who are diagnosed with AIDS; at autopsy, 80 to 90 percent are found to have neurological abnormalities. (See also AIDS DEMENTIA COMPLEX.)

Some of these complications occur in early stages of the disease, while others do not show up until late in the course of the condition. They include MENINGITIS, ENCEPHALOPATHY, AIDS dementia complex, cytomegalovirus encephalitis, TOXOPLASMOSIS, STROKE, MYELOPATHY, and PERIPHERAL NEUROPATHIES.

NEUROLOGICAL COMPLICATIONS IN AIDS	
AIDS dementia complex	5–33%
Cryptococcal meningitis	2–10%
Cytomegalovirus poly-radiculomyelopathy	2% (approx.)
Cytomegalovirus encephalitis	< 1% (approx.)
Lymphoma (primary CNS)	2–13%
Meningitis (aseptic)	< 5% (approx.)
Meningitis lymphomatosis	0.5–3%

AIDS dementia complex (ADC) A marked mental deterioration that has been reported in up to 30 percent of AIDS patients. Some AIDS patients in advanced stages of the disease also develop symptoms of an organic mental disorder due to the direct infection of the brain by the human immunodeficiency virus (HIV). Symptoms of ADC include disturbances in thinking, behavior, and motor performance.

Human immunodeficiency virus (HIV) was established as the cause of AIDS in 1983; by 1985, it was understood that it was a type of virus that primarily infects macrophages and leads to chronic disease such as ENCEPHALITIS. Researchers believe that infection of the nervous system occurs in most cases and that it takes place very early—perhaps at the time when the blood first tests positive for the HIV virus—although the infected person may not show symptoms for quite some time. About one fourth of all AIDS patients first seek help when they experience symptoms of the AIDS dementia complex.

The disease was first described in 1986, but the diagnostic criteria for AIDS devised by the U.S. Centers for Disease Control was modified to allow a diagnosis of AIDS solely on the basis of dementia in a person who is HIV-positive, without any evidence of other opportunistic infection or Kaposi's sarcoma.

Dementia is found at increasing rates throughout the course of an AIDS infection—

from about 3 percent at the time AIDS is first diagnosed to 8 to 16 percent of HIV positive outpatients to more than 60 percent in AIDS patients who die; some estimates place the occurrence closer to 90 percent at time of death.

Many neuroscientists believe that the N-methyl-D-aspartate (NMDA) receptor on nerve cells plays a role in AIDS dementia; the receptor triggers nerve-cell death when overexcited by NMDA or by glutamate (see TOXIC ENCEPHALOPATHY). Some experts suspect that HIV may destroy nerve cells indirectly by prompting the overproduction of a brain chemical called *quinolinic acid,* which can cause toxic effects at high levels.

Still, experts point out that most AIDS patients develop dementia despite pentamidine treatment, although they admit that the inhaled form of the drug that is usually given may not reach the brain as efficiently as an injection would. On the other hand, injected pentamidine can cause seizures in some people.

Diagnostic studies have revealed that the brains of people with ADC typically show cortical atrophy and enlarged ventricles.

Symptoms Early symptoms of AIDS dementia include forgetfulness, poor concentration and confusion, movement problems (unsteady gait, leg weakness), apathy, depression, agitation, and mania. Patients become apathetic and lose interest in the environment, becoming socially withdrawn. Motor symptoms include clumsiness, tremors, poor balance, unsteady gait, and slowed movements. Some patients may become overtly psychotic.

Most studies suggest that even if the brain is infected early, cognitive ability remains relatively unimpaired until the later stages of the disease. Although dementia is fairly common in *advanced* stages of AIDS, scientists aren't sure whether people who test positive for HIV but who have no symptoms are already mentally impaired; it is clear that otherwise asymptomatic HIV carriers do not generally exhibit signs of AIDS dementia. Studies have shown that less than one percent of those who are HIV carriers but have no symptoms have AIDS dementia.

Children with AIDS experience a much higher percentage of AIDS dementia. About 60 percent go on to develop the disorder, probably because children better resist opportunistic infections and live long enough to develop dementia.

Course The development and course of ADC have not been clearly defined; its incidence has declined since the introduction of zidovudine (AZT).

Treatment AZT is the best treatment so far for ADC. Able to cross the BLOOD-BRAIN BARRIER, AZT has been associated with a decrease in ADC since it was introduced. Moreover, a drug now taken by most AIDS patients to prevent pneumonia may also protect against AIDS dementia. The widely used drug, pentamidine, can help prevent brain cells from succumbing to the deadly effects of HIV. Preliminary data on dideoxyinosine also suggest that it is effective in improving cognitive deficits in HIV-infected children, but its usefulness in adults is controversial.

alcohol and the brain Alcohol is a central nervous system depressant that in higher concentrations is a NEUROTOXIN; it acts on the brain's RETICULAR FORMATION and spinal cord, depressing brain activity and thus reducing anxiety, tension, and inhibitions. In moderate amounts, alcohol can impart feelings of relaxation and confidence because the alcohol loosens the control exercised by higher brain centers. However, tests show that alcohol also interferes with the brain's activities, slowing reactions; even a few drinks four times a week can affect the brain.

Whether moderate social drinking (no more than one or two drinks per day) *damages* the brain is not clear, but most physicians agree that limited quantities of alcohol do not usually produce nerve-cell damage (unless the person is already an alcoholic).

Chronic drinking and alcoholism can cause a variety of neurological problems, including mental deterioration and muscle damage; alcohol withdrawal can cause minor tremors to DELIRIUM TREMENS (DTs), a potentially fatal syndrome characterized by extreme agitation, hallucinations, and a very high fever. Alcoholism is one of the most serious and prevalent medical problems in the United States; at least 12 to 15 percent of the population may be alcoholics. As many as 70 percent of known alcoholics display neurological abnormalities, according to the National Council on Alcoholism and Drug Dependence, Inc., a nonprofit educational organization.

Blood levels The more alcohol in the bloodstream, the more it impairs concentration and judgment and the more the drinker's false confidence is increased. Excess amounts of alcohol are toxic to the brain, causing possible unconsciousness and even death. Blood alcohol level is determined by the amount of alcohol consumed, whether or not there is food in the stomach, and how physically large the drinker is. A drinker begins to feel less inhibited when the level of alcohol reaches 0.05 percent. When the blood concentration reaches 0.1 percent, the drinker becomes clumsy; in most states, this is considered the legal limit of sobriety. As blood-level content increases, more and more brain control centers are affected. At a blood level above 0.2 percent, the motor area of the brain is significantly depressed and the drinker begins to stagger and become uncoordinated. Emotional centers including the LIMBIC SYSTEM are also affected, leading to unpredictable outbursts.

As the blood level increases, effects become more serious: at 0.3 percent, the drinker is completely confused and may fall into a stupor; anything above 0.4 percent induces coma; and a level of 0.5 percent

depresses activity in the MEDULLA OBLONGATA, the part of the BRAINSTEM that controls breathing. This will lead to death from respiratory failure in two to three hours (lower blood alcohol levels of about 0.4 percent can be fatal if they rise suddenly, such as when a drinker drinks an entire bottle of alcohol in a few minutes).

How alcohol affects the brain Exactly how alcohol affects individual brain cells is not completely understood. Alcohol works on the reticular formation, the part of the brain that plays a major role in attention and awareness, and coordinates information from the sensory systems to the brain's higher centers. It also can impair function of the CEREBELLUM, producing many of the symptoms of cerebellar disease such as slurred speech, jerky gait, and posture and movement problems.

Habitual drinkers experience a tolerance for alcohol so that nerve cells in the brain become less and less responsive to a given amount of alcohol. Paradoxically, however,

EFFECTS OF BLOOD ALCOHOL LEVELS

Percent concentration	Observable effects
.05	Flushed face, euphoria, false confidence
0.1	Disturbed thinking, coordination, irritability, reduced self-control, irresponsible behavior
0.2	Marked confusion, unsteady gait, slurred speech, unpredictable behavior
0.3–0.4	Extreme confusion and disorientation, drowsiness, delayed or incoherent reaction to questions progressing to coma
0.5	Risk of death due to breathing arrest (habitual drinkers may survive such high levels)

after years of drinking, many alcoholics experience a reduced tolerance.

One theory is that long-term alcohol abuse damages the right frontal lobe of the CEREBRAL CORTEX, which is responsible for spatial skills and perception. This could be the reason why verbal skills (controlled mainly by the *left* side of the cortex) are relatively unharmed.

Genetic link Some research suggests that some individuals seem predisposed to become alcoholics; the inherited trait appears to be a decreased reaction to the effects of drinking during the first three to five drinks. Because the person's brain doesn't quickly indicate drunkenness, the drinker consumes more alcohol. Asians and Native Americans are genetically inclined to experience drunkenness earlier and more powerfully than drinkers of other races; it is unclear whether this puts them at higher risk for alcoholism.

Long-term effects Prolonged alcohol abuse can permanently impair brain function, causing visible changes in the brain. For example, the brain actually shrinks in size because the brain cells begin to waste away. CAT SCANS can measure the shrinkage by detecting an *increase* in the size of VENTRICLES, the fluid-filled cavities in the central part of the brain lying beneath the cerebral cortex. The ventricles enlarge because alcoholics have less brain and more empty space. Another measure of brain shrinkage is the size of the sulci—the valleys in the folds of the cortex. As the brain atrophies, the valleys widen.

This wasting of the brain can cause loss of some mental capabilities in nonverbal skills, such as the ability to solve problems involving shapes and space, to reason abstractly, and to perform physical tasks that require eye-hand coordination. On the other hand, often-repeated verbal skills such as vocabulary and word comprehension tend to be retained.

Short-term memory loss is a classic problem among alcohol abusers who have problems remembering new information.

People over age 40 experience the most short-term memory problems after drinking—but even people age 21 to 30 experience some short-term memory loss, according to research at UCLA. Women in particular appear to be more susceptible to the toxic effects of alcohol; women alcoholics seem to experience both verbal and spatial cognitive problems, whereas men only seem to have spatial cognitive problems.

Even social drinkers have memory problems of the same kind, albeit milder, related to the amount of alcohol they drink. Occasional drinkers are less affected than those who drink often.

Not all the damage experienced by alcoholics is caused directly by alcohol, however. The most severe brain condition found in chronic alcoholism is related to vitamin deficiency; in this way, chronic alcohol abuse may lead to WERNICKE'S ENCEPHALOPATHY, a condition characterized by sudden confusion as well as impaired coordination, sensory perception, and REFLEXES. Untreated, this syndrome may lead to coma and death. Administration with large doses of thiamine, a vitamin, can reverse some of these symptoms. If treatment is not begun early enough, Wernicke's encephalopathy can escalate into KORSAKOFF'S SYNDROME, a syndrome characterized by severe amnesia, apathy, and disorientation. While most alcohol-induced memory problems seem to disappear when the person stops drinking, chronic abuse may cause irreversible damage. Most Korsakoff's patients must be institutionalized for life.

Pregnancy Drinking alcohol during pregnancy can be especially harmful to a woman's unborn baby because alcohol readily crosses the placenta, where it can enter the vulnerable developing nervous system of the fetus. Heavy or chronic alcohol abuse by pregnant women can lead to FETAL ALCOHOL SYNDROME, a condition found in infants when alcohol interferes with normal brain development. These infants have abnormally small heads, with a smaller-than-normal brain size, usually with some degree of MENTAL RETARDATION. However, recent research suggests that even light to moderate drinking probably affects the developing fetus. Many authorities advise pregnant women not to drink at all because only a few glasses of alcohol can be harmful if taken during a critical period of fetal brain development, causing slight but measurable mental deficits.

Treatment In addition to the administration of thiamine, the central nervous system effects of alcohol abuse can be reversed in most cases except for the most severe. As soon as an alcoholic stops drinking, brain size begins to increase; both the ventricles and SULCI grow smaller, causing the brain to grow larger. At the same time, performance tests begin to improve. Verbal abilities, if impaired, appear to improve fastest, followed by sensory and motor function. The more complex abilities of short-term memory, visuo-spatial learning, and abstract thinking improve at slower rates. Still, even years after giving up drinking, alcoholics may have some cognitive deficits.

alexia The inability to recognize and name written words, severely interfering with the ability to read; this is caused by damage to the language areas of the brain to a part of the CEREBRUM from STROKE or HEAD INJURY.

See also AGRAPHIA; APHASIA; APRAXIA; BROCA'S AREA; DYSPHASIA; DYSLEXIA; WERNICKE'S AREA.

alpha waves A type of brain wave that occurs when the brain is "at rest" and not receiving sensory input. One of the four main types of brain waves, alpha (together with beta) rhythms are the most often found in healthy waking adults, usually with eyes closed; slower rhythms are found during sleep, in early childhood and during serious illness.

Brain waves are recorded by ELECTROEN-CEPHALOGRAPHY; the alpha waves are in the 8–13 hertz range. According to British researchers in the 1940s, alpha waves may reveal a person's personality based on the type of activity of this wave. Type R (for "responsive") people have alpha rhythms that predominate when their eyes are closed and their minds are relaxed. The waves are blocked when the eyes are open or during mental effort. About two-thirds of all people tested were Type R.

Type P ("persistent") subjects exhibited alpha rhythms with eyes open or closed or when struggling with mental problems. About one-sixth of subjects were type Ps, who seem to perceive by sound or touch much better than by forming visual images.

Type M ("minus") subjects showed no noticeable alpha rhythms at any time, whether or not their minds were busy or at rest or whether their eyes were open or shut. About one-sixth of all adults are type M, who always think in visual images.

ALS Forbes Norris Research Center A clearinghouse for lab and clinical research into neuromuscular diseases, primarily AMYO-TROPHIC LATERAL SCLEROSIS (Lou Gehrig's disease). The center conducts monthly support groups for ALS patients and families in the San Francisco Bay area and sponsors the ALS Research Center at the California Pacific Medical Center in San Francisco. The center also maintains an extensive bank of ALS patient information. Founded in 1981, the center publishes a monthly newsletter. For address, see Appendix A.

Alzheimer's Association A national, nonprofit organization dedicated to research for the prevention, cure, and treatment of ALZHEI-MER'S DISEASE and related disorders and to providing support and assistance to afflicted patients and their families. In 1980, seven independent caregiver groups joined to form the Alzheimer's Disease and Related Disorders Association to help families who endure the financial, physical, and emotional tolls of

Alzheimer's disease. The association has become the nation's leading nonprofit health organization with an annual $30-million budget concerned with the disease. In 1988, the organization changed its name from ADEDA to the Alzheimer's Association.

The goals of the group include research into the cause, prevention, treatment, and cure; education of the public; and information to health-care professionals. The group also helps set up chapters at the local level, advocate for improved public policy and legislation, and provide patient and family service to help present and future victims and caregivers.

Through its national chapter and volunteer network, the association sponsors 1,600 support groups and other services for American's four million patients, families and caregivers. A nationwide 24-hour hotline (800) 272-3900 provides information and referrals to local chapters.

The association publishes *Alzheimer's Association Newsletter* quarterly for 650,000 concerned readers nationwide and produces educational brochures, books, and publications for patients, family members, and professionals.

Through its medical and scientific advisory board, the association promotes and funds research; its Autopsy Assistance Network helps families make the difficult decision about autopsy to confirm the diagnosis of Alzheimer's disease.

In addition to its Chicago headquarters, the association maintains an office in Washington, D.C., to ensure that the needs of patients and families are taken into consideration as legislation and public policy are developed. Each year, the association presents Congress and the President with a National Program to Conquer Alzheimer's Disease.

For more information, contact the Alzheimer's Association (for address, see Appendix A).

Alzheimer's disease A chronic condition characterized by irreversible memory loss, disorientation, speech and balance problems, and decline of the intellect. Alzheimer's disease is the most common form of dementia in which cognitive functions are progressively lost. This fatal disorder affects the cells of the brain, producing intellectual impairment in up to four million Americans who are usually in the sixth decade of life; about 60,000 patients are between 40 and 60. The disease kills about 120,000 Americans each year and is the fourth leading cause of death among the elderly (behind heart disease, cancer, and stroke).

About half of the elderly men and women with severe intellectual impairment have Alzheimer's disease; another fourth suffer from vascular disorders (especially multiple STROKES), and the rest have a variety of problems, including BRAIN TUMOR, abnormal thyroid function, infections, pernicious anemia, adverse drug reactions, and abnormalities in the cerebrospinal fluid. An early diagnosis is important because most of these other disorders can be treated.

Alzheimer's disease, which is the most common of the more than 70 forms of dementia, is characterized by abnormal fibers in the brain that appear under the microscope as a tangle of filaments (neurofibrillary tangles). These tangles were first described in 1906 by German neurologist Alois Alzheimer, M.D., who discovered them after performing an autopsy on the brain of a 51-year-old woman afflicted with dementia. Newer diagnostic techniques indicate there are other brain cell changes common in Alzheimer's disease, including groups of degenerated nerve endings (called plaques) that disrupt the passage of electrochemical signals in the brain. The larger the number of plaques and tangles, the greater the disturbance in intellectual functioning and memory.

Etiology Alzheimer's disease is a disorder of the brain that is linked to a gene pair in susceptible families. Scientists don't know why some people with the gene don't develop the disease, and some do. However, the disease is *not* caused by hardening of the arteries or stress, and it's not contagious. A wide range of causes have been studied, although no clear conclusions have been reached.

Genes The early onset form of the disease has been linked to genes on chromosomes 21 and 14; a cholesterol-processing gene pair called apolipoprotein E-type IV (apo E-IV) has been identified as the carrier of a 90-percent risk of the disease by age 80. This gene is located on chromosome 19; a person may have up to two copies of the gene pair—and the more copies, the higher the risk of contracting Alzheimer's, according to researchers, and the earlier in life individuals are affected. The gene is fairly common; 15 percent of the overall population has one of this gene pair, and one percent has two. But not everyone with apo E-IV will develop the disease.

In recent research, scientists have discovered that apo E promotes the formation of amyloid plaques in the brain. Apo E-IV is the most aggressive stimulator of this plaque formation; apo E-III causes fewer plaques and apo E-II can even slow plaque formation.

But while researchers have made great strides in untangling the mystery, scientists still don't know how to prevent or cure Alzheimer's disease. However, some scientists suspect that an imbalance between different kinds of apo E proteins may cause plaque formation. If Alzheimer's is related to a specific protein imbalance, it may be possible to alter diet or lower the protein that is too high. Researchers believe they will be able to develop a diagnostic tool that could screen for the gene pair, enabling counselors to make judgments about whether a person's likelihood of contracting the disease is high or low, early or late. Researchers cautioned that their conclusions about the gene can be applied only to families where members have late-onset Alzheimer's, the most common form of the disease.

In addition to the apo E-4 cholesterol-processing gene found on chromosome 19 (which must be inherited from both parents in order to produce the disease), British researchers have identified a genetic defect associated with an inherited form of Alzheimer's disease that occurs in only a fraction of Alzheimer's patients.

The defective gene, located on chromosome 21, causes cells to insert a single incorrect amino acid while manufacturing a substance called *amyloid precursor protein* (APP). Family members not affected by the disease and 100 unrelated, normal individuals from the local population lacked the genetic error. DNA analysis of 18 individuals with early-onset Alzheimer's in 16 other families revealed two members of one family bearing the same mutation. The finding adds fuel to the assumption that there are many underlying causes of Alzheimer's disease.

The link between chromosome 21 and Alzheimer's disease was discovered because nearly all Down's syndrome people (with a defect on the same chromosome) who live to their late 30s develop brain degeneration similar to that seen in Alzheimer's disease.

Other studies suggest that the gene for amyloid precursor protein is on chromosome 21, and a few cases of Alzheimer's disease are linked to a defective APP gene.

However, there are also a large number of Alzheimer's disease patients with no family history of the disease; these sporadic cases suggest there must be other factors influencing the development of the disease. In addition to the Alzheimer's gene, there is some evidence that some forms of the disease may be due to a "slow virus;" it's also possible that the disorder is caused by an accumulation of toxic metals in the brain or by the absence of certain kinds of endogenous brain chemicals.

Toxins Research has found accumulated amounts of aluminum within the affected nerve cells of subjects having the classic neurofibrillary tangles of Alzheimer's disease. Other studies have shown high amounts of aluminum, iron and calcium in the brains of Chamorro natives of Guam, who had died of AMYOTROPHIC LATERAL SCLEROSIS or PARKINSONISM-dementia. This population is adversely affected by these two chronic disorders, both of which were previously suspected to be transmitted by a slow-acting virus. But now scientists suspect that there is a link between their environmental deficiency in calcium and magnesium and the excess of aluminum and other metals. The studies are important because of the similarity between parkinsonism-dementia and Alzheimer's disease.

Mercury, selenium, zinc, and other elements have also been studied to see whether there is a link with Alzheimer's disease, but so far no proof has been found.

Other investigations are looking at excitotoxins, chemicals that overstimulate nerve cells to the point of killing them. Some excitotoxins are found in certain food, such as the cycad seed eaten on the island of Guam; others occur naturally within the body. Under certain conditions, the neurotransmitters glutamate and aspartate (contained in the artificial sweetener aspartame) can become toxic to nerve cells.

Chemical abnormality Most brain function depends on messages transmitted from cell to cell by a chemical carrier (or neurotransmitter). Scientists have identified in Alzheimer's patients a striking reduction of up to 90 percent in a brain enzyme called *choline acetyltransferase*. This enzyme is critical in the biosynthesis of acetylcholine. In addition, scientists have found low levels of the neurotransmitter ACETYLCHOLINE important in the formation of memories in the same areas of the brain where plaques and tangles occur.

Some scientists focused on proteins such as beta-amyloid, a major component of neuritic plaques, but more recent research has found these proteins in the brains of healthy subjects—not just those with Alzheimer's disease. Beta-amyloid is a fragment of a normal protein, amyloid precursor protein. Researchers showed that beta-amyloid is used in the cells' ordinary activities and that the levels of the protein in the cerebrospinal fluid of healthy subjects was no different than in the fluid of those with Alzheimer's disease. Before this, scientists thought the protein was present only in the brains of people with Alzheimer's, and they thought the protein caused the massive slaughter of brain cells that characterize the condition. Now scientists wonder if Alzheimer's might be caused by a danagerous mutation of beta-amyloid or an abnormal reaction to normal P-amyloid.

Slow virus Some researchers believe that the disease could be caused by a slow-acting virus that produces symptoms years after a person is exposed. Unlike most viral diseases, however, Alzheimer's disease is not transmissible, and it is not similar to other viral disease patterns. If it is caused by a virus, then it is not a conventionally-recognized one.

There are other rare dementias that are caused by unusual viruses, including CREUTZFELDT-JAKOB DISEASE, KURU, and Gerstmann-Straussler syndrome. Because these dementias have similar brain changes to Alzheimer's disease, scientists hope that studying them may reveal clues about how a slow-acting virus may play a role in brain disease.

Symptoms The disease can affect anyone, and its symptoms vary from patient to patient. In the early stages, the patient notices increasing memory loss that may be selective, often accompanied by some loss of previously well-established memory and a worsening short-term memory. The forgetfulness soon becomes a far more profound memory loss than simply misplacing keys or forgetting a name. If a patient misplaces eyeglasses, that's normal forgetfulness; if he or she can't remember that he or she *wears* glasses, it could be a sign of Alzheimer's. The person may compensate by writing lists or asking others for help. Patients may feel anxious and depressed because of the memory problems, but these symptoms are often unnoticed.

The patient may have a problem with remembering recent events; the patient may neglect to turn off the oven, may recheck to see if jobs are done, and may repeat already-answered questions.

As the disease worsens, the signs become more pronounced. This early forgetfulness gradually evolves into a second stage of severe memory loss (especially for recent events). Patients may remember things that happened long ago, but they can't remember yesterday's dinner menu or what they heard on television. They may become disoriented in time or place and begin to lose their way even in familiar territory. Their concentration and ability to calculate numbers worsens, and they may begin to have trouble finding the right word (dysphasia). The patient's conversation becomes more and more senseless, and judgment begins to be affected.

As their problems deepen, patients begin to experience sudden unpredictable mood changes; personality changes begin to appear as well. As mental ability declines, daily activities become more difficult—and then impossible. Patients can't concentrate, and they begin to forget about bathing, dressing, brushing their teeth, and shaving.

In the third stage, the patient becomes seriously disoriented and confused and may suffer from psychosis, HALLUCINATIONS, and paranoid delusions. Symptoms are usually worse at night. Some people become demanding, unpleasant, and even violent, forgetting everything they ever knew about social behavior. Other patients become docile and helpless; many wander from home and may not be able to find the way back. Others get lost inside their own house.

Patients forget to eat and can't remember where they are or even who they are. They no longer recognize friends or members of their own family.

Eventually, even the most dedicated family members can no longer care for the person, and hospitalization is necessary.

While the symptoms are progressive, there is a great deal of variation in the rate of change from person to person. In some patients, there may be a rapid decline, but more commonly many months pass with little change. In later stages, the patient's immobility may result in pneumonia, bedsores, and feeding problems, shortening the remaining life expectancy by as much as one-half. The disease may last between 3 to 15 years before the patient dies.

AAMI and Alzheimer's There is a difference between age-associated memory impairment (AAMI) and Alzheimer's disease. AAMI may remain unchanged for years, but Alzheimer's disease is progressive, interfering with the normal activities of daily life. In addition, Alzheimer's disease affects more than memory; it affects the ability to use words, compute figures, solve problems, and reason. It results in changes in mood and personality.

Diagnosis Preliminary findings have suggested that it may soon be possible for doctors to screen for Alzheimer's by monitoring pupil dilation after exposure to a chemical commonly used by eye doctors. In tests of the chemical tropicamide, which blocks transmission of the neurotransmitter acetylcholine (deficient in Alzheimer's disease patients), pupils dilate about 23 percent in those with Alzheimer's disease, as compared to about 5 percent for those without the disease—including patients with other types of dementia. Scientists also note that pupils appear to become sensitive to tropicamide very early in Alzheimer's disease.

In addition, with the discovery of the apo E-IV genetic pair in late onset Alzheimer's disease, scientists believe they will be able to screen for the defect and predict with precision who will go on to develop the disease. Otherwise, the only way to make a *definite* diagnosis is by examining brain tissue at autopsy, looking for the characteristic tangles and plaques.

Researchers studied skin cells from 50 subjects and were able to pick out the 15 individuals who had Alzheimer's disease. However, researchers at the National Institute of Neurological Disorders and Stroke in Bethesda, Maryland, caution that tests must verify their findings in many more people before it can be used with confidence. Scientists don't expect any clinical test based on the findings to be available for several years.

As it is now, short of autopsy, the only way a physician can diagnose Alzheimer's is to rule out other diseases. It must be clear that the memory problems are not the result of mild, occasional forgetfulness caused by normal aging. Depression, which can affect memory, must also be ruled out. Any patient suspected of having Alzheimer's disease should have physical, neurological, and psychiatric tests.

If other diseases have been ruled out, a diagnosis of Alzheimer's disease can usually be made based on medical history, mental status and consistent symptoms. An electroencephalogram may show a general slowing of certain brain waves or patterns that may help confirm the presence of Alzheimer's. Periodic neurological exams and psychological testing help evaluate the progress of the disease.

Risk factors   Age is the most clearly established risk factor; most victims of Alzheimer's disease are over 65. Family history is another risk factor; many studies show that those with relatives with Alzheimer's disease are more likely to develop the disease than someone with no such family history. Other potential risk factors include toxins, head injury, and gender.

Treatment   It is imperative that patients be under the care of a physician who can consult with a neurologist. As yet, doctors can neither prevent nor cure Alzheimer's disease, although it's possible to ease some of the symptoms with a new drug, TACRINE, or THA (TETRAHYDROAMINOACRIDINE; brand name: COGNEX), that has recently been FDA-approved. Although tacrine is not a cure for the disease, it is the first drug that has proved to have some effect on the diseases's devastating symptoms. It has been shown to provide small but meaningful improvement in memory and cognitive ability for some patients suffering from mild to moderate Alzheimer's. Studies show that 40 percent of patients with mild cases who took the drug experience a brief slowing of progressive memory loss. Tacrine blocks the function of acetylcholinesterase that normally breaks down acetylcholine in the synaptic cleft, making the neurotransmitter last longer during neurotransmission. Its manufacturer, Warner-Lambert Co. of Morris Plains, New Jersey, began to sell the drug in late 1993 at a cost of about $1,500 a year.

Anti-inflammatory drugs may put off or slow down the development of Alzheimer's, according to a new study of aging twins. At present, there is no way to stop the progressive deterioration of the brain. The anti-inflammatory study adds encouraging data to suggest that inflammation plays some role in the development of the disease. The study found that twins who had used anti-inflammatory drugs regularly for at least one year were four times more likely than twins who hadn't used these drugs to remain healthy or develop the disease later than expected. Doctors warn that this information is still not proven; self-medication of anti-inflammatory drugs can also cause internal bleeding and ulcers.

Most drugs being tested today attempt not to cure but to treat the cognitive symptoms, including memory loss, confusion, and problems in learning, speech, and reasoning. A number of these drugs are being tested in multicenter clinical trials in the United States.

Other drug researchers are excited about a substance called HYPERZINE A, a chemical found in a type of tea brewed with club moss (*Huperzia serrata*) that the Chinese have insisted for hundreds of years improves memory. Chemists at the Mayo Clinic in Jacksonville, Florida, have been studying hyperzine A, a potent and selective acetylcholinesterase inhibitor. Acetylcholinesterase is an enzyme that breaks down acetylcholine, a key chemical messenger in the brain involved in awareness and memory; an acetylcholinesterase inhibitor like hyperzine A blocks acetylcholinesterase. Like the drug tacrine, hyperzine A prevents acetylcholinesterase from breaking down acetylcholine, thus raising synaptic levels of acetylcholine in the brain and possibly improving memory. Researchers say hyperzine A is a more effective, more specific agent than tacrine, but the drug has not been approved by the FDA.

Other treatments target behavioral problems, including anxiety, aggression, wandering, depression, and sleep problems. While no drug has yet been found that will cure the disease, judicious use of tranquilizers can lessen anxiety, agitation, and unpredictable behavior, improve sleeping patterns, and treat depression.

Recent trends in behavioral management are moving away from the use of drugs and focusing on non-drug management, including better environmental design, patient monitoring systems, organized activities, and programs tailored to individual needs. Proper nutrition is very important, although special diets are not usually needed.

Other experimental strategies include the use of certain substances such as an infusion of the protein NERVE GROWTH FACTOR directly into the brain; this protein is found in healthy brains but is deficient in Alzheimer's patients. In animal studies, a catheter is surgically implanted under the skin and scalp, leading into a hole drilled in the skull to allow a catheter tip to enter the brain. The catheter infuses the drug directly into the brain at a set rate from a refillable pump implanted under the skin in the abdomen. The pump is powered by a battery that lasts about two years.

While it's helpful if the patient can continue a daily routine and be encouraged to do a little more than the patient feels can be done, when the condition becomes severe, a special setting with professional staff and full-time care may be required. See also ALZHEIMER'S DISEASE INTERNATIONAL.

Alzheimer's Disease International A support group for health professionals, scientists, caregivers, families of those with ALZHEIMER'S DISEASE, and others concerned with discovering the cause, treatment and cure of Alzheimer's disease and providing support to families affected by the condition. Founded in 1984, the group has 25 members and publishes a quarterly newsletter. For address, see Appendix A.

amblyopia A permanent loss of visual acuity caused by a failure in the link of nerve connections in the visual pathway between the retina and the brain; the eye is functionally sound. If normal vision is to develop during infancy and childhood, it is important that clear, corresponding visual images are formed on both retinas so that compatible nerve impulses pass from the eyes to the brain. If no such images are received, normal vision cannot develop. If images from the two eyes are very different, one will be suppressed to avoid double vision, and normal vision may not develop in one of the eyes.

The primary cause of the failure to develop a normal visual pathway is a squint in very young children, in which only one eye focuses on a selected object while the brain suppresses a different image from the other eye. The problem could also develop as a result of congenital cataracts or severe focusing errors in a young child (such as when one eye is normal and the other has a severe astigmatism that causes a blurry image).

Treatment Amblyopia must be treated as soon as possible; after age eight, it is physiologically too late for the brain to make proper connections in the visual pathway. For amblyopia caused by squinting, the patient must cover the good eye to force the poor eye to function normally. Glasses or surgery to place the deviant eye in the correct position may also be required. Glasses may also help correct severe focusing errors, and congenital cataracts may be removed surgically.

American Academy for Cerebral Palsy and Developmental Medicine

A professional organization of physicians, diplomates of specialty boards, PhDs, and allied healthcare individuals concerned with diagnosis, care, treatment, and research of CEREBRAL PALSY and developmental disorders and with acceptance of the handicaps caused by these conditions. Founded in 1947, the academy has 1,800 members and publishes a biennial newsletter and a monthly journal. For address, see Appendix B.

See also CENTER FOR FAMILY SUPPORT; FEDERATION FOR CHILDREN WITH SPECIAL NEEDS; NATIONAL ASSOCIATION OF DEVELOPMENTAL DISABILITIES COUNCILS; YOUNG ADULT INSTITUTE AND WORKSHOP.

American Academy of Neurological and Orthopaedic Surgeons

A professional organization of neurological and orthopaedic surgeons, neurologists, and professionals in allied medical or surgical specialties. The group provides information about neurological and orthopaedic medicine and surgery and seeks to improve patient care. It maintains the American Board of Neurological and Orthopaedic Medicine and Surgery and the American Board of Medical-Legal Analysis in Medicine and Surgery.

The group maintains an audiovisual library and a complete collection of recordings of scientific meetings since 1977 and operates 40 colleges of experts in individual disciplines related to neurological and orthopaedic surgery and medicine.

The group publishes the quarterly *Journal of Neurological and Orthopaedic Surgery* and holds an annual scientific meeting in Las Vegas. For address, see Appendix B.

American Academy of Neurological Surgery

A professional society for leaders in the field of neurological surgery interested in neurosurgical education. The group, which was founded in 1938 and has 168 members, bestows an award for the best research by a young investigator and holds an annual convention. For address, see Appendix B.

American Academy of Neurology

A professional society of physicians specializing in nerve and nervous system diseases that presents annual research awards, maintains a placement service, and funds research and educational programs. Founded in 1948, the group has 11,500 members and sponsors an annual conference with exhibits and seminars.

The group also publishes a quarterly newsletter, *AAN Governmental Report*; a bimonthly newsletter, *AANews*; the bimonthly placement publication *The Dendrite*; career brochure *Medical Specialty of Neurology*; patient brochure *Neurologist*; monthly scientific journal *Neurology*; handbook for patients *Patient Information Guide for Neurology*. The academy also sponsors an annual conference with exhibits and seminars.

American Academy of Somnology

A professional group for clinicians, researchers, and students who study sleep and sleep disorders. The academy advocates standardization of university programs in somnology and a multidisciplinary approach to the study and treatment of sleep disorders. The academy sponsors the American Board of Somnology, which evaluates qualifications of applicants, administers exams, and confers diplomate status on qualified individuals. Founded in 1986, the academy publishes the annual *Journal of Somnology* and the quarterly *The Somnologist*. For address, see Appendix B.

American Association of Neurological Surgeons A professional organization of neurological surgeons interested in promoting excellence in neurological surgery and its related sciences. The group, which was founded in 1931 and has 3,470 members, funds research and conducts specialized education. It maintains an archives and a 300-volume library and bestows a fellowship.

Its publications include a quarterly bulletin, *American Association of Neurological Surgeons Bulletin*; the monthly *Journal of Neurosurgery*; a quarterly *Neurosurgical Topics*; and a triennial *Self-Assessment in Neurological Surgery*. The group also publishes the *Neurological Topics* book series. It holds an annual convention. For address, see Appendix B.

American Board of Neurological Microsurgery A professional group of neurological microsurgery specialists that promotes scientific advancement and provides educational courses in the field. Its 175 members hold an annual convention. For address, see Appendix B.

American Board of Neurological and Orthopaedic Medicine and Surgery A professional group of physicians proficient in neurological and orthopaedic medicine and surgery who have previous board certification and who have made significant contributions to the field.

Founded in 1977, the group has 500 members and strives to demonstrate expertise and capability in the field of neurological and orthopaedic medicine and surgery through written and oral certification exams. The group also conducts research and educational programs on neuromusculoskeletal disorders of the limbs and spine, and it maintains a library, biographical archives, and a hall of fame. It is allied with the AMERICAN ACADEMY OF NEUROLOGICAL AND ORTHOPAEDIC SURGEONS.

The board publishes a quarterly journal, *American Board of Neurological and Orthopedic Medicine and Surgery Journal* and sponsors an annual scientific congress. For address, see Appendix B.

American Board of Neurological Surgery A certification board that administers exams and certifies physicians who specialize in neurological surgery. The board also tries to help develop adequate training facilities and helps evaluate residencies under consideration by the Accreditation Council on Graduate Medical Education of the American Medical Association. It publishes an annual newsletter for members and sponsors a semiannual board meeting and oral examination. For address, see Appendix B.

American Board of Orthopaedic Microneurosurgery A professional group of orthopaedic microneurosurgeons that seeks to advance scientific knowledge and provide educational opportunities in the field. The board sponsors an annual convention. For address, see Appendix B.

American Epilepsy Society A professional group for physicians and researchers engaged in practice and research in EPILEPSY or closely related fields such as ELECTROENCEPHALOGRAPHY. The society fosters treatment of epilepsy in its biological, clinical, and social phases and promotes better care and treatment of patients. For address, see Appendix B.

American Mental Health Association
Professional group dedicated to increasing
public awareness of the facts and warning
signs of mental illnesses. The group raises
funds to support expanded research into the
causes and cures of mental illness, conducts
programs in public education, and sponsors
Understanding Mental Illness, an educational campaign in conjunction with the Advertising Council, which focuses on raising
the public's awareness of the warning signs
of mental illness and where to turn for help.
Founded in 1983, the group publishes a quarterly report and brochures. For address, see
Appendix A.

American Narcolepsy Association A support group for those suffering from NARCO-
LEPSY, SLEEP APNEA, or both, plus physicians,
researchers, and other interested people. The
association helps to improve through education and information programs, the quality of
life for those who have narcolepsy. The
group also supports and conducts research
on the detection, prevention, treatment, and
cure for these illnesses. It also works to
reduce average time between onset of symptoms and diagnosis and to assist patients
with personal, community, and business
problems arising from their illness. The
group also hopes to improve awareness and
understanding of the syndrome and its treatment within the medical profession. It conducts programs of mutual support and self-
help and operates a grant program for
narcolepsy research.

Founded in 1975, the group has 4,000
members and publishes a quarterly newsletter. For address, see Appendix A.

See also ASSOCIATION OF SLEEP DISORDERS CEN-
TERS; NARCOLEPSY AND CATAPLEXY FOUNDATION OF
AMERICA.

**American Network of Community
Options and Resources** A network for
agencies that provide services and support to

those with MENTAL RETARDATION and other developmental disabilities and to others interested in the field. The network is committed
to enhancing the quality of life for individuals
who have developmental disabilities, with a
direct concern for all living situations. The
group supports each person's need to enhance his or her independence and chosen
lifestyle. The network works with others to
develop a total array of options and resources
necessary for the fulfillment of other human
needs and supports activities to develop standards and guidelines, while also conducting
studies and offering a placement assistance,
workshops, and seminars. Founded in 1970,
the group has 620 members and publishes a
monthly *Executives' Notebook,* a periodic *Legislative Alert,* a monthly newsletter, and a quarterly *Ps & Qs News.* For address, see Appendix A.

See also ASSOCIATION FOR CHILDREN WITH DOWN
SYNDROME; ASSOCIATION FOR CHILDREN WITH RE-
TARDED MENTAL DEVELOPMENT; ASSOCIATION FOR RE-
TARDED CITIZENS; CENTER FOR FAMILY SUPPORT; FED-
ERATION FOR CHILDREN WITH SPECIAL NEEDS; JARC;
MENTAL RETARDATION ASSOCIATION OF AMERICA; NA-
TIONAL ASSOCIATION OF DEVELOPMENTAL DISABILI-
TIES COUNCILS; NATIONAL DOWN SYNDROME CON-
GRESS; NATIONAL DOWN SYNDROME SOCIETY;
PARENTS OF CHILDREN WITH DOWN SYNDROME; PILOT
PARENTS; VOICE OF THE RETARDED; YOUNG ADULT IN-
STITUTE AND WORKSHOP.

American Neurological Association A
professional group of physicians and scientists interested in the form, functioning, and
disorders of the nervous system. Founded in
1875, the group has 960 members and conducts research programs and bestows
awards.

It publishes the monthly *Annals of Neurology* and sponsors an annual conference.
For address, see Appendix B.

American Pain Society A professional
group for health-care professionals interested

in the study of pain to promote the control, management, and understanding of pain through scientific meetings and research. Founded in 1977, the group has 2,500 members and publishes a journal and other periodic publications. For address, see Appendix B.

American Paralysis Association A national support group for spinal-cord-injured patients, their families, and other interested people to encourage and support research aimed at finding a cure for paralysis caused by spinal-cord injury, head injury, or STROKE. The group compiles statistics on spinal cord injuries and operates research seminars. Founded in 1979, the group has 10,000 members and publishes a quarterly newsletter and a bimonthly bulletin. For address, see Appendix A.

American Parkinson Disease Association National support group that works to find the cure for PARKINSON'S DISEASE and to alleviate the suffering of its patients by subsidizing information and referral centers and providing funds for research. The association offers counseling services to patients and their families and maintains 46 information and referral centers. Founded in 1961, the association publishes a quarterly newsletter, an annual report, and a wide variety of informational pamphlets and booklets. For address, see Appendix A.

American Schizophrenia Association A national support group for health professionals, patients, and their families that seeks the cure and prevention of SCHIZOPHRENIA through research into its biochemical and genetic causes. Supports research, seeks to educate the public, and encourages formation of local support groups (Schizophrenic Anonymous). For address, see Appendix A.

American Society for Clinical Evoked Potentials A group of physicians in physical medicine and rehabilitation, neurology,

neurosurgery, ophthalmology, and anesthesiology who gather for the purpose of studying the central nervous system's transmissions and to teach electrodiagnostic reading of evoked potentials, a test of brain response to certain stimuli.

The group, founded in 1981, has 410 members and conducts seminars and workshops, maintains a speakers' bureau, and sponsors an annual convention. For address, see Appendix B.

American Society for Stereotactic and Functional Neurosurgery A professional group for neurosurgeons practicing stereotactic surgery, a technique for inserting delicate instruments in precise areas of the nervous system. The group compiles statistics, maintains a biographical archives, and plans to establish a museum.

Founded in 1968, the group has 200 members and is affiliated with the AMERICAN ASSOCIATION OF NEUROLOGICAL SURGEONS and the CONGRESS OF NEUROLOGICAL SURGEONS.

The group publishes the bimonthly *Stereotactic and Functional Neurosurgery* and holds a biennial scientific meeting and a semiannual congress. For address, see Appendix B.

American Spinal Injury Association A professional organization for health-care professionals who have been trained in the care of spinal paralytic patients. They are either actively engaged in the field and acknowledged to be competent or have made a significant contribution to the advancement of the basic sciences or one of the clinical fields of practice as they are applicable to the treatment of the spine.

The purposes of the association are to develop knowledge and investigation of the causes, cure, and prevention of spinal injury and related trauma; to pursue excellence in patient care; to promote and exchange ideas; to standardize medical terminology in spinal cord injury; to coordinate basic research; to develop teaching material; and to provide specialized training. Founded in 1973, the association has 500 members and publishes a semiannual bulletin and other publications. For address, see Appendix A.

amino acids The fundamental building blocks of protein, this term refers to any of a number of organic compounds containing an amine and a carboxyl group. The body uses amino acids as the basic ore from which to construct not only proteins but NEUROTRANS-MITTERS as well.

Individual amino-acid molecules are linked together by chemical bonds (called PEPTIDE BONDS) to form short chains of peptides called *polypeptides*. In turn, hundreds of these polypeptides are linked together to form a protein molecule. One protein differs from another in the way their amino acids are arranged.

A total of 20 different amino acids make up all the proteins found in the human body; 12 can be made within the body (known as *nonessential amino acids*). The other eight (called the *essential amino acids*) must be obtained from the diet and can't be produced by the body. In addition, there are about 200 other amino acids not found in proteins but which play an important part in chemical reactions within cells.

Animal sources usually provide a wider range of amino acids than do plant sources, so people on a vegetarian diet must be especially careful that their selection of food includes all of the essential amino acids.

Because the amino acids are responsible for producing neurotransmitters, some researchers suggested that boosting the brain's supply of certain amino acids should also increase the production of neurotransmitters, affecting both mood and cognition. Two amino acids have been singled out for particular study: TRYPTOPHAN and TYROSINE.

Some studies have suggested that tryptophan may ease depression and boost effec-tiveness of antidepressants. In addition, several controlled trials have suggested that tyrozine appears to improve alertness and cognitive performance in the face of stress.

On the other hand, increasing the pool of amino acids does not necessarily mean more end-product will be made.

amnesia Loss of the ability to memorize and/or recall stored information. In most cases of amnesia, the patient has problems storing information in long-term memory and/or recalling this information. There are many theories that explain the underlying mechanism of amnesia and many different causes, including brain damage from injury or disease. Anterograde amnesia is the loss of memory for events following trauma; retrograde amnesia is a loss of memory for events preceding the trauma. Some patients experience both types of amnesia.

Amnesia following trauma (such as a concussion) in areas of the brain concerned with memory function is known as *traumatic amnesia*. Degenerative disorders such as ALZHEIMER'S DISEASE or other types of DEMENTIA may also cause amnesia, as can infections such as ENCEPHALITIS or a thiamine deficiency in alcoholics. Amnesia could also be caused by a BRAIN TUMOR, a STROKE or a SUBARACHNOID HEMORRHAGE, or certain types of mental illness for which there is no apparent physical damage.

Transient global amnesia This type of uncommon amnesia refers to an abrupt loss of memory for a few seconds to a few hours without loss of consciousness or other impairment. During the amnesia period, the subject can't store new experiences and suffers a permanent memory gap for the period of time during the amnesic episode. There may also be loss of memory encompassing many years prior to the amnesia attack; this retrograde amnesia gradually disappears, although it leaves a permanent gap in memory that does not usually extend backward more than an hour before onset of the attack. These attacks, which may occur more than once, are believed to be caused by a temporary reduction in blood supply in certain brain areas. Sometimes, they act as a warning sign of an impending stroke.

The attacks, which usually strike healthy, middle-aged patients, may be set off by many things, including sudden temperature changes, stress, overeating, or sexual intercourse. While several toxic substances have been associated with transient global amnesia, it is believed that the attacks are usually caused by a TRANSIENT CEREBRAL ISCHEMIA to regions of the brain involved in memory.

Posthypnotic amnesia Amnesia may also occur after HYPNOSIS either spontaneously or by instruction, making the memory of an hypnotic trance vague and unclear, much the way a person has trouble recalling a dream. If a hypnotized subject is told that he or she will remember nothing after awakening, the subject will experience a much more profound posthypnotic amnesia. However, if the patient is rehypnotized and given a countersuggestion, he or she will awaken and remember everything; therefore, experts believe this phenomenon is clearly psychogenic.

The amnesia may include all the events of the trance state or only selected items—or it may occur in matters unrelated to the trance. Memory for experiences during the hypnotic state may also return (even after a suggestion to forget) if the subject is persistently questioned after awakening. It was this observation that led Sigmund Freud to search for repressed memories in his patients without the use of hypnosis.

Psychogenic amnesia Several types of amnesia belong to a different class of amnesia than those types caused by injury or disease; called *psychogenic amnesia,* they are induced by hypnotic suggestion or occur spontaneously in reaction to acute conflict or stress (usually called *hysterical*). This type of amnesia may also extend to basic knowledge learned in school (such as mathematics), which is never seen in organic amnesia unless there is an accompanying APHASIA or dementia. These types of amnesia are completely reversible, although they have never been fully explained.

In one type of "mixed amnesia," organic factors may also be involved in the development of psychogenic amnesia, and an accurate diagnosis may be difficult. This complex intermingling of a true organic-memory defect with psychogenic factors can prolong or reinforce the memory loss. It is quite common for a brain-damaged person to experience an hysterical reaction in addition to brain problems. For example, one patient who developed a severe amnesia that impaired the formation of new memories after carbon-monoxide poisoning went on to develop an hysterical amnesia that continued to sustain the memory loss.

In psychogenic amnesia, there is no fundamental impairment in the memory process or in the consolidation or retention of information. Instead, the problem lies in *accessing* stored or repressed (usually painful) memories. This inability to recall painful memories is a protection against bringing into consciousness ideas associated with profound loss or fear, rage, or shame.

This type of amnesia usually can be treated successfully by procedures such as hypnosis. A normal, mentally healthy person is assumed to be integrated within a unified personality. But under traumatic conditions, memories can become detached from personal identity, making recall impossible. Modern accounts of hysterical amnesia have been heavily influenced by Sigmund Freud, who attributed the problem to a need to repress information injurious to the ego.

With this theory, the memory produces a defense reaction for the individual's own good. This explains why psychogenic amnesia occurs only in the wake of trauma and is consistent with the high incidence of depression and other psychiatric disorders in those who go on to develop psychogenic memory problems.

There are four types of psychogenic amnesia: localized, selective, generalized, and continuous. Localized amnesia is the failure to recall all the events during a certain period of time, usually the first few hours after a disturbing event. Selective amnesia is the failure to recall some but not all of the events during a certain time period. Generalized amnesia is the inability to recall any events from a person's entire life, and continuous amnesia is the failure to recall events subsequent to a specific time up to and including the present.

amphetamines and the brain Also known as uppers or "pep pills," this group of stimulant drugs facilitate the release of certain NEUROTRANSMITTERS, in particular norepinephrine and dopamine. Amphetamine also blocks the reuptake mechanisms for neurons using these neurotransmitters. Consequently, higher levels of transmitter that remain longer in the synaptic cleft tend to overactivate postsynaptic neurons. This is the cause of the amphetamine "high." Because of this ability, amphetamines are often abused for their stimulant effects. Their manufacture and distribution are governed by the Controlled Substances Act.

The short-term effects of amphetamine use include reduced appetite and increased heart rate and blood pressure. Long-term effects include malnutrition and psychological dependence and psychosis. Withdrawal symptoms range from excessive sleep to large appetite and depression.

amygdala Term for the amygdaloid complex, a group of related nuclei located at the base of the temporal lobe whose primary function may be its responsibility for bringing emotional content to memory. Sensory information from certain cortical areas enters the LIMBIC SYSTEM directly through the amygdala.

Because the amygdala connects to the HIPPOCAMPUS, it has been believed for a long time to play a role in memory. While most now believe the amygdala does not itself process memory, it is believed to be a source of emotions that imbue memory with meaning. For example, the remembrance of a memory or a whole stream of recollection often brings with it a burst of emotion—evidence that the amygdala is most likely involved.

amyotrophic lateral sclerosis (ALS) The most common of the rare MOTOR NEURON DISEASES, also known as *Lou Gehrig's disease*, is characterized by the degeneration of nerves in the brain and spinal cord that control muscular activity.

The diagnosis is confirmed by a measure of muscle electrical activity and muscle biopsy, blood studies, myelography, CT scanning, and MRI.

Symptoms Weakness beginning in hands and arms (and more rarely, legs), together with wasting and quivering of muscles together with stiffness and cramping. Eventually, all limbs are affected equally. There is no loss of sensation, and bladder function remains normal.

Weakness usually spreads to include the muscles involved in breathing and swallowing, leading to death within four years. However, a few people have lived more than 20 years after the diagnosis. The final stages of the disease leave the patient unable to speak, swallow, or move, but the intellect and awareness remain untouched by disease.

Treatment There is no way to slow the nerve degeneration, although physical therapy can improve the disability. Care is usually aimed at relieving discomfort.

Amyotrophic Lateral Sclerosis Association National support group for patients, relatives and friends, health professionals, and professional organizations dedicated to finding the cause, prevention, and cure for AMYOTROPHIC LATERAL SCLEROSIS (ALS). The association offers help and information to patients and families and funds ALS research at major medical institutions. The group also works with other agencies, including the government, to increase their involvement on a priority basis in ALS research. Founded in 1985, the group has 250,000 members and publishes a quarterly newspaper, fact sheets, and pamphlets. For address, see Appendix A.

analgesics See PAINKILLERS.

anencephaly Congenital absence of the brain, top of the skull, and spinal cord; this is an extreme form of SPINA BIFIDA. Most infants born with this condition are stillborn or live only a few hours after birth. This birth defect is detectable early in pregnancy by measurement of alpha-fetoprotein, by ultrasound scanning, and by amniocentesis. If anencephaly is detected, the parents may want to consider termination of the pregnancy.

Anencephaly occurs in about 5 out of every 1,000 pregnancies, but only in about one-third does the pregnancy continue to term. For more information, see SPINA BIFIDA ASSOCIATION OF AMERICA (for address, see Appendix A).

Causes The lack of brain development is caused by a failure in the development of the NEURAL TUBE, the nerve tissue in the embryo that eventually develops into the spinal cord and brain. While doctors don't know why this occurs, cases have been linked to low levels of folic acid in the mother's diet. There may also be a genetic component to the problem. Maldevelopment of the neural tube may also cause spina bifida or HYDROCEPHALUS. Collectively, these birth defects are known as NEURAL TUBE DEFECTS and are assumed to have similar causes.

aneurysm, brain Ballooning of an artery leading to the brain due to pressure of blood

flowing through a weakened area. The weakening may be caused by disease, injury, or a defective artery wall. A cerebral aneurysm (or "berry" aneurysm) often occurs as a swelling where the arteries branch at the brain's base, which is usually caused by a congenital weakness.

Pressure from the aneurysm may cause a wide range of symptoms (see below). If the arteries rupture, they may cause a fatal blood loss or severe damage to the local brain tissue.

CAT or MRI SCANS can provide critical information about this type of aneurysm.

Causes There are several reasons why an aneurysm would form in a blood vessel. First, the muscular middle layer of an artery might have a congenital weakness, and normal blood pressure can cause a ballooning at the weak point. Aneurysms of smaller vessels may occur in blood poisoning as a result of local infection on the artery wall.

Symptoms Cerebral aneurysms may last for many years without causing any symptoms, but because they are located in the brain, they are extremely dangerous. Sudden enlargement or bursting of an aneurysm in the brain will produce immediate signs much like those of a stroke—dilated pupils, drooping eyelid, rigid neck, severe headache, and unconsciousness.

Treatment If a cerebral aneurysm causes symptoms, surgery is recommended if the patient is otherwise healthy enough to withstand the procedure and the aneurysm is in an accessible location. Drugs may also lower cerebral blood pressure.

angiography A type of diagnostic technique that enables blood vessels to be seen on X-ray film after a deep artery has been injected with a contrast medium.

The procedure can detect brain tumors (see TUMORS, BRAIN) and help the surgeon see the pattern of blood vessels and the amount of blood that is feeding a tumor. By detecting a cerebral blood vessel with an unnatural appearance, an angiogram can help detect diseases that affect cerebral blood flow. *Carotid angiography* sometimes is performed on patients suffering from TRANSIENT ISCHEMIC ATTACKS (brief symptoms of stroke lasting less than 24 hours) to see whether there is a block or a narrowing in one of the carotid arteries in the neck supplying blood to the brain. *Cerebral angiography* can demonstrate the presence of an aneurysm within the brain or reveal a brain tumor before surgery.

Technique First, contrast dye is usually injected into the vessel to be examined through a fine catheter inserted into the carotid artery deep in the neck. Then, skin and tissues around the artery are numbed with local anesthetic, followed by a needle inserted through the skin into the artery; a long thin wire with a soft tip is inserted through the needle, the needle is removed, and the catheter is then threaded over the wire into the blood vessel. Using an X ray for guidance, the tip of the catheter is guided into the vessel to be examined, and contrast dye is injected so that a rapid sequence of X rays are taken to study the flow of dye along the vessels.

Risks There are some risks involved with this procedure. While it is possible to experience an allergic reaction to the dye, new contrast agents have lowered the risk of a severe reaction to less than one in 80,000 exams. Blood vessels may be damaged at the puncture site, anywhere along the vessel during passage of the catheter, or at the dye injection site.

Techniques have been modified recently to allow for treatment in addition to diagnosis; for example, small balloons can be inflated at the tip of a catheter to expand a narrowed or blocked segment of artery, called *balloon angioplasty*. Other material can be injected to reduce or shunt blood supply away from a tumor, and medication to control bleeding or treat tumors can be infused directly into the local blood supply targeted at individual organs.

aniracetam   One of a class of NOOTROPIC drugs that some studies suggest may be capable of improving cognitive performance on a number of intelligence and memory tests. Its chemical structure is similar to PIRACETAM, a drug being investigated in the treatment of ALZHEIMER'S DISEASE.

Aniracetam's mechanism of action is unknown, although it does not seem to act directly upon the CATECHOLAMINE, SEROTONIN, or ACETYLCHOLINE NEUROTRANSMITTER systems. It appears to be a general enhancer of transmitter release for a number of transmitter systems.

Aniracetam is not approved for distribution in any country. Other names for aniracetam include Draganon, RO 13-5057, and Sarpul.

anomia   A type of APHASIA involving the inability to verbalize the names of people, objects, and places. It appears to relate to speech output, since patients usually have no problem comprehending when the object is named for them.

anoxia   The complete disruption of oxygen supply to a given cell. This loss of oxygen causes a disruption of cell metabolism and can be fatal to the cell unless it is corrected within a few minutes. Anoxia refers to oxygen deprivation, as opposed to ischemia, which produces a loss of oxygen and other blood constituents, such as glucose. See also HYPOXIA.

anterior commissure   A collection of nerve cells that connects the brain's two hemispheres. It is smaller and appeared earlier in evolution than the CORPUS CALLOSUM. Recent research has suggested that in men, this part of the brain is smaller than in women, even though men's brains are generally larger than women's brains. The larger commissure in women may help explain, at least in part, why the two hemispheres of the female brain seem to work together on activities ranging from language to emotional responses.

See also CEREBRAL COMMISSURE.

anterior communicating artery A short artery located in the FOREBRAIN that connects the two arteries in the front of each hemisphere. Aneurysms often occur along this artery, which can cause a type of AMNESIA when the aneurysm bursts, damaging the forebrain.

See also ANEURYSM, BRAIN; ANTERIOR COMMUNICATING ARTERY.

anticholinergics An agent that disrupts acetylcholine transmission by blocking cholinergic receptors, preventing acetylcholine release or completely depleting cholinergic neurons of acetylcholine.

anticoagulant drugs and the brain This group of drugs prevents abnormal blood clotting and is used to prevent and treat STROKE or TRANSIENT ISCHEMIC ATTACKS. If the drugs are given by injection, they begin to work within a few hours; those given by mouth work within a day. They increase the effect of an enzyme that blocks the activity of coagulation factors that are needed for blood to clot.

By interfering with the blood-clotting mechanism, these drugs can prevent an abnormal blood clot from forming; if a clot already exists, the drugs can stop it from growing larger and reduce the risk of a piece of it breaking off (embolus) and blocking another blood vessel. Unlike thrombolytic drugs, these drugs do not dissolve clots that already exist.

anticonvulsant drugs and the brain This group of drugs is used to prevent SEIZURES or to interrupt a seizure taking place by inhibiting the excess electrical activity in the brain and blocking its spread. (See also EPILEPSY). Anticonvulsants include carbamazepine, clonazepam, diazepam, ethosuximide, phenobarbital, phenytoin, primidone, and valproic acid.

The choice of drug is determined by the type of seizure; in long-term seizure prevention, more than one type of drug may be needed.

Adverse effects include reduced concentration, memory problems, poor coordination, and fatigue.

antidepressant drugs and the brain Antidepressants appear to correct a chemical imbalance or dysfunction in the brains of depressed people by boosting the level of NEUROTRANSMITTERS that may be too low in depressed people. Each of the major classes of antidepressants—MONOAMINE OXIDASE (MAO) INHIBITORS, TRICYCLICS and SEROTONIN inhibitors—affect different neurotransmitter systems in different ways.

Most of these drugs usually take at least 10 days before they begin to work and up to two months before they are fully effective; they all carry some type of side effects of varying intensity.

The complex array of various brain chemicals and processes that influence depression tend to differ from one patient to the next; because there's no foolproof way to identify what's causing depression, prescribing antidepressants may be a trial-and-error process until the right one is found.

For many people, the first antidepressant is often not the *right* antidepressant. In fact, only a little more than half of all patients who are given antidepressants find relief with their first prescription. No one is quite sure how or why antidepressants work, and no one can predict who will respond to which drug. The best a physician can do is to look at a person's symptoms and try to match those symptoms with an antidepressant.

There is no one miracle antidepressant that works better than any other, all the time, for everybody. Because depression itself is a complex disease with many causes, doctors must choose among a wide range of antidepressants that work on different brain systems and affect different processes.

Tricyclic antidepressants are a class of traditional drugs that treat depression by boosting the level of several different neurotransmitters (NOREPINEPHRINE, EPINEPHRINE, serotonin, and DOPAMINE) by blocking their reabsorption. *MAO inhibitors* destroy enzymes responsible for breaking down monoamine neurotransmitters, boosting the neurotransmitter levels. In general, MAOIs are used to treat those who don't respond to tricyclics. Some of the newest antidepressants (called *selective serotonin reuptake inhibitors*, including Prozac) interfere with the reuptake of one specific neurotransmitter (serotonin).

Antidepressants include the tricyclics amitriptyline, amoxapine, clomipramine, desipramine, doxepin, imipramine, nortriptyline and protriptyline; the tetracyclic maprotiline (Ludiomil); monaamine oxidase inhibitors (MAOIs) isocarboxazid (Marplan), phenelzine (Nardil) and tranylcypromine; the selective serotonin reuptake inhibitors (SSRIs) fluoxetine, paroxetine, and sertraline; and the structurally unrelated compounds bupropion, venlafaxine and trazodone. LITHIUM is another antidepressant used to treat manic depression.

Adverse effects Side effects from antidepressants generally fall into three categories: Sedation; dry mouth, blurry vision, constipation, urinary problems, increased heart rate, and memory problems; and dizziness on standing up (orthostatic hypotension). Drugs that block norepinephrine uptake can produce rapid heartbeat, tremor, and sexual problems (loss of interest or inability to reach orgasm). Those that interfere with dopamine (such as Wellbutrin and Asendin) may produce movement disorders and endocrine system changes. Blocking serotonin may create stomach problems, insomnia, and anxiety.

Those that work on the other side of the synapse, blocking receptors that pick up neurotransmitters, have other side effects, depending on which receptors are affected. Blocking histamine H1 receptors produces weight gain and sedation; muscarinic receptor blockade causes dry mouth, constipation, blurry vision, and memory problems.

This is why a tricyclic such as amitriptyline (Elavil) causes so many side effects—it blocks the absorption of both norepinephrine and serotonin, plus four different receptors (Alpha$_1$, Dopamine D$_2$, Histamine H$_1$, and muscarinic).

Each drug has a profile of its own particular side effects. *Tricyclics* often cause dry mouth, constipation, sedation, nervousness, weight gain, and diminished sex drive. *MAOIs* interact with certain foods and other medications to produce potentially fatal high blood pressure. Newer antidepressants like the *SSRIs* (such as Prozac, Paxil, and Zoloft) produce fewer side effects than MAOIs or tricyclics because they affect fewer brain pathways, but nausea and headache may occur.

Still, even though a drug is characterized by certain side effects, it doesn't mean a patient will experience any of them. In addition, many antidepressants can be taken before bed so that the side effects will occur during sleep. If a bedtime dose makes a patient too sleepy the next morning, a dose at dinner may be a better idea. A physician can work with a person's schedule to find the dosage timetable that works best.

Many antidepressants lower sex drive; they might cause impotence or interfere in orgasm. These side effects an be eliminated by adding another drug or changing the antidepressant.

antiemetic drugs A group of drugs used to treat nausea and vomiting; many work by reducing nerve activity at the base of the brain, suppressing the vomiting reflex. (Antihistamine drugs and anticholinergic drugs also reduce the vomiting associated with vertigo by suppressing nerve activity in the balance center in the inner ear. Some antiemetics cause drowsiness, and some should not be taken during pregnancy because they may cause birth defects.

antioxidant A substance that chemically neutralizes FREE RADICALS (potentially harmful, highly-charged atoms on molecules). The most common free radical is a species of oxygen. In the brain, it can chemically interact with lipids (main component of a cell wall), harming the neuron. New research suggests that antioxidants can neutralize free radicals *before* they begin to damage the brain's cells.

While a certain amount of free radicals are necessary to maintain proper body function, high levels are toxic to brain (and body) cells. Each day, the body generates thousands upon thousands of these free radicals in response to ultraviolet (UV) light, smoke, or pollution. Once activated, they destroy the cells in the brain and elsewhere in the body.

Some of the most common of the antioxidants include vitamins C (found in citrus fruits) and E (found in eggs, butter, and vegetable oil).

antipsychotic drugs A group of drugs used to treat psychoses (mental disorders involving loss of contact with reality) that block the action of certain NEUROTRANSMITTERS in the brain. These drugs are especially helpful in the treatment of SCHIZOPHRENIA and MANIC-DEPRESSIVE ILLNESS and are also used to calm or sedate patients with other mental disorders (such as DEMENTIA). The antipsychotic drugs include the phenothiazines (such as chlorpromazine, fluphenazine, perphenazine, thioridazine, and trifluoperazine) and various other medications including haloperidol, thiothixene, or LITHIUM, which is used specifically to treat the symptoms of mania.

Most antipsychotics block the action of DOPAMINE, a neurotransmitter found in the brain. Excess dopamine activity has been associated with many forms of psychoses. Lithium may control symptoms of mania by reducing activity in certain nerve impulse transmitters (SEROTONIN and NOREPINEPHRINE) that influence emotional status and behavior.

Adverse effects While these drugs have been helpful in controlling irrational thinking, aggressive behavior, and HYPERACTIVITY, serious side effects have appeared with increasing prominence. Especially troublesome is TARDIVE DYSKINESIA, which began to appear in large numbers of people during the 1970s. This movement disorder is caused by high doses of neuroleptic drugs for more than six months and appears primarily in adults and the elderly, although children can also be affected. Certain areas of the body are especially affected, including lips, eyes, jaw, arms, legs, and trunk; movements are usually involuntary and irregular and may be confused with PARKINSONISM (a disorder with symptoms similar to those of PARKINSON'S DISEASE). Protruding tongue, lip and facial contortions with eye blinks and unplanned opening of the jaw are common. Slow, writhing movements and rapid, jerky expressions are also found, together with a rocking movement of the trunk. In some adults, the condition is irreversible.

Most of the antipsychotics also can cause drowsiness or lethargy; other possible side effects include dry mouth, blurry vision, and urinary problems.

anxiety An unpleasant emotional state ranging from mild discomfort to intense fear that some scientists believe may be the result of an elevated level of arousal in the CENTRAL NERVOUS SYSTEM. This excess arousal would lead a person to react more excitedly and adapt more slowly to events surrounding him or her.

While a certain amount of anxiety is normal, it can become a symptom when the anxious feelings interfere with normal daily activities.

Symptoms The most common symptoms of anxiety center around the chest, including palpitations (more forceful, irregular heartbeat), throbbing or stabbing pains, air hunger (inability to take in enough air), feelings of tightness in the chest, and a tendency to hyperventilate (sigh or overbreathe).

Other symptoms include headaches, neck spasms, back pain, and an inability to relax, together with restlessness, tremors, and sense of tiredness. The symptoms of anxiety may include a feeling of impending doom in the absence of any particular threat.

Stomach symptoms include dry mouth, feelings of distention, diarrhea, nausea, appetite changes, swallowing problems, and constant belching.

Treatment Effective treatment may include reassurance, counseling, and therapy, together with antianxiety drugs (such as the BENZODIAZEPINES).

aphasia A neurological condition in which language comprehension or expression is disturbed due to brain dysfunction, affecting the ability to speak and write and/or the ability to comprehend and read the written word. *Aphasia* is a complete absence of these skills, while *dysphasia* refers to a disturbance in these abilities. A STROKE or a HEAD INJURY are the most common causes of brain damage leading to aphasia.

The speech problems caused by brain damage are different from speech problems caused by dysfuntion in other parts of the body. Related disabilities with aphasia include word blindness (ALEXIA) or writing problems (AGRAPHIA).

Language functions within the brain are situated in the dominant cerebral hemisphere, especially in the Broca's and Wernicke's areas, and in the pathways that connect the two. Damage in this area is the most common cause of aphasia. A patient with damage to BROCA'S AREA will experience problems in expressing language; speech is labored, slow, and dysrhythmic. However, the few words that are uttered are meaningful. A patient with a damaged WERNICKE'S AREA will experience problems in comprehending language; speech is fluent, but because of the comprehension problems, the meaning is disturbed. The patient will have problems choosing the right word or the correct grammatical form; writing is affected, and spoken or written commands may not be understood.

In *global aphasia*, the patient has an almost or complete inability to speak, write, or understand spoken or written words, usually with widespread damage to the dominant cerebral hemisphere. Patients with *nominal aphasia* have problems naming objects or finding words, although the person may be able to choose the correct name from several offered. This condition may be caused by general cerebral dysfunction or damage to a specific language area. In *developmental aphasia*, the problem is caused by delayed development of the central nervous system. (For more information about aphasia, contact the National Institute of Neurological Disorders and Stroke; see Appendix A for address)

Treatment While aphasia may improve after a stroke or head injury, the more severe the aphasia, the less chance for improvement. Speech therapy is the primary treatment.

apnea A prolonged cessation of breathing that can be caused by a brainstem damage from STROKE, TRANSIENT ISCHEMIC ATTACK, or HEAD INJURY.

Breathing is an automatic process that is controlled by the respiratory center in the brainstem; these breathing centers send nerve impulses to the muscles of the chestand diaphragm that regulate lung expansion and deflation.

apoplexy An outdated term for STROKE. Symptoms include sudden loss of consciousness, paralysis, or loss of sensation. The usual cause of apoplexy is the rupture of a brain artery or blockage by a clot.

appestat Outdated term referring to the region of the brain within the HYPOTHALAMUS that controls food intake. It is believed that appetite suppressants probably decrease the sense of hunger by altering the chemical characteristics in this area. Stimulating the appestat with electrodes provokes overeating in satiated lab animals.

appetite The desire for food that can be a pleasant sensation in anticipation of eating (as compared to HUNGER, an unpleasant feeling triggered by a physiological need for food). A person's appetite is regulated by two parts of the brain—the HYPOTHALAMUS and the CEREBRAL CORTEX—and is a sensation learned by enjoying a variety of food that smells and tastes good. When combined with hunger, it can provide the body with enough foods to maintain health.

How hungry a person feels at any one time is dependent on the amount of glucose circulating in the blood, which is monitored in the brain. Temporary appetite loss (known medically as anorexia) can be caused by a range of illnesses or minor emotional upsets. A more chronic loss of appetite may be the sign of a more serious illness or mental disorder. Physical causes of loss of appetite could include STROKE, BRAIN TUMOR, or brain injury causing damage to the hypothalamus or cerebral cortex. Other possible physical problems linked to appetite loss include stomach problems, gastric ulcers, or liver disorders (such as hepatitis).

In addition, some youngsters between ages two and four may refuse food; this is usually considered to be a normal phase of child development (if there are no other symptoms).

Under normal conditions, healthy people can go hungry for a day or two without causing harm to the brain, as long as plenty of fluids are consumed.

appetite stimulants Although a variety of drugs have been prescribed (including alcohol and iron-containing elixirs), there are no known drugs that safely and effectively stimulate the APPETITE.

See also APPETITE SUPPRESSANTS; HUNGER.

appetite suppressants A group of drugs that suppress the APPETITE, probably by affecting the HYPOTHALAMUS, the part of the brain that controls the desire to eat. Common appetite suppressants include diethylpropion, fenfluramine, mazindol, phenmetrazine, phentermine, and phenylpropanolamine.

Side effects Common side effects include dry mouth, insomnia, dizziness, palpitations, and restlessness. Taking an appetite suppressant for more than six weeks may lead to dependence; however, newer drugs are less addictive than the amphetamines that used to be prescribed for appetite control.

Taking appetite suppressants with alcohol may cause increased sedation; taking them with CAFFEINE may cause excessive stimulation. Taken with food or drinks containing tyramine (such as Chianti, robust red wines, vermouth, ale, or beer) can cause an increase in blood pressure.

See also APPETITE STIMULANTS; HUNGER.

apraxia The inability to make purposeful movements despite normal muscles and coordination because of nerve tract damage within the CORTEX (the main mass of the brain). People with apraxia usually know what they want to do, but they seem to be unable to remember the sequence of actions necessary to make the movement. The cortical damage may be caused by HEAD INJURY, infection, STROKE, or brain tumor that results in nerve tract damage within areas of the cortex responsible for translating the idea for a movement into the movement itself.

There are several different types of apraxia, depending on the part of the brain that has been damaged. A person who can't carry out a spoken command to make a particular movement but who can unconsciously make that movement has *ideomotor apraxia*. *Agraphia* (writing problems) and *expressive aphasia* (severe speaking problems) are both special forms of apraxia.

Treatment Recovery from head injury or stroke varies widely from one patient to the next; degree of recovery often depends on severity of the initial injury. Even in the best of situations, however, there is usually some deficit that remains, and it may require considerable effort for the patient to relearn the lost skill.

aprosodia A condition caused by damage to certain sections of the right brain hemisphere in which speech can become flat and emotionless or in which the emotional qualities of speech and gestures are not completely comprehended or executed.

arachnoid membrane The middle of the three layers (MENINGES) of connective tissue surrounding and protecting the brain and the spinal cord.

arachnoiditis A fairly rare condition characterized by chronic inflammation and thickening of the ARACHNOID MEMBRANE that may develop for several years after MENINGITIS or bleeding beneath the arachnoid. It may also be caused by a variety of diseases, such as SYPHILIS, from head injury, or errors in diagnostic procedures such as MYELOGRAPHY. Usually, however, no cause is ever found.

Although symptoms vary with the severity of the disorder, they can include epileptic seizures, headache, blindness, or spastic paralysis. There is no treatment.

archicortex Older region of the CEREBRAL CORTEX that includes the LIMBIC SYSTEM, although usually refers to the HIPPOCAMPUS only.

Aretaeus of Cappadocia (A.D. 81?–138) This Greek physician from Cappadocia made the distinction between mental and nervous diseases and described the characteristics of EPILEPSY. He led a revival of the teachings of HIPPOCRATES and is believed to be second only to Hippocrates in his keen observational abilities. He adhered to the pneumatic school of medicine, believing that health was maintained by "vital air." Pneumatists felt that an imbalance of the humors (blood, phlegm, choler, and melancholy) disturbed the pneuma (breathing), which is characterized by an abnormal pulse. Actually, however, Aretaeus practiced the methods of several different schools of medical thought.

His contributions were forgotten until the discovery of two of his manuscripts in 1554 that described pleurisy, diphtheria, tetanus, pneumonia, asthma, and epilepsy. He gave diabetes its name and gave the earliest clear description of that disease.

See also BRAIN IN HISTORY.

Arnold-Chiari malformation A congenital disorder characterized by a distortion of the base of the skull; the lower BRAINSTEM and parts of the CEREBELLUM protrude through the opening for the spinal cord at the base of the skull. This condition is commonly associated with NEURAL TUBE DEFECTS and HYDROCEPHALUS.

arteriogram Another term for angiogram. See ANGIOGRAPHY.

arteriography, cerebral Also known as carotid artery angiography, this is an X-RAY examination of an artery that has been outlined by the injection of a radiopaque contrast medium used to detect diseases of the vascular system, such as carotid artery disease or aneurysms. There are two types of arteriography: *digital arterial angiography* and *magnetic resonance angiography*. Digital arterial angiography allows computer-enhanced views of the carotid arteries, but it was not used as often in the past to evaluate carotid disease. Magnetic resonance angiography is being used more often and may replace conventional angiography in the future.

ascending reticular activating system Diffuse and complex net of cells in the BRAINSTEM concerned with attention, sleep, and wakefulness. It is called "ascending" because of its widespread flow of information into the neocortex.

association areas Areas in the NEOCORTEX that are not concerned with primary sensory processing but that have a secondary role in integrating sensory information with other brain systems. Many scientists suspect that these areas play a large role in thinking and memory.

Association for Brain Tumor Research A volunteer organization dedicated to funding research that will lead to improved treatment for patients with brain tumors, the group was founded in 1973 by two Chicago families who lost young daughters to brain tumors. The group raises and grants funds for specific brain tumor research projects, and supports fellowships for promising medical investigators. It also provides information for patients and their families, offering a range of booklets and brochures to provide basic information about different types of tumors, methods of treatment, how to cope, how to deal with a child who has a brain tumor, etc.

The association also provides computerized listings of major research and treatment centers as well as information about the closest brain tumor support groups; in addition, trained volunteers are available by telephone to offer reassurance and understanding. For address, see Appendix A.

Association for Children and Adults with Learning Disabilities Educates and disseminates information on special programs in schools and camps, offers referral services, and publishes materials. For address, see Appendix A.

Association for Children with Down Syndrome A national support group for parents of children with DOWN SYNDROME and for health professionals. The association acts as a resource and information center about Down syndrome and works to maintain contact with the medical community and with parents of children with Down syndrome. The organization seeks to ease children into the mainstream through social, recreational, and educational programs, encourages parental advocacy, seeks to educate the public, conducts research, and publishes materials. The association also administers infant, toddler, and preschool programs in New York and offers recreational and socialization programs and support groups for children over age 5 and young adults. Founded in 1966, the association has 1,000 members and publishes a bimonthly newsletter and an annual journal. For address, see Appendix A.

Association for Children with Retarded Mental Development A national support group for professionals, parents, siblings, and others interested in MENTALLY RETARDED and developmentally disabled children and adults. Membership is centered in the New York City area. The group offers professionally supervised programs for developmentally disabled young adults, including vocational rehabilitation centers, dual-diagnosis programs, job placement, rehabilitation workshops, social centers, activities for daily living, day treatment, day training, supported work, and family support programs. The association also operates the Lubin Center for Independent Living, an apartment complex for gainfully employed adults capable of independent living, and operates community residences, supportive apartments, and intermediate care facilities.

In addition, the association acts as an advocate for the developmentally disabled in all phases of life in the city of New York. It sponsors conferences and training regarding developmental disability. Founded in 1951, the group has 5,000 members and publishes a quarterly newsletter and several brochures. For address, see Appendix A.

See also AMERICAN NETWORK OF COMMUNITY OPTIONS AND RESOURCES; THE ASSOCIATION OF RETARDED CITIZENS, THE ASSOCIATION FOR CHILDREN WITH DOWN SYNDROME; CENTER FOR FAMILY SUPPORT; FEDERATION FOR CHILDREN WITH SPECIAL NEEDS; JARC; MENTAL RETARDATION ASSOCIATION OF AMERICA; NATIONAL ASSOCIATION OF DEVELOPMENTAL DISABILITIES COUNCILS; NATIONAL DOWN SYNDROME CONGRESS; NATIONAL DOWN SYNDROME SOCIETY; PARENTS OF CHILDREN WITH DOWN SYNDROME; PILOT PARENTS; VOICE OF THE RETARDED; YOUNG ADULT INSTITUTE AND WORKSHOP.

Association for Retarded Citizens (ARC)

A national support group for parents, professionals, and others interested in individuals with MENTAL RETARDATION. The group works on the local, state, and national levels to promote services, research, public understanding, and legislation for mentally retarded persons and their families. Founded in 1950, the group has 140,000 members and publishes a semimonthly *ARC Government Report,* a monthly *The ARC NOW,* and the bimonthly *The ARC today.* For address, see Appendix A.

See also ASSOCIATION FOR CHILDREN WITH DOWN SYNDROME; AMERICAN NETWORK OF COMMUNITY OPTIONS AND RESOURCES; ASSOCIATION FOR CHILDREN WITH RETARDED MENTAL DEVELOPMENT; CENTER FOR FAMILY SUPPORT; FEDERATION FOR CHILDREN WITH SPECIAL NEEDS; JARC; MENTAL RETARDATION ASSOCIATION OF AMERICA; NATIONAL ASSOCIATION OF DEVELOPMENTAL DISABILITIES COUNCILS; NATIONAL DOWN SYNDROME CONGRESS; NATIONAL DOWN SYNDROME SOCIETY; PARENTS OF CHILDREN WITH DOWN SYNDROME; PILOT PARENTS; VOICE OF THE RETARDED; YOUNG ADULT INSTITUTE AND WORKSHOP.

Association of Sleep Disorders Centers

A professional organization of specialists in sleep disorders that encourages high standards and training and ethics; the center also serves as the accrediting agency for sleep-disorder clinics and publishes various materials, including a quarterly newsletter and the journal *SLEEP.*

See also AMERICAN NARCOLEPSY ASSOCIATION; NARCOLEPSY; NARCOLEPSY AND CATAPLEXY FOUNDATION OF AMERICA.

astrocytoma A usually malignant brain tumor, the most common type of GLIOMA (arising from supportive cells around neurons called GLIAL CELLS). This type of tumor is most often found in the CORTEX. Although all types of this tumor are serious, they are divided into four grades according to their growth rate and malignancy, with grade I the slowest tumor that may spread throughout the brain without showing symptoms for many years. The so-called benign astrocytoma is slow growing, but it may spread to large areas of the brain and may be encapsulated in a cyst.

The astrocytoma may occur in the cerebral hemispheres of adults or in the cerebellum, brain stem, or optic nerve of children.

Symptoms Symptoms are similar to other types of tumors and depend on the area affected.

Treatment The usual treatment is surgery, but very few astrocytomas can be completely surgically removed. Usually, radiation therapy and possibly chemotherapy follows surgery.

asymmetry in the brain Many parallel areas (especially in the CORTEX) are larger in one hemisphere than in the other. For example, the PLANUM TEMPORALE, an important component in the understanding of speech, is larger in the left hemisphere in most healthy people.

The normal asymmetry of the brain appears to be reversed in the brains of those with SCHIZOPHRENIA. In these patients, for example, the planum temporale is much larger in the right hemisphere, which may help to explain their garbled speech.

ataxia Shaky movements and unsteady gait caused by the brain's failure to regulate the body's posture and the strength and direction of limb movements. Ataxia is usually the result of brain damage in the CEREBELLUM or spinal cord, resulting from infection, head injury, brain tumor, toxins, multiple sclerosis, etc. In cerebellar ataxia, there is a clumsiness in intentional movements, including walking, speaking, and eye movements. Sensory ataxia (unsteady movements that are exaggerated when the patient closes the eyes) occurs from a lack of sensory feedback.

Friedreich's ataxia is a fatal genetic disease characterized by the degeneration of the motor nerves of the spinal cord and the cerebellum, causing a loss of coordination and a disturbance in gait. It may be inherited as a recessive or dominant trait and may strike persons from a very early age up to and beyond age 50. While it is similar to MULTIPLE SCLEROSIS, MS is not inherited and has a different origin.

See also NATIONAL ATAXIA FOUNDATION; FRIEDREICH'S ATAXIA GROUP IN AMERICA.

atherosclerosis A disease of the arteries characterized by buildup of fat deposits on the inner walls, eventually obstructing blood flow. Atherosclerosis is one of the primary causes of STROKE, the third most common cause of death (after cancer), which occurs when blood flow to the brain is reduced or cut off.

Risk factors The probability that this condition will occur is increased with certain risk factors, such as cigarette smoking, high blood pressure, obesity, physical inactivity, high serum cholesterol level, family history, anxious or aggressive personality, and male gender. The risk is also increased as patients age, since more plaques develop with each passing year.

Prevention Moderating or eliminating the risk factors (especially early in adult life) can significantly reduce the probability that a person will develop atherosclerosis—or at least delay its onset. Diet should be low in saturated fat and salt; patients should stop smoking, treat high blood pressure, get regular exercise, control cholesterol and maintain control of diabetes.

Symptoms Atherosclerosis produces no symptoms until the arteries are so clogged that blood flow begins to slow down. Narrowing of the arteries supplying blood to the brain may cause TRANSIENT ISCHEMIC ATTACKS (TIAs) which temporarily mimic the signs and symptoms of a stroke.

Diagnosis Medical history, ANGIOGRAPHY (X rays after injection of radiopaque dye), ultrasound or plethysmography (pulse pattern tracing).

Treatment Once the damage has been done, medication alone can't unclog the arteries. However, anticoagulant drugs may minimize the development of secondary blood clots, and vasodilators can ease symptoms. Balloon angioplasty can open narrowed vessels and improve blood supply to the brain. Large blocks can be removed by endarterectomy, and entire segments of disease peripheral vessels can be replaced by woven plastic tube grafts.

athetosis Slow writhing movements made involuntarily, often as a result of a dysfunction deep within the brain. When associated with the jerky movements of chorea, it is called *choreoathetosis*. This condition is often found in those with HUNTINGTON'S DISEASE, CEREBRAL PALSY, ENCEPHALITIS, or other brain disorders. It also may occur as a side effect to certain medications.

(See TARDIVE DYSKINESIA).

attention and the brain The brain is capable of paying attention to relatively few outside events at the same time. What we think of as "attention" is in fact a highly directed process that depends on a person's alertness, concentration, and interest.

Scientists have learned about attention by studying patients who have suffered from brain damage and experienced a subsequent inability to pay attention. For example, a patient who has injured one side of the brain may ignore anything that happens on the opposite side of the body. Another may wave only one hand when commanded to "wave both hands."

Such problems are known as *neglect* and may result in bizarre behavior such as applying makeup on only one side of the face or ignoring food on one side of the plate. The problem does not involve paralysis, however; the person is physically capable of the required activity but has a neurological malfunction that affects selective attention.

According to research, focused attention is a process distributed throughout the brain that begins with a "red alert" in the reticular structures, progressing within an interlocking system involving sensation, movement, and emotion. The degree of our attention is mediated by a variety of factors, including interest, internal state (hunger, etc.), and emotional significance. Brain damage anywhere along this system can result in attention disorder.

Although some parts of the brain—especially the right hemisphere—are more important in the process than others, there is no one "attention center" in the brain.

attention deficit hyperactivity disorder (ADHD) A group of behavioral problems marked by inattention, hyperactivity, and impulsiveness, formerly called attention deficit disorder (ADD), hyperactivity, hyperkinetic syndrome and/or minimal brain dysfunction.

ADHD's wide variety of names and definitions occurs primarily because the symptoms of this syndrome are complex and varied; many times, all these behaviors do not appear in one child at any one time.

Symptoms In general, children with ADHD have problems following instructions, organizing work, finishing a task—even sitting still long enough to watch an entire TV program. These children are often impulsive, acting without thinking about consequences. These behaviors all interfere with education and may lead to low self-esteem, emotional instability, and mood swings. Boys are three times more likely to have ADHD.

In addition, ADHD behaviors are often found in children with other problems, such as TOURETTE'S SYNDROME, MENTAL RETARDATION, CEREBRAL PALSY, EPILEPSY, or SCHIZOPHRENIA.

Cause ADHD has been linked to many causes, but its development is still poorly understood. It is presumed to result from damage or dysfunction in the brain and central nervous system, although children do not exhibit major brain damage. In fact, many ADHD patients are at or above average intelligence. The behaviors may be triggered in an unsettled or chaotic environment, especiallyone involving neglect or abuse; they may sometimes be linked to a family history of alcohol abuse and psychiatric problems. But many children with ADHD have no such troubled family experiences. Also implicated in the etiology of ADHD are genetics, biochemical problems, injury or damage during birth, and allergy to foods or additives.

Treatment The stimulant RITALIN may be administered to help those youngsters whose hyperactivity interferes with learning; paradoxically, it has a calming effect on many ADHD youngsters, decreasing distractibility and increasing attention and coordination.

auditory agnosia A defect, loss, or failure in development of the ability of comprehend spoken words, caused by disease, injury, or malformation of the hearing centers of the brain. A person with auditory agnosia may or may not be able to reliably respond to an audiometric test or may give very different results at different times.

auditory brainstem response (ABR) test A diagnostic test that determines how well certain portions of the auditory system in the brain respond to a presented stimulus. As nerve impulses pass through the lower levels of the brain from the auditory nerve on their way to higher brain centers, they make connections in the brainstem.

The ABR measures this electrical activity in the brainstem. This test is useful for detecting hearing loss in newborns, to diagnose auditory disorders, and for confirming nonorganic hearing loss. This test can be performed on individuals of any age—even the youngest infant.

The test consists of a brief tone that causes a small variation in electrical potentials that can be recorded from the scalp. Clicks or tone pips are fed into the ear, and a computer analyzes the results to see if the brain activity changes. Rather than a true test of the entire process of hearing, the AGBR determines whether auditory signals are reaching higher brain centers.

By repeating the stimulus up to 100 times and averaging the response by computer, the responses can be enhanced while eliminating random background electrical activity. Auditory thresholds can be established that are quite close to those that can be obtained in conventional audiometry.

Development of new stimulus-delivery systems and recording electrodes now allow the use of ABR for the audiometric monitoring of people with head injuries.

auditory cortex An area of the brain situated in the TEMPORAL LOBE that is critical to HEARING. The auditory cortex connects to the cochlear nerve fibers that respond to a specific sound frequency.

auditory-evoked potentials Slight electrical signals in the brain read from an electroencephalogram that have a characteristic pattern and occur in response to repetitions of identical sounds. The characteristic pattern (or wave form) indicates that the brain has responded to the test sound and that the sound must therefore have been heard by the client. Tests of auditory-evoked potentials are useful for those who can't participate in hearing tests, such as the very young or mentally retarded patients.

See AUDITORY BRAINSTEM RESPONSE TEST.

auditory nerve See ACOUSTIC NERVE.

autism A condition that appears in early childhood (usually before age three) that is characterized by lack of normal social interaction, resistance to physical or eye contact, and impaired development of social, communication, and self-help skills. Children affected by autism usually retreat within themselves and fail to form relationships with others. The severity of the condition differs from one child to the next, but in general the child's activities and interests are often restricted, with an insistence on sameness and repetition. Some autistic children are also retarded, and some of the most severely affected youngsters tend to develop EPILEPSY. At present, this disorder is characterized as a type of pervasive developmental disorder known as *autistic disorder*, but it has previously been known as *atypical development*, *symbiotic psychosis*, *childhood psychosis*, and *childhood schizophrenia*.

Symptoms After a normal first month or two, autistic infants become increasingly unresponsive, screaming when cuddled and growing more aloof. Later on, the child will avoid eye contact and will be extremely resistant to change. Any attempt at altering the routine will cause severe tantrums; rituals develop in play, and often the child becomes attached to unusual objects or collections, or is obsessed with a particular idea. This hysterical need for "sameness" makes it very difficult to teach an autistic child new skills. There are usually delays in speech; when the child does speak, it is usually immature, unimaginative and robotic, with frequent echoing of words or phrases. Behavioral abnormalities include rocking, self-injury, flicking or twiddling fingers, walking on tiptoe, hyperactivity or sudden screaming fits. Sometimes, the child may have one outstanding special skill (such as rote memory, artistic or musical talent).

Cause In the past, autism was assumed to be caused by poor parenting, but today scientists believe parenting styles have no effect on the development of the disorder. While the true cause is not known, it is believed to be related to some type of brain dysfunction. It has been associated with various physical disorders, including maternal rubella, untreated PHENYLKETONURIA, celiac sprue, ENCEPHALITIS, TUBEROUS SCLEROSIS, FRAGILE X SYNDROME or a lack of oxygen at birth.

See also AUTISM NETWORK INTERNATIONAL; AUTISM SERVICES CENTER; AUTISM SOCIETY OF AMERICA.

Treatment There is no known treatment that is reliably effective at all times for all children, although special schooling, behavioral therapy, support and counseling for parents and families may help. Medication may be useful to treat the accompanying epilepsy or hyperactivity.

Autism Network International A self-help and advocacy group run by autistics for autistic individuals that seeks to provide a forum to share information and tips for coping with AUTISM. The group advocates for appropriate services and civil rights for autistic people at all levels of functioning. The network provides information and makes referrals for parents and teachers of autistic people and sponsors group lobbying and educational campaigns. Founded in 1992, the group has 100 members. For address, see Appendix A.

See also AUTISM SERVICES CENTER; AUTISM SOCIETY OF AMERICA.

Autism Services Center An informational clearinghouse that works to improve the processes by which appropriate professional training, consulting, advocacy, and information are provided to those responsible for the welfare and care of autistic people and others with developmental disabilities. The center also maintains a roster of autism professionals, researchers, therapists, and educators. For address, see Appendix A.

See also AUTISM NETWORK INTERNATIONAL; AUTISM SOCIETY OF AMERICA.

Autism Society of America National support organization for parents, teachers, psychologists, speech therapists, pediatricians, neurologists, and others interested in the welfare of children with AUTISM or other severe disorders of communication and behavior. The group is committed to the alleviation of this disorder through support of research, public and professional education, and development of rehabilitative services. Founded in 1965, the group has 12,000 members and publishes a bimonthly newsletter, brochures, booklets, books, and pamphlets. For address, see Appendix A.

See also AUTISM NETWORK INTERNATIONAL; AUTISM SERVICES CENTER.

autonomic nervous system A system of nerves running to smooth muscles or glands that controls such involuntary functions as heart rate, blood pressure, hormone flow, etc. It consists of a network of nerves divided into two parts: the SYMPATHETIC NERVOUS SYSTEM and the PARASYMPATHETIC NERVOUS SYSTEM.

The sympathetic nervous system boosts activity in the body, increasing the heart and breathing rates as part of the body's "fight or flight" response.

In normal conditions, these two systems balance each other, but during exercise or when facing stress, the sympathetic system takes over. During sleep, the parasympathetic system asserts more control.

Physicians can treat certain disorders by administering drugs that affect the autonomic nervous system; for example, anticholinergic drugs block the effect of ACETYLCHOLINE, reducing muscle spasms. Beta-blockers can slow the heart rate by blocking the action of EPINEPHRINE and NOREPINPHRINE on the heart.

averaged evoked response An EVOKED RESPONSE repeated and averaged over time to help discriminate a specific response from other unrelated brain activity.

axon A long unbranched fiber emerging from a neuron that carries nerve impulses to other cells. In some exceptional cases, an axon may also receive input.

B

balance The ability to remain upright and not fall over when walking is a complex process that depends on a continuing flow of information to the brain about the position of the body. The body maintains its balance due to a complex integration of this information combined with a constant flow of instructions from the brain to various parts of the body, performing the necessary changes to keep the body in balance.

The brain receives information about body position from many sources: eyes, sensory nerves in skin, muscles and joints, and the three semicircular canals of the labyrinth in the inner ear that detect placement and speed of head movements. The CEREBELLUM is the part of the brain mainly responsible for collecting and integrating this information and conveying data to other motor centers to coordinate body movement.

Anything that affects the cerebellum—such as a tumor or a STROKE—may cause clumsiness, speech disorders, and other features of impaired muscular coordination.

See VESTIBULAR SYSTEM.

barbiturates A group of sedative drugs properly known as "downers" or tranquilizers, that work by mimicking brain chemicals related to sedation, depressing activity in the brain. Barbital was the first of the barbiturates that appeared at the turn of the century; it was originally widely prescribed for anxiety, insomnia, and seizures. More than a dozen different barbiturates are currently on the market, although their use has rapidly declined in the past 10 years and is strictly controlled because they are habit forming and widely abused. Overdoses can be fatal. Common barbiturates include amobarbital, pentobarbital, phenobarbital, secobarbital, and thiopental. Phenobarbital is still used to treat EPILEPSY, and thiopental is used to induce anesthesia. Barbiturates also are sometimes used to reduce cerebral blood pressure. However, BENZODIAZEPINES and other drugs have replaced barbiturates in treating insomnia and anxiety.

See also CENTRAL NERVOUS SYSTEM DEPRESSANTS.

Action Barbiturates slow down the activity of nerves that control many mental and physical functions, such as emotions or heart rate.

Adverse effects If used longer than four weeks, barbiturates can produce dependence. Withdrawal effects (insomnia, twitching, nightmares, convulsions) may occur if treatment is stopped abruptly. In addition, higher and higher doses of the drug (tolerance) are needed to produce the same effect. Other adverse effects include drowsiness, staggering, and excitability. *Taking alcohol with barbiturates will dangerously depress brain activity*, which can depress breathing. Like all other central-nervous system depressants, barbiturates can lead to coma when taken in overdose. They are especially dangerous when combined; most drug-related hospital emergency admissions involve overdoses of these depressants.

basal forebrain Nuclei in the deep regions of the forebrain that primarily contain neurons that release the NEUROTRANSMITTER called ACETYLCHOLINE. The basal forebrain includes the medial septum, which projects to the HIPPOCAMPUS, the band of Broca, which projects to the hippocampus and AMYGDALA, and the nucleus basalis of Meynert, which projects to the NEOCORTEX and amygdala. Damage to these structures of the brain is believed to contribute to organic AMNESIA. It is also a primary focus of ALZHEIMER'S DISEASE.

basal ganglia Clusters of nuclei deep within the CEREBRUM and the upper parts of the

BRAINSTEM that play an important part in producing smooth, continuous muscular actions and in stopping and starting movement. They may also help mediate the development of skills and habits, and—according to recent research—may help coordinate thinking. Fibers pass from almost every region of the cerebral CORTEX (especially the motor cortex) to the basal ganglia. After processing in the basal ganglia, nerve signals are then transmitted back to the supplementary motor area and premotor cortex of the frontal lobe. The three major nuclei of the basal ganglia are the CAUDATE, putamen, and the globus pallidus. The SUBSTANTIA NIGRA and the AMYGDALA are also considered as part of the basal ganglia.

Diseases or degeneration of the basal ganglia and their connections may lead to the appearance of involuntary movements, trembling, and weakness such as those found in PARKINSON'S DISEASE. In fact, much of what scientists know about this part of the brain was learned during the study of Parkinson's disease.

PARKINSONISM, a neurologic disorder characterized by a masklike face, rigidity, and slowed movements, is caused by neuron damage in the SUBSTANTIA NIGRA of the basal ganglia. These neurons normally release the neurotransmitter DOPAMINE. As these dopaminergic neurons die, brain levels of dopamine decrease. As such, the drug LEVODOPA (which is transformed into dopamine in the brain) is used to treat Parkinson's disease. Malfunctions in this area may also be associated with SCHIZOPHRENIA.

See also BRAIN DAMAGE; CARBON MONOXIDE POISONING; CAUDATE NUCLEUS; HUNTINGTON'S DISEASE.

basilar membrane A flexible membrane in the cochlea of the ear that is attached to the bony shelf and divides the coil of the cochlea lengthwise into two compartments. On one side of the membrane is the perilymph fluid of the scala tympani; on the other side is the organ of Corti. As sound vibrations disturb the perilymph fluid, they are transferred through the basilar membrane to the organ of Corti and on, to the hair cells inside.

The movement of the hair cells is translated into electrical activity which eventually reaches the auditory cortex for final processing.

See also HEARING.

Batten's disease A degenerative neurological disease affecting children, characterized by progressive seizures, dementia, intellectual failure, loss of motor skills and blindness. The condition is usually fatal by age 20. Also known as neuronal ceroid lipofuscinoses, this condition is subtyped by age of onset into *infantile* (Haltia-Santavouri), *late infantile* (Bielschowsky-Jansky), *juvenile* (Spielmeyer-Vogt) or *adult* (Kufs') disease.

Afflicting about one in every 25,000 newborns, it is the most common neurodegenerative disorder of childhood. In the past, the only way physicians were able to distinguish Batten's disease from other conditions was by noting the accumulation of certain pigments and proteins within neurons and many other cell types, which may either have caused the illness or been a byproduct of the true problem. Often the diagnosis was completely missed.

Recently, the International Batten Disease Consortium has tracked down the mutant gene responsible for the devastating brain disorder, which appears to be located on chromosome 16. Most of the patients have an identical chunk missing. Identification of this gene could help physicians diagnose the disease quickly, and scientists hope that a treatment may be found if they can determine how the protein encoded by the gene works in healthy people.

See also BATTEN'S DISEASE SUPPORT AND RESEARCH ASSOCIATION.

Batten's Disease Support and Research Association A national support group for families of children afflicted with BATTEN'S

DISEASE, health-care professionals, and others. The association represents the interests of those with the condition and provides information to the public and professional community. The association also provides referral services and conducts support-group activities. Founded in 1987, the group has 300 members and publishes a bimonthly newsletter. For address, see Appendix A.

B-complex vitamins   See VITAMINS, B-COMPLEX.

Bell's palsy   Also known as facial palsy, this condition is caused by a paralysis of the muscles that control one side of the face caused by damage to the facial nerve that runs beneath the ear to the muscles of the face of the same side. While the cause is not known, scientists suspect that the facial nerve becomes swollen and injured (perhaps by a viral infection such as herpes zoster); with no room to expand in its bony channel, the nerve becomes damaged.

Full paralysis leaves the patient without facial expression; the corner of the mouth may droop and drool. The eye of the affected side may close only partially, and tears may leak. There may be changes in salivation and in the sense of taste, with heightened sensitivity to sound, or problems in speaking or eating.

Bell's palsy is most common between ages 30 and 60 and may be associated with a middle-ear infection; each year about 40,000 Americans contract the disorder. Usually a temporary problem, recovery begins within a few weeks and may be complete within a few months. If the paralysis partially improves by the end of the first week, there will probably be a good outcome. Recovery from total paralysis may not be complete; if the damage to the facial nerve is quite severe, the fibers may be irreversibly damaged.

Treatment   Treatment is controversial. Some physicians believe that no treatment is necessary, although the eyes must be protected if they do not close. A temporary patch or ointment may be recommended for sleeping; eyedrops may also help. Sometimes, corticosteroids may be prescribed to reduce the swelling of the facial nerve; facial massage may prevent long-term contracture.

benzodiazepines   These tranquilizers are among the best-known and most widely prescribed drugs in the world and are used primarily to control symptoms caused by anxiety or stress. They work by depressing brain function, relieving anxiety, and promoting sleep. The drugs slow down the activity of nerves that control many mental and physical functions, such as emotions or heart rate.

The first benzodiazepine was marketed as an antianxiety drug in 1960 under the trade name Librium; three years later, its relative, Valium (DIAZEPAM), was put on the market. By the mid-1970s, one out of every seven Americans was taking Librium or Valium and more than a hundred million prescriptions a year were being written for them. While in terms of sales they were among the most successful drugs in history, they were beginning to be overprescribed for a range of emotional problems that might have been better treated without drugs. Finally, by the mid-1980s prescriptions for these two drugs dropped after repeated warnings of overdose.

Still, the benzodiazepines are still widely used because they can relieve anxiety while being much less sedating and dangerous than BARBITURATES. They are also fairly safe drugs; while it is possible to commit suicide by overdosing on either Valium or Librium, it is not easy.

Benzodiazepines can strengthen the sedating effects of alcohol or barbiturates and can also increase their depressant effects on important brain centers (especially the areas that control breathing).

Scientists believe that benzodiazepines, barbiturates, and alcohol all act on the same synapses in the brain, although benzodiazepines act in a slightly different site than the others.

Adverse effects Daytime drowsiness, dizziness and forgetfulness, unsteadiness, slowed reactions. Drowsiness usually wears off after a few weeks. Chronic users may become dependent when used for more than three or four weeks, and tolerance can develop in time. Stopping benzodiazepines abruptly may lead to withdrawal symptoms (anxiety, nightmares, restlessness), but these are less severe than with other addictive drugs.

beta-endorphins See ENDORPHINS.

beta waves Brain waves are characterized by their intensity, indicating brain activity. Beta I waves, like alpha waves, show the brain's readiness for action; beta II waves show intense mental activity.

Binet, Alfred (1857–1911) French psychologist known as the "father of modern intelligence testing" and who played a major role in the development of experimental psychology.

Originally intending to become an attorney, Binet became interested in medicine and eventually served as director of a research lab at the Sorbonne. He began to develop experimental techniques to measure reasoning ability and other mental processes through a variety of tests. His early diagnostic techniques often supplemented formal tests with observations of handwriting, body type, and other characteristics. In 1903, he published an experimental study of the mental characteristics of his two daughters, and by 1911 he and Theodore Simon developed scales to measure intelligence in children.

biofeedback A technique to gain mental control over the AUTONOMIC NERVOUS SYSTEM, such as decreasing blood pressure, controlling heart rate, and preventing stress or disorders such as migraine HEADACHES.

Some form of electronic device is used to monitor a biologic function (such as skin conductance with a galvanic skin responder). This information is sent to the patient, who then tries consciously to alter the output of the machine in some way. For example, by relaxing and decreasing the sweating of the palms, the person tries to alter the tone generated by the machine. The activity that produces an altered tone in the machine alters the biologic functioning.

With practice, the person can learn to alter the autonomic activity without a machine.

biological clocks See CIRCADIAN RHYTHM; JET LAG; MELATONIN.

birth injury to the brain Any problem that occurs during the birth process that carries the risk of anoxia (loss of oxygen) can have a potentially devastating effect on the newborn's brain. Damage to the brain may either be localized or diffuse (a much more serious problem); loss of oxygen during birth for longer than about five minutes will likely cause serious damage.

Brain problems linked to birth trauma can include CEREBRAL PALSY, MENTAL RETARDATION, EPILEPSY, AUTISM, ATAXIA, LEARNING DISABILITIES, SCHIZOPHRENIA, and MICROCEPHALY.

blood-brain barrier A protective filtering mechanism of the blood vessels of the brain that keeps out (or slows down) many substances in the blood. The barrier utilizes a semipermeable membrane separating circulating blood from fluid surrounding brain cells. This barrier serves to protect the brain from some poisons and unwanted chemicals.

Blood vessels have small windows to allow for the passage of food and oxygen into all parts of the body and the return to the blood of cellular waste products. But the blood vessels of the brain are highly selective, which is helpful when it comes to keeping out harmful chemicals but not so beneficial when it also excludes substances such as chemotherapy drugs.

Fortunately, blood vessels near tumors are often damaged, with enlarged, leaky windows. This damage may allow drugs and lymphocytes into the tumor area. Research is currently looking at the possibility of further disrupting this blood-brain barrier by certain drugs or by hyperthermia (increased temperature of brain tissue).

Normally a helpful mechanism, the blood-brain barrier can also have a negative impact, such as when it keeps certain drugs from reaching dysfunctional portions of the brain. In these cases, drugs may be injected directly into the cerebrospinal fluid or directly into an artery feeding into a brain tumor.

In addition, some medications given first can temporarily allow passage of other drugs through the blood-brain barrier.

Boe, Franz de la (1614–1672) A Dutch professor also known as Franciscus Sylvius, for whom the fissure of Sylvius was named. This fissure is a large groove in each side of the CEREBRAL CORTEX.

See also BRAIN IN HISTORY.

botulism A serious form of food poisoning that selectively affects the CENTRAL NERVOUS SYSTEM. The toxins are rapidly absorbed by the gastrointestinal tract and bind to brain tissue; in fatal cases, death is often caused by a failure of the cardiac and respiratory centers in the brain. The food poisoning is caused by contamination with the toxin *botulin* produced by the bacterium *Clostridium botulinum* that thrives in improperly preserved foods (especially canned raw meat).

Because the toxin is not stable when heated, it is generally destroyed when boiled at 100°C. for one minute (or if the food is sterilized by pressure cooking at 250°F. for 30 minutes).

C. botulinum is found in air, water, and food as harmless inactive spores; when the spores are deprived of oxygen, however (such as inside a sealed can or jar), they begin to grow, producing one of the most deadly toxins known to humans—7 million times more deadly than cobra venom. Still, even inside a sealed jar, the spores will not grow if the food is very acidic, sweet, or salty (such as canned fruit juice, jams, and jellies, sauerkraut, tomatoes, and heavily salted hams). Canned foods that *are* susceptible to contamination include green beans, beets, peppers, corn, and meat.

Although the spores are invisible, it is possible to tell if food is spoiled by detecting a broken vacuum seal (when the spores grow, they give off gas that makes cans and jars lose their seal so that jars will burst or cans will swell). Any food that is spoiled or whose color or odor doesn't seem right inside a home-canned jar should be destroyed without tasting or even sniffing because the spores can be fatal in even small amounts.

Botulism is more common in the United States than anywhere else in the world, due to the popularity in this country of home canning. The name originates from the Latin word for *sausage* (*botulus*) after some people in the 1800s were poisoned after eating contaminated sausages. Cases of botulism from commercially canned food are rare because the U.S. Food and Drug Administration enforces strict health standards.

Botulism also can occur if the bacteria in the soil enters the body through an open wound.

Symptoms Onset of symptoms may vary from 12 to 36 hours, although they can appear as soon as three hours or as late as two weeks after ingestion of contaminated food. The earlier the symptoms, the more severe the reaction and the higher rate of fatality. Cranial nerve symptoms include double or blurred vision, drooping eyelid, difficulty or pain on swallowing, or slurred speech. This is followed by a descending paralysis that affects all the muscles. Throughout the course of the illness, the patient's mind remains clear, but almost all patients have breathing problems. Other symptoms include nausea and vomiting, diarrhea, stomach cramps, and headache.

Death usually occurs in untreated cases from suffocation as a result of the paralysis of breathing muscles.

Infant botulism (often caused by eating contaminated honey) may include constipation, facial-muscle flaccidity, sucking problems, irritability, lethargy, and floppy limbs.

Prognosis Botulism is very rare (only about 20 cases per year), which is fortunate because two thirds of those who are poisoned will die; the rest face a long recovery period.

Treatment Prompt administration of the antitoxin (type ABE botulinus) lowers the risk of death to 25 percent. The Centers for Disease Control in Atlanta, Georgia, is the only agency with the antitoxin; this is the agency that makes the decision to treat the problem. Local health departments should be called first.

The patient should vomit immediately after ingestion of food known to contain botulism toxin, but because vomiting may not be complete and the disease can occur in the presence of only a small amount of toxin, botulism may still develop.

In infant botulism, if symptoms are present, it is often too late to administer the antitoxin because the damage has probably already been done by the toxin, although it is possible to try.

brain The jellylike major organ of the human NERVOUS SYSTEM, part of a complex network of nerve cells and fibers, that is responsible for controlling all the processes in the body in addition to thought, speech, emotion, and memory. Sensations from nerves extending from CENTRAL NERVOUS SYSTEM to every other part of the body are received, sorted, and interpreted by the brain.

Nervous system The nervous system is broken down into three main divisions: the central nervous system, which includes the brain and spinal cord; the PERIPHERAL NERVOUS SYSTEM, which comprises the entire nervous system outside the brain and spinal cord; and the AUTONOMIC NERVOUS SYSTEM, which is that portion of the peripheral nervous system that regulates the involuntary functions of internal smooth muscles and glands, such as the heart rate. In addition, the nerve pathways that carry sensations to the brain from sense organs and messages from the brain to movement muscles, make up the SOMATIC NERVOUS SYSTEM. Although some brain functions are performed entirely within the central nervous system, many others are closely linked with the elements of the peripheral or autonomic nervous systems.

Structure The brain is made up of three main structures: the BRAINSTEM (the extension of the SPINAL CORD), the CEREBELLUM, and the FOREBRAIN, which includes the two large cerebral hemispheres. The most obvious features of the brain are the two wrinkly lobes of the hemispheres that together form the CEREBRUM; the hemispheres are made up of the outer layer (CORTEX) and the inner areas. Each hemisphere is bent into folds (called *gyri*) separated by fissures (called *sulci*). The two hemispheres are linked by the CORPUS CALLOSUM, a thick bundle of nerve fibers.

Below the cerebrum in front of the cerebellum lies the brainstem, which merges into the top of the spinal cord. Deep within the forebrain in front of the brainstem are a variety of structures of crucial importance to maintaining body functions, including the

THALAMUS, HYPOTHALAMUS, BASAL GANGLIA, and PITUITARY GLAND, part of the body's hormonal system.

The four lobes of the brain are broad surface regions in each hemisphere that are named after the bones of the skull lying above them: the frontal, parietal, temporal, and occipital lobes.

Each part of the brain is associated with separate functions, including regulation, consciousness, sensation, voluntary acts, emotions, and higher mental processes.

The brain interprets sensory impulses that it receives from a variety of sensory organs (such as the eyes, ears, nose, taste buds, skin, etc.) that lead to sensations (sight, hearing, smell, taste, and touch).

Moreover, feelings, drives, or urges that make up behavior are all dependent on brain activity, from which all voluntary acts are initiated. Perception, understanding, thought, reasoning, judgment, memory, and learning are all possible only through the activity of the brain. These activities make up the basis of intelligence.

Meninges The brain itself is protected by three layers of membrane coverings called the MENINGES within the skull. CEREBROSPINAL FLUID circulates between two of these layers and within the four main brain cavities, called VENTRICLES. (There is a ventricle in each cerebral hemisphere, a third in the forebrain, and a fourth in the brainstem). This fluid helps feed the brain and protect it from injury.

Nourishment The brain is kept alive by a constant flow of blood from a circle of arteries fed by the internal carotid arteries, which run up each side of the front of the neck through the base of the skull, and from two vertebral arteries running parallel to the spinal cord. The brain receives about 20 percent of all the blood pumped by the heart; if it is deprived of oxygen for two or three minutes or of glucose for 10 to 15 minutes, serious brain damage may result.

brain cells There are two kinds of brain cells: NEURONS and GLIA. While the majority of brain cells (85 percent) are glia, it is the remaining 15 percent—the neurons—that make the brain the most important organ in the body.

Glial cells play a supportive role in brain function, helping to remove waste products, supplying nutrients, aiding in electrical balance, and guiding the brain's development. The neurons, on the other hand, control the body's emotions, activities—and the ability to think.

Neurons (or nerve cells) in the brain are structurally the same as nerve cells in the SPINAL CORD and throughout the body, with a main cell body composed of a nucleus and cytoplasm. (The nucleus contains the genetic material that allows a cell to reproduce); the cytoplasm provides energy for the cell. Neurons have very long extensions called AXONS that allow neurons to communicate with each other. At the end of each axon are many branches that touch a neighboring neuron. One neuron has more than 10,000 "antennae," called DENDRITES, that receive impulses from the axons of other neurons.

The human brain has more than 10 billion neurons.

brain damage Degeneration or death of nerve cells within the brain that may be centered in one area, causing specific defects, or may occur in a diffuse pattern, bringing mental problems or severe physical handicap.

Localized brain damage can occur as a result of a head injury or from a STROKE, TUMOR, or BRAIN ABSCESS. It may also be caused by damage to the brain at birth. The BASAL GANGLIA may be damaged by CARBON MONOXIDE POISONING. *Diffuse brain damage* is more severe and may be caused by lack of oxygen at birth from cardiac or respiratory arrest or from poisoning, drowning, electric shock, or prolonged convulsions. It may also be caused by toxic substances or environmental poisons, brain infections, or as a rare reaction to immunization.

Unlike nerves in the limbs or trunk, nerve cells and tracts in the brain and spinal cord do not recover their function if they have been destroyed. However, there may be some improvement after brain damage as certain parts of the brain take over the function of damaged cells, for the loss. It is not fully understood how this occurs. The ability of a brain-damaged patient to recover depends on the cause and site of the damage and the individual's personality and motivation.

brain death   Total absence of all brain activity, usually measured by lack of electrical signals on ELECTROENCEPHALOGRAMS taken over a period of at least 12 to 24 hours, even if the heart and lungs continue to function with help from a machine. This time period is important because brain activity may be depressed by some forms of drug reactions or poisons. If there is a suspicion of intoxication with CENTRAL NERVOUS-SYSTEM DEPRESSANTS, the diagnosis of brain death cannot be made.

The concept of brain death does not apply to patients who exist in a persistent vegetative state or to other severe degrees of brain damage. Decisions concerning these patients must be made based on other criteria.

While the legal definition of brain death (also called *irreversible coma*) may vary from state to state, it is usually taken to mean the absence of REFLEXES, movements, and independent breathing.

This legal definition may become important when considering whether the patient's organs should be donated and in determining whether or not to turn off a ventilator. Because blood supply to organs is important if they are to be transplanted with the best chance for success, they should be taken after the brain is dead but while the heart and lungs are still functioning.

The American Bar Association, the American Medical Association, the National Conference of Commissioners on Uniform State Laws and the President's Commission for the Study of Ethical Problems in Medicine have proposed a model statute to come up with a more standard definition of death. This proposed statute (called the "uniform determination of death act") says:

> An individual who has sustained either (1) irreversible cessation of circulation and respiratory functions or (2) irreversible cessation of all functions of the entire brain, including the brainstem is dead. A determination of death must be made in accordance with acceptable medical standards.

The concept of brain death has been accepted by the Roman Catholic Church and by those attending the First World Meeting on Transplantation of Organs. In 1972, the American Neurological Association accepted brain death as a definition of death.

brain development in childhood   Recent research has discovered that the environment in which children aged three and younger were raised affected their brain structure. A lack of intellectual stimulation in childhood could interfere with development of brain cells and synapses. Researchers also suspect that early childhood stress could activate hormones that limit a child's learning and memory, adversely affecting intellect and behavior.

See also DEVELOPMENT OF THE BRAIN.

brain disorders   See GENETIC DISORDERS OF THE BRAIN.

brain food   Ever since the dawn of time, people have been searching for foods that will boost their brain power. In biblical times, the lentil was thought to have the power to improve the brain; by medieval days, eagle hearts or crushed lizard was thought to be the magic elixir. Asians during this period swore by ginkgo tea. By the time of France's

Louis XI, hopeful savants ate gold leaf, an early Greek practice, in hopes that the substance would improve the function of the brain.

By far, the most popular brain food of all has been fish, a high-protein food that will indeed improve health and neuron growth. However, experts warn that amounts of protein in excess of the recommended daily allowance (44 grams for women and 56 grams for men) won't boost the brain's power.

VITAMINS and minerals are also important to brain function. In recent studies, those children who were given a vitamin-and-mineral supplement showed improvement in non-verbal intelligence scores compared to students taking a placebo. Scientists discovered that it is particularly important to consume enough minerals for optimum brain efficiency because most Americans are deficient in this area. Peak brain performance requires adequate levels of selenium, iron, zinc, iodine, chromium, molybdenum, boron, copper, and manganese. Because minerals are the first nutrients lost in food processing, a mineral supplement may help to make up the difference.

brain function tests   See ELECTROENCEPHALO-GRAPHY; PET SCAN.

brain hemorrhage   See HEMORRHAGE, BRAIN.

Brain Information Service   A cooperative effort of the UCLA Brain Research Institute and the Biomedical Library to provide rapid, accurate, and complete information in the basic brain sciences to aid investigators and teachers in the field. Subject area of the service includes alcohol and sleep research; it does not cover the literature of diagnosis and treatment of neurological diseases.

The service provides bibliographies using an automated retrieval system and manual searching. It publishes a quarterly journal *Alcohol, Drugs, and Driving*; a quarterly *Bibli-ography of Recent Literature in Sleep Research*; and an annual compilation of sleep research abstracts, *Brain Information Service-Sleep Research*. For address, see Appendix A.

brain in history   While modern thinkers today revere the brain as the most important and irreplaceable organ in the body, ancient physicians and scientists did not share such deep respect for this structure. In ancient Egypt, the heart was esteemed as the pinnacle of complexity, the seat of the soul and all mental functioning. Others at the time thought that the liver was probably the location for intellectual abilities.

By the sixth century B.C., scientists had changed their minds, now deciding that the brain was the repository of the soul, and the fourth VENTRICLE its likely home. Herophilus described the "marvelous net" (*rete mirabile*) of brain localization, a point of view later endorsed by the great anatomist GALEN. In Galen's time, the MOTOR and SENSORY NERVES had been identified and traced to the CERE-BELLUM and CEREBRUM respectively.

Still, agreement on neurophysiology was far from widespread. Later in the sixth century and on through the Middle Ages, physicians found themselves constantly at odds as to whether the soul was found in the brain or heart.

By the fourth century B.C., however, medicine had made strides toward a more modern understanding of brain function, and Hippocrates identified the brain (which he thought was a gland) as the interpreter of consciousness. He was among the first to believe that the various forms of insanity originate in an unhealthy brain. On the other hand, Aristotle delegated the brain to the third-rate job of cooling the body.

In the time of the early Christians, scientists understood more about the complexity of the brain, believing that mental ability was located in the ventricles proceeding from the front toward the back of the head. Sensation and imagination was located in the front ventricle, they believed; reason and intellect in the next ventricle; and memory, the most selective ability, in the rear-most ventricle.

By about 1505, LEONARDO DA VINCI was the first to make a wax cast of the brain ventricles, using the brain of an ox. He believed that the site of sensory analysis was in fact found in the second ventricle, which had formerly been the site of reason. By 1543, the Belgian ANDREAS VESALIUS wrote the first "modern" anatomy of the brain that was based on detailed drawings of corpses. He laid to rest the formerly popular medieval idea that the ventricles houses separate mental abilities.

By the 18th century, the pseudoscience of phrenology had become popular, in which personality traits were assigned by the shape and protuberances of the skull.

brain injury See BRAIN DAMAGE.

brain mapping See BRAIN SCANS.

brain scans A group of specialized tests that track brain function using a variety of chemical, electrical, or magnetic technologies. Each type of brain scan has its strengths and weaknesses; some can distinguish the smallest structures; others can track brain function but can't resolve structures less than 0.5 inches apart.

Diagnostic neurology has been revolutionized by the introduction of computerized scanning equipment during the past 15 years. The most popular scans include computed axial tomographic (CAT) scanning and magnetic resonance imaging (MRI)—also known as nuclear magnetic resonance (NMR).

The computerized scanning techniques of CAT and MRI rely on two distinct methods of producing an image: CAT scans use an ultra-thin X-RAY beam, and MRI uses a very strong magnetic field. During CAT scans, an x-ray beam passes through the brain, and the intensity of the emerging beam is measured by an X-ray detector. On the scan, the brain appears as various shades of gray; bones of the skull appear white, and air appears black.

During an MRI scan, each hydrogen atom in the brain responds to the magnetic field produced by the device; a magnetic field detector measures the responses of the atoms. There is no radiation in an MRI scan, but the magnetic field may affect metallic objects such as heart pacemakers, inner-ear implants, brain-aneurysm clips, or embedded shrapnel.

Both CAT and MRI scans involve taking measurements from thousands of angles; these data are then processed by computer to create a composite three-dimensional representation of the brain. Any particular slice can be selected from this representation and displayed on a TV screen; photos can also be produced from this screen.

CAT shows internal brain structures much better than conventional X rays. It is particularly useful for diagnosing brain disorders such as STROKE, HEMORRHAGE, TUMOR, injury, abscesses, cysts, swelling, fluid accumulation, and dead tissue. MRI scans are good at imaging areas affected by stroke that can't be seen well on a CAT scan and to diagnose nerve-fiber disorders (such as MULTIPLE SCLEROSIS).

Other brain scan technology includes PET (positron emission tomography). This imaging technique can track brain activity of the living brain, pinpointing the source of heightened activity. These data are sent to computers that produce two-dimensional drawings showing neural "hot spots" of brain activity. PET accurately tracks brain function but can't resolve brain structures less than 0.5 inches apart. This type of scan evaluates cerebral blood flow and brain metabolism and may provide useful information on functional pathology.

SPECT (single-photon emission computerized tomography) is another type of brain scan that tracks blood flow and measures brain activity. Less expensive than PET (positron emission tomography) scans, SPECTs may be used to identify the subtle injury following mild head injury.

Other brain-scanning devices include SQUID (superconducting quantum interference device).

brainstem Located at the top of the SPINAL CORD, the brainstem connects the FOREBRAIN and MIDBRAIN to the spinal cord. It controls such functions as heartbeat and breathing and is the source for the CRANIAL NERVES serving the eyes, ears, mouth, and other areas of the face and throat. The oldest (most primitive) part of the brain, the brainstem is almost identical to the brain of a reptile, which is why it earned the nickname "reptilian brain." Evolutionary studies show that in complex animals, the brainstem was one of the first parts of the brain to develop.

The brainstem is one of three major divisions of the brain responsible for monitoring muscular movement and also for receiving NERVE IMPULSES through the cranial nerves. The brainstem connects with 10 of the 12 pairs of cranial nerves and controls basic functions such as breathing, vomiting, and eye reflexes. This part of the brain also acts as a conduit for messages traveling between other parts of the brain and the spinal cord.

From the spinal cord upward, the brainstem includes the MEDULLA, the PONS, and the midbrain. The *medulla* looks a bit like a thicker continuation of the spinal cord and contains the nuclei of the ninth, tenth, eleventh, and twelfth cranial nerves. It's responsible for relaying taste sensations from the tongue and signals to muscles controlling speech, tongue, and neck movements. The medulla also houses groups of nerve cells that regulate heartbeat, breathing, blood pressure, and digestion and relaying information about these activities via the VAGUS (TENTH CRANIAL) NERVE.

The *pons* is much wider than the medulla and contains bundles of nerves connecting with the CEREBELLUM lying behind the brainstem. The pons receives information from ear, face, and teeth via its nuclei for the fifth through eighth cranial nerves and also receives signals controlling the jaw, facial expression, and eye movement. The pons is also important for breathing regulation.

The *midbrain* is the smallest part of the brainstem, located above the pons and containing the nuclei of the third and fourth cranial nerves, which control eye movement and pupil size.

Scattered throughout the brainstem are groups of nerve cells known collectively as the RETICULAR FORMATION, which is believed to control incoming sensory information and governs such basic activities as awareness, attention, sleep, and waking, breathing, and heart rate.

The cerebellum is a separate brain organ that is attached directly to the back of the brainstem and is concerned mostly with balance and coordinated movement.

Running through the middle of the brainstem is a canal that widens into the fourth ventricle of the brain, home of the circulating CEREBROSPINAL FLUID.

Disorders The brainstem is susceptible to the same type of problems that can beset the rest of the CENTRAL NERVOUS SYSTEM; damage to different parts of the brainstem will result in different problems. Any sort of damage to the vitally important centers in the medulla can be quickly fatal; damage to the reticular formation can result in COMA. Likewise, damage to a specific cranial nerve can have particular effects; for example, damage to the seventh (facial) cranial nerve will result in facial palsy. Degeneration of the SUBSTANTIA NIGRA in the midbrain is linked to the development of PARKINSON'S DISEASE.

brain syndrome, organic See ORGANIC BRAIN SYNDROME.

brain tissue transplants Fetal brain tissue that is used to repair brain damage by implanting cerebral tissue from aborted fetuses into the impaired brain. Scientists agree that one of the greatest problems in treating BRAIN DAMAGE and a range of degenerative brain diseases is that up to now, brain tissue has not been able to regenerate itself. When the brain is damaged, other regions don't always take over.

Rat studies have shown that grafted brain tissue can become effective parts of the animal's brain and can even improve age-related learning impairments. Scientists have also shown improvement in some PARKINSON'S DISEASE patients after transplanting fetal brain cells to produce DOPAMINE, a key brain chemical lacking in the disease.

In 1992, a Swedish team from the University of Lund performed a fetal tissue transplant on two Americans who had destroyed their SUBSTANTIA NIGRA after injecting themselves with tainted synthetic heroin. For seven years the two had not been able to use their voluntary muscles; after receiving brain tissue from more than one fetus, both recovered enough to be able to live independently.

In the United States, scientists have implanted fetal tissue into the brains of 10 patients with Parkinson's disease and reported that patients showed improvement in movement examinations. Scientists hope that someday they will be able to treat a range of other brain diseases with this technique. However, the moral and philosophical issues surrounding the use of tissue implants presents problems. Moreover, the fact that successful transplants require the use of fetal tissue adds to the ethical and legal dilemma.

Genes and genetically altered cells also can be injected into brains to combat or reverse damage caused by degenerative diseases. The new approaches rely on the same basic strategy: using living tissue instead of drugs to supply chemicals necessary for brain function.

Brain Tumor Foundation for Children A national support organization that sponsors local support groups and publishes a newsletter for parents of children with BRAIN TUMOR. For address, see Appendix A.

See also ASSOCIATION FOR BRAIN TUMOR RESEARCH.

brain waves Patterns of brain activity traced on an ELECTROENCEPHALOGRAM. On an ongoing basis—even during sleep—electrical signals are constantly flashing over the brain; these signals can be detected and measured by an encephalograph.

Because the tissues of the body conduct electricity well, metal sensors attached to the skin of the head can detect the signals passing from the brain through the muscles and skin. The signals are amplified within the device and displayed on a monitor or paper chart. These devices show that electrical signals in the brain don't come steadily, but are produced in short bursts like a series of waves; the shape of the waves change with the activity level of the brain.

Brain waves are measured in up to 30 cycles per second; one cycle (or one hertz) is one complete oscillation. *Brain-wave frequency* is a measurement of oscillations per second; the more there are, the higher the frequency of the wave. *Amplitude* refers to half the height from the peak to the trough in a single oscillation.

During wakefulness, the waves are fast and small (called ALPHA WAVES); intense thoughts or walking around will produce faster, sharper, more-jagged rhythms characteristic of BETA WAVES. In deep sleep, the brain produces large, slow DELTA WAVES, and THETA WAVES are seen in babies and during sleep.

Measurements of brain waves can help diagnose brain abnormalities, although there are no waveforms that are clearly abnormal in and of themselves. However, the site of brain damage following STROKE may be determined by recording brain waves from different locations on the scalp. Brain-wave evaluations are especially helpful in evaluating EPILEPSY, brain tumors, brain infections, COMA, and BRAIN DEATH. Serial brain-wave recordings can be used to trace recovery after head or brain injuries.

brain weight The weight of the human brain depends on age, stature, body weight, sex, race, blood-vessel congestion, degenerative changes, and atrophy. At birth, the brain weighs about 13 ounces and makes up about 12.4 percent of the body weight. The entire brain of an adult male weighs about three pounds; a female adult brain weighs about 2.78 pounds. When factors of size and weight are considered, the size and weight of the brain in both sexes are about equal. At adulthood, the brain makes up less than 2 percent of the body's weight but uses up 20 percent of the body's energy.

Age has a considerable influence on brain weight; the brain grows rapidly during the first three years and then slows down up to the seventh year, when it is almost its full weight. After this, the increase is very gradual; prime weight is usually achieved by age 20 in males and somewhat earlier in females. From this period onward, in both sexes there is a continuous gradual lessening of the brain's weight by about a gram (0.03 of an ounce) each year.

Tall people in general have heavier brains than shorter folks, but relative to their height, short people have larger heads and brains than tall people. While many people of conspicuous ability have had large brains, averages calculated for groups (such as scholarship winners) show there is really only a slight correlation between head size and intelligence.

The heaviest known normal human brain belonged to the Russian writer Ivan Turgenev, who died in 1883. His brain weighed 4.43 pounds, more than a pound heavier than the average male brain. The smallest known normal brain belonged to a woman who died in 1977; her brain weighed just 2.41 pounds.

breathing center Breathing is an automatic process that is controlled by the respiratory center low in the BRAINSTEM. This breathing center sends nerve impulses to the muscles of the chest diaphragm that regulate lung expansion and contraction.

Broca, Pierre-Paul (1824–1880) A French surgeon whose study of brain lesions contributed significantly to the understanding of the origins of APHASIA (the loss or impairment of the ability to form or articulate words).

Broca founded the anthropology lab in the École des Hautes Études in Paris in 1858 and the Société d'Anthropologie de Paris in 1859, where he developed his research into the comparative study of the craniums of the races of mankind. In this work, he used original techniques to study the form, structure, and topography of the brain.

In 1861 he announced his discovery of the seat of articulate speech located in the left frontal region of the brain, since known as the *convolution of Broca.* With this discovery, Broca had provided the first anatomical proof of the localization of brain function.

See also BROCA'S APHASIA.

Broca's aphasia An expressive language disorder that affects both written and spoken speech, producing nonfluent, slow, labored,and arrhythmic speech. There is, however, reasonably good comprehension of some words, such as nouns, and the few words that can be uttered do tend to be meaningful.

Broca's aphasia is caused by a lesion in the left frontal CORTEX, although a lesion serious enough to produce a permanent disorder probably also includes parts of the BASAL GANGLIA.

See also APHASIA; BROCA, PIERRE-PAUL; WERNICKE'S APHASIA.

Broca's area   Language center in the left CEREBRAL HEMISPHERE that controls the output aspects of language, such as speech and writing.

Brown-Sequard, Charles Edouard (1817–1894)   British physiologist and neurologist who made major discoveries involving the SPINAL CORD and endocrine glands and whose work foreshadowed the later discovery of NEUROTRANSMITTERS. Brown-Sequard taught at Harvard for four years and practiced briefly in New York, eventually moving to France to serve as professor of experimental medicine at the Collège de France.

See also BRAIN IN HISTORY.

C

caffeine and the brain Caffeine affects the BRAINSTEM'S RETICULAR FORMATION (which controls consciousness) and affects coordination, concentration, sleep patterns, and behavior. While it may improve simple motor tasks, more complex problems involving fine motor coordination and quick reactions may be slightly disrupted. Of course, any drug's effect depends on the amount consumed, how often, how much was absorbed by the body, and how quickly it was metabolized. However, small amounts of caffeine may not greatly affect the body; some research has shown that administering small amounts (such as two or more cups of regular coffee) did not affect performance when compared with subjects who drank the same amount of decaffeinated coffee.

The gastrointestinal tract absorbs almost all of the caffeine and within minutes distributes it to all tissues and organs; maximum blood levels are reached within 45 minutes.

Too much caffeine (and the exact amount varies from person to person) can bring on the jitters, insomnia, and memory problems. For a habitual user, however, omitting this stimulant will have the same negative effect, in addition to dizziness and headaches. This is because regular intake of caffeine (a cup or more per day) conditions the brain to await the caffeine stimulus before it responds with wakefulness.

A study of healthy college students found that their ability to remember lists of words they just heard was diminished following the administration of caffeine. Also, a 1983 study found that combining caffeine and alcohol actually slowed the reaction time of eight subjects, making subjects more drunk than alcohol alone.

In any case, caffeine may be hard to avoid. It is contained in a staggeringly large number of products in the United States; in addition to food and beverages, caffeine is contained in over-the-counter stimulants, analgesics, cold preparations, antihistamines, and prescription drugs. In fact, there are more than 2,000 nonprescription drugs and 1,000 prescription drugs that contain caffeine or caffeine-type stimulants.

Cajal Club A professional group for neuroanatomists who meet to discuss and present papers on research, techniques, and history of neurology. The group bestows annual awards for research on the CEREBRAL CORTEX. The club, which was founded in 1947, was named after Don Santiago Ramon y Cajal, a founder of and Nobel laureate for the science of NEUROANATOMY.

It has 450 members and sponsors an annual convention in conjunction with the American Association of Anatomists; it publishes the quinquennial *History of Cajal Club*. For address, see Appendix B.

calcium One of the most abundant elements in the body, calcium is necessary for conducting messages from one neuron to another. The main dietary sources of calcium are milk and dairy products, eggs, fish, green vegetables, and fruit.

Calcium has been indicated as a possible cause of brain disorders; high levels have been associated with memory problems. When excess calcium is blocked by drugs in the part of the brain associated with memory and learning, scientists have been able to improve memory loss in STROKE victims. Similarly, conditions that increase the level of calcium in the brain cause memory problems. At the same time, normal levels of calcium are associated with the release of a substance called CALPAIN, which seems to improve memory by improving cell-to-cell communication.

New research has identified a potential link between calcium and HANDEDNESS. A team of Canadian and U.S. researchers found crucial chemical differences between left- and right-handed people. The left-handed subjects had far fewer cells that produce a protein called *parvalbumin*, which plays a key role in regulating calcium in the brain. In some cases, left-handed people had only half as many parvalbumin-producing cells as right-handers.

The inability to regulate neuronal levels of calcium has been implicated in ALZHEIMER'S DISEASE.

calpain One of several brain chemicals currently being studied by their role in memory. Released by CALCIUM within neurons, calpain can alter proteins and actually changes the structure of nerve terminals, letting neurons communicate more easily with each other. It could be that low calcium levels in older patients may be one reason behind the memory loss of old age.

cancer, brain See ACOUSTIC NEUROMA; ASTROCYTOMA; CRANIOPHARYNGIOMA; EPENDYMONA; GLIOBLASTOMA; GLIOMA; HEMANGIOBLASTOMA; MEDULLOBLASTOMA; MENINGIOMA; NEUROBLASTOMA; NEUROECTODERMAL TUMORS; OLIGODENDROGLIOMA; PINEALOMA; PITUITARY ADENOMAS; PITUITARY TUMOR; RETINOBLASTOMA.

carbon monoxide A colorless, odorless gas that is a potent NEUROTOXIN and can cause serious brain damage and death. Carbon-monoxide poisoning is the leading cause of death by poison in the United States.

Brain damage (particularly to the BASAL GANGLIA) is caused by a lack of oxygen to the brain. Several minutes or exposure to 1,000 ppm (0.1 percent) may cause fatal poisoning.

The developing fetus is very vulnerable to carbon-monoxide poisoning. For this reason, mothers who smoke more often deliver low birth-weight babies.

LEVELS OF CARBON MONOXIDE POISONING

Carbon monoxide concentration	Symptoms
Less than 35 ppm (cigarette smoke)	None, or mild headache
0.005% (50 ppm)	Slight headache
0.01% (100 ppm)	Throbbing headache
0.02% (200 ppm)	Severe headache, irritability, fatigue
0.03%–0.05 (300–500 ppm)	Headache, confusion, lethargy, collapse
0.08–0.12% (800–1200 ppm)	Coma, convulsions
0.19% (1900 ppm)	Rapidly fatal

Sources The primary source is exposure to exhaust from car engines, but the gas is emitted from any flame or combustion device (such as kerosene heaters or stoves). Other sources include faulty or poorly ventilated charcoal, kerosene or gas stoves; paint stripper (hobbyists and film processors are especially at risk); and cigarette smoke. Fire victims are often affected by carbon monoxide, and burning natural gas or petroleum fuels emits the gas. Smoke from cigarettes pipes and cigars is another common source, and smokers have a significantly higher blood level; those who inhale secondary smoke are also exposed to and show elevated blood levels of carbon monoxide. Workers exposed to high levels in the environment are also at risk.

Symptoms Carbon monoxide may be either inhaled or absorbed through the skin. People exposed to carbon monoxide complain of headache, dizziness, lethargy, irritability, increased breathing rate, chest pain, confusion, impaired judgment, shortness of breath, fainting, and nausea. Patients with heart problems may experience angina or heart attacks. Exposure to more concentrated levels may lead to impaired thinking, HYPER-

ACTIVITY, bizarre behavior, COMA, and convulsions and may be fatal. Chronic exposure may lead to poor memory and mental deterioration and has been linked with hearing loss. Delayed effects (between two and four weeks after a significant exposure) may include visual loss, DEMENTIA, retardation, memory loss, lack of speech coordination, personality changes, loss of bladder control, and problems in walking). Survivors may suffer numerous neurological problems such as PARKINSONISM, personality problems, and memory disorders.

Treatment The administration of oxygen in the highest possible concentration (100 percent); some experts support the use of hyperbaric chambers, which can enhance the elimination of carbon monoxide. Such treatment may be useful to patients exposed to very high levels of carbon monoxide and who are reasonably close to a chamber (found in hospitals).

carotid artery Any of the four main arteries of the neck and head that supply the brain with blood. There are two common carotid arteries (left and right), each of which divides into two main branches (internal and external). The right common carotid artery arises from the subclavian artery, which branches off the heart, up the neck on the right side of the windpipe; just above the level of the larynx, it divides into two, forming the right internal and external carotid ardors. The left common carotid arises from the aorta above the heart and then follows a similar path.

The internal carotid arteries enter the skull to supply the brain with blood via its cerebral branches. At the base of the brain, branches of the two internal carotids and the basilar artery join to form a ring of blood vessels called the CIRCLE OF WILLIS. When these arteries become narrowed, they can cause a TRANSIENT ISCHEMIC ATTACK (TIA); if blocked, they cause a STROKE.

carotid endarterectomy The most commonly performed surgical technique to remove plaque from inside the carotid artery. This plaque can interfere with blood flow to the brain or be the source of particles that break off and flow to the brain. Such plaque formation is a common disease called ATHEROSCLEROSIS that often occurs in the neck arteries to the brain, especially where the two branches meet. There are two carotid arteries supplying blood to the brain; if fatty plaques clog one of them, it can shut off blood flow, causing brain tissue damage and STROKE. Obstructed carotid arteries that cause no symptoms are usually diagnosed during a physical exam; the physician hears a rushing sound when holding the stethoscope to the person's neck.

Carotid endarterectomy is usually performed after TRANSIENT ISCHEMIC ATTACKS to prevent a stroke; it is sometimes performed during the first few hours of an evolving ischemic stroke.

Blockage may recur after surgery, but this is uncommon; the operation is usually successful because it eliminates further transient ischemic attacks and reduces the chance of stroke.

Procedure In the procedure, surgeons make an incision in the neck and cut away the fatty plaque blocking blood flow. However, carotid endarterectomy is not recommended for everyone with narrowed carotid arteries. Once a possible block has been identified by a physician, more tests (ultrasounds or angiograms) must chart the extent of the problem.

While scientists have long understood that such surgery benefits people who show symptoms of, or who have suffered, a stroke, it has only recently been shown to be valuable in treating patients with no symptoms despite a severe constriction. People with no symptoms who underwent carotid endarterectomy had only a 4.8 percent chance of stroke five years later; this is significantly lower than the 10.6 percent risk for those patients who had received standard treatment for narrowed carotid arteries with no surgery. This surgery has now been shown to be superior to medical treatment in patients with arteries that are narrowed by 70 percent or more.

Risks While the procedure has a high success rate, it also has risks. Active heart disease may make the risks of this operation too great; chronic high blood pressure should be corrected before surgery begins. Experts point out the importance of seeking an experienced surgeon to perform the surgery. An inexperienced surgeon could sharply increase a patient's risk of suffering a stroke or of dying as a result of the procedure, according to Robert Hobson II of the New Jersey Medical School in Newark. For that reason, the National Institute of Neurological Disorders and Stroke recommends that patients have the operation only at medical centers with complication rates of 3 percent or less.

The timing of the procedure is controversial. In the past, scientists were concerned that a sudden restoration of blood flow to the brain might cause a more serious hemorrhage; often, surgery was delayed for days or weeks after a stroke. However, many surgeons are now comfortable with operating immediately, and early surgical intervention could prevent a more serious stroke.

In some people, the combined risk of diagnostic ARTERIOGRAPHY plus the surgical procedure may be higher than nonsurgical therapy (such as blood-thinning medication). Risk is highest for those with acute stroke or a stroke in evolution. It is lowest for those with no stroke symptoms at the time of surgery.

cataplexy Recurrent condition in which a person suddenly collapses to the ground without loss of consciousness. It can be provoked by any strong emotion (particularly laughter). This rare cause of sudden involuntary falling is almost exclusively found among people suffering from NARCOLEPSY and other sleep disorders. Cataplexy usually lasts for just a few seconds.

See NARCOLEPSY AND CATAPLEXY FOUNDATION OF AMERICA.

catecholamine A class of NEUROTRANSMITTER, including NOREPINEPHRINE, *epinephrine*, and *dopamine*, that affects the nervous and cardiovascular systems, the metabolic rate, and body temperature.

CAT scan This quick and accurate diagnostic technique utilizes a computer and X-RAYS passed through the body at different angles to produce clear cross-sectional pictures of the tissue being examined, allowing greater differentiation among normal soft tissues.

The CAT scan provides a clearer and more detailed picture of the body than X rays by themselves, and it tends to minimize the amount of radiation exposure. It is the preferred initial examining procedure in the diagnosis of STROKE; approximately 70 percent of strokes will be visible within seven days. Although a stroke does not usually require an emergency CAT scan, it can provide valuable information about the presence of hemorrhage if bloodthinners are being considered as a possible treatment. MAGNETIC RESONANCE IMAGING is less accurate in diagnosing acute hemorrhage and may miss the presence of blood in the SUBARACHNOID SPACE.

Before the scan is performed, a contrast dye may be injected to make blood vessels, organs, or abnormalities show up more clearly. A number of low-dose X-ray beams are passed through the brain at different angles as the scanner rotates around the patient.

Using the information produced by the scanner, a computer constructs cross-section pictures of the brain, which are then displayed on a TV screen and can reveal soft tissue, including tumors, more clearly than normal X rays. They are particularly useful in scanning the brain because they sharply define the ventricles (fluid-filled spaces). Technical advances in imaging and processing have dramatically decreased the time required to acquire data and reconstruct an image. Likewise, spatial resolution has been improved to 1 to 2 mm.

The first scanner was developed as a brain research tool and was used clinically in 1973. Since then, CAT brain scans have improved the diagnosis and treatment of STROKE, HEAD INJURY, tumors, abscesses, and so forth and have superseded plain skull X rays and PNEU-MOENCEPHALOGRAPHY. However, the development of MAGNETIC RESONANCE IMAGING (MRI) has become the preferred technique for brain imaging. CAT scans remain in use, however, because they are cheaper and faster than MRI.

caudate nucleus A part of the BASAL GAN-GLIA often referred to as the NEOSTRIATUM. The deterioration of this part of the brain results in HUNTINGTON'S DISEASE.

cell body The core of the cell that contains the nucleus, where genetic material is found.

cells, brain See BRAIN CELLS; NEURONS; GLIA.

cellular phones and brain tumors Although a Florida lawsuit raised questions in 1993 about certain types of cellular phones (those with built-in antennas), there has been no proof that these phones are connected to BRAIN CANCER.

Unlike an ordinary phone, a cellular phone does not transmit calls through a wire. Instead, its signals are encoded in radio waves that are broadcast by an antenna to a receiving tower. Often, the consumer holds the antenna close to the head. Cellular phones are different from cordless phones, which broadcast much weaker radio signals to household receivers that route calls along conventional phone lines.

Like television, cellular phones operate at the lowest end of the microwave portion of the electromagnetic spectrum. They conform to guidelines set by the Federal Communications Commission for acceptable emission levels of electromagnetic radiation. The signals emitted by cellular phones have a frequency between 840 mH and 880 mH, located at the high end of the radio band (also called high-frequency radio waves).

Most experts do agree that there is a general lack of scientific knowledge about the health effects of the low-level radiation leaked by all sorts of household appliances. Only a few studies have been performed that explore the high-frequency radio waves generated by cellular phones. It is true that at high power, high-frequency radio waves can burn the skin; although cellular phones operate at low power, many brands carry warnings against pressing the antenna against the skin.

The scare began when researchers at the Medical College of Virginia found that brain tumors as well as healthy red blood cells grow faster when exposed to high-power microwave radiation. Despite the lack of further studies, most scientists expressed confidence that cellular phones will not prove harmful.

The concern began when a Florida man appeared on a TV talk show to say that his wife had died of brain cancer caused by a cellular phone. The tumor, he said, was where the antenna had rested; he was seeking damages from three companies involved in the phones. His assertion prompted several other claims; at the time of the lawsuit, about 10 million Americans owned such phones.

Despite the lack of proof, the lack of thorough long-term studies has prompted the U.S. Food and Drug Administration to work with other federal agencies and industries to resolve the question over the safety of these phones.

See also TUMORS, BRAIN.

cellular rhythms See CIRCADIAN RHYTHM.

Center for Family Support A service agency devoted to the physical well-being and development of the mentally retarded child and the sound mental health of the parents. The center helps families with retarded children with all aspects of home care, including counseling, referrals, home-aide service, and consultation. The center also offers intervention for parents at the birth of a retarded child with in-home support, guidance, and infant stimulation. The emphasis is on working with entire families and keeping families together whenever possible; the center sponsors parents' groups and pioneered training of nonprofessional women as home aides to provide support services in homes. Founded in 1953, the group has a staff of 50. For address, see Appendix A. See also ASSOCIATION FOR CHILDREN WITH DOWN SYNDROME; ASSOCIATION FOR CHILDREN WITH RETARDED MENTAL DEVELOPMENT; ASSOCIATION FOR RETARDED CITIZENS; FEDERATION FOR CHILDREN WITH SPECIAL NEEDS; MENTAL RETARDATION; MENTAL RETARDATION ASSOCIATION OF AMERICA; NATIONAL ASSOCIATION OF DEVELOPMENTAL DISABILITIES COUNCILS; NATIONAL DOWN SYNDROME CONGRESS; NATIONAL DOWN SYNDROME SOCIETY; PARENTS OF CHILDREN WITH DOWN SYNDROME; PILOT PARENTS; VOICE OF THE RETARDED; YOUNG ADULT INSTITUTE AND WORKSHOP.

Center for Hyperactive Child Information A national informational and support group that disseminates information on diagnosis and medical/education needs, publishes brochures, etc. For address, see Appendix A.

See also HYPERACTIVITY; LEARNING DISABILITIES.

Central Linguistic Auditory Milestones Scale (CLAMS) A screening instrument that is easily administered and indicates delay in expressive and receptive language up to the age of three years.

See also EARLY LANGUAGE MILESTONE SCALE (ELM).

central nervous system (CNS) The collective term for the brain and the SPINAL CORD, which is the two-way highway for messages between the brain and the rest of the body. The CNS is responsible for integrating all nervous activities and works together with the PERIPHERAL NERVOUS SYSTEM (PNS), which consists of all the nerves that carry signals between the CNS and the rest of the body.

The CNS receives sensory information from all sensory organs in the body; analyzes this information; and triggers appropriate motor responses.

The CNS consists of neurons cells and supporting cells. Injury or disease involving the CNS usually causes permanent disability.

central nervous system depressants A group of drugs that cause sedation or diminish brain activity. These drugs include alcohol, aminoglutethimide, anesthetics, anticonvulsants, antidepressants, antidyskinetics (except amantadine), antihistamines, apomorphine, baclofen, BARBITURATES, BENZODIAZEPINES, buclizine, carbamazepine, chloral hydrate, chlorzoxazone, clonidine, cyclizine, difenoxin and atropine, diphenoxylate and atropine, disulfiram, dronabinol, ethchlorvynol, ethinamate, etomidate, fenfluramine, flavoxate, glutethimide, guanabenz, guanfacine, haloperidol, hydroxyzine, interferon, loxapine, magnesium sulfate, matprotiline, meclizine, meprobamate, methyldopa, methyprylon, metoclopramide, metyrosine, mitotane, molindone, opioid (narcotic) analgesics, oxybutynin, paraldehyde, paregoric, pargyline, phenothiazines, pimozide, procarbazine, promethazine, propiomazine, rauwolfia, scopolamine, skeletal muscle relaxants, thioxanthenes, trazodone, trimeprazine, and trimethobenzamide.

central nervous system stimulants Drugs that cause anxiety, excitation, or nervousness or that otherwise stimulate the brain and central nervous system. These drugs include amantadine, amphetamines, anesthetics, appetite suppressants (except fenfluramine), bronchodilators (xanthine-derivative), CAFFEINE, clophedianol, COCAINE, doxapram, methylphenidate, pemoline, and sympathomimetics.

central sulcus The main fissure that separates the FRONTAL LOBE from the PARIETAL LOBE behind it.

centrophenoxine (Trade name: Lucidril) This drug is believed to improve cognitive function and may remove deposits of LIPOFUSCIN (the material precursor to "age spots"). Lipofuscin accumulates in the brain cells with age, and decreased deposits have been correlated with improved learning ability. In some studies, centrophenoxine appears to remove these lipofuscin deposits; other studies suggest that centrophenoxine can protect the brain against lack of oxygen and may be of value in treating diseases caused by lack of oxygen in the brain.

cerebellar astrocytoma See ASTROCYTOMA.

cerebellum This small, two-lobed wrinkled structure actually originated as an outgrowth of the HINDBRAIN, as suggested by its position directly behind the BRAINSTEM to which it is linked, tucked under the cerebral hemispheres. Its primary function is to coordinate movement and balance, helping the body to assume postures and maintain muscle coordination. It is also responsible for certain subconscious activities and—new research suggests—for coordinating thinking as well. It is also where simple, learned motor responses (such as yanking a finger away from a hot stove) are believed to be stored.

The arrangement of nerve cells in the cerebellum is different from other parts of the brain; here, the cells are positioned with mathematical precision, much like an electrical wiring diagram.

The cerebellum is the second-largest portion of the brain, and it fits inside the skull by a process of many foldings that give it a sort of pleated look.

Structure Latin for "little brain," the cerebellum looks very much like the CEREBRUM and makes up about 11 percent of the entire brain weight. The CORTEX (surface) of the two hemispheres are made up of many parallel ridges marked with deep ridges. Each hemisphere sports three nerve-fiber stalks from its inner side, linked to different parts of the brainstem. It is along these nerve tracts that all of the signals flash back and forth between the cerebellum and the rest of the brain.

The right and left hemispheres of the cerebellum each connect with the fibers coming from nerve tracts from the SPINAL CORD on the same side of the body and with the opposite cerebral hemisphere. Therefore, nerve impulses governing movement of the right hand start off in the left cerebral hemisphere; details about the speed and orientation of the movement are transmitted back to the left cerebral hemisphere through the right half of the cerebellum. As such, the cerebellum "updates" movement as it occurs.

Nerves in the outer edges of the cerebellum govern the ends of the arms and legs, whereas nerves embedded near the center of the cerebellum monitor the body's orientation in space and help to maintain posture in response to data about balance sent via nerve impulses from the inner ear.

The cerebellum collects information about balance and movement from other organs through its connections with the brainstem, and working together with the thalamus and BASAL GANGLIA, the cerebellum integrates movement signals sent to the MOTOR CORTEX, which transmits them to the spinal cord; from there they are sent to designated muscle groups. At the same time, the cerebellum receives impulses from the muscles and joints that are being activated, somehow compares them with instructions sent from the motor cortex, and makes adjustments via the THALAMUS. This part of the brain helps modify direction, force, rate, and steadiness of intentional movements. Movement is not initiated within the cerebellum, but it does not serve simply as a sort of transmission device, either; rather, the cerebellum continually reroutes and refines instructions for movement and may store instructions for oft-used movements and for skilled repetitive movements (those that are learned "by rote").

Damage Any damage to this part of the brain can interfere with proper posture or movement ranging from jerky eye movements of nystagmus to hand tremor or slurred speech. It may also, according to research, be linked to the development of SCHIZOPHRENIA. It is this area of the brain that is impaired during excess alcohol intake, producing symptoms mimicking diseases of the cerebellum (slurred speech, jerky gait, posture and balance problems). This area is also vulnerable to STROKE, often associated with functional problems of the CRANIAL NERVES.

See CEREBELLUM, DISEASES OF.

cerebellum, diseases of the The CEREBELLUM may be damaged by tumors, injuries, vascular lesions, infection, intoxicants, and metabolic diseases. The cerebellum is also involved in a number of hereditary degen-erative diseases (the most common is FRIEDREICH'S ATAXIA). Malfunction in the cerebellum may also contribute to the development of SCHIZOPHRENIA.

Among the disorders that are linked with diseases of the cerebellum are ATAXIA, DYSARTHRIA, and aberrant nystagmus. In addition, MEDULLOBLASTOMA, a brain tumor of childhood, often grows in the cerebellum.

cerebral blood-flow studies Tests that measure blood flow to determine areas of blood supply. In one method for determining total cerebral blood flow, the patient inhales a mixture of 15 percent nitrous oxide and air for 10 minutes; after this, blood is drawn to measure the clearance of the gas from cerebral tissue. Another method continuously measures carotid blood flow in order to assess the capacity of cerebral collateral circulation. Regional studies can help determine areas of aberrant mental activity in the brain.

cerebral commissures The bundles of fibers connecting sites in the two hemispheres of the brain. See ANTERIOR COMMISSURE; CORPUS CALLOSUM.

cerebral cortex The furrowed, outer surface of the CEREBRUM that carries out many cerebral functions. From a word meaning "bark," this outer layer of the brain is made up of cell bodies of neurons called GRAY MATTER that cover the cerebrum like bark on a tree. Under the pinkish gray cortex lies the WHITE MATTER, tissue made up only of nerve fibers.

The home of the most lofty abilities in the brain, the cortex is a quarter-inch-thick pad of grooved tissue with a right and left hemisphere and four distinct lobes each: the FRONTAL LOBE (controlling decision making, problem solving, and will), the PARIETAL LOBE (receiving sensory information), the OCCIPITAL LOBE (where vision is processed), and the TEMPORAL LOBE (hearing, memory and language). The lobes are connected by a pathway of fibers called the CORPUS CALLOSUM.

Within the cortex, research studies have pinpointed scores of regions that seem to specialize in different jobs, especially in the diffuse storing of memories. The cortex stores a person's abstract memory, a huge jumble of events and objects. Damage to the temporal, parietal, or occipital cortex affects abstract memory in different ways. For example, damage to the left temporal or parietal lobes produces problems in reading, writing, speaking, and simple arithmetic skills, but other mental abilities and memory remain intact. However, damage to the right temporal or parietal lobes causes subjects to easily become lost even in familiar surroundings; they cannot negotiate simple mazes, use or draw maps, match or copy the slant of a line, copy simple shapes or arrange blocks to form required patterns, or judge size, distance, and direction of objects.

The sensory and motor areas of the cortex take up relatively little space, compared with the huge areas occupied by the association parts of the brain. The SENSORY AREAS of the brain receive sensations from the muscles, skin, and organs, such as temperature or touch. MOTOR AREAS of the cortex send out messages that control muscles or muscle groups, which make the body move. The ASSOCIATION AREAS of the cortex link the sensory areas with motor areas; the association areas are the true seat of the personality, intelligence, language, judgment, emotions, and memory. The association areas of the brain allow the brain to think.

The cortex varies in thickness from about 2 to 4 mm. (about a quarter of an inch), lying in deep folds and creases so that many more nerve cells can be packed in tightly. If the cortex were flattened out, it would stretch out about as big as a pillowcase or a newspaper page. This large brain surface may be one reason why humans, with their wrinkled cortices, are more capable of complex thoughts than are animals, with smoother cortices.

The cortex is really what makes us human; it is the center of neurons involved in thinking, learning, remembering, and planning and functions as a sort of control center for the rest of the brain.

cerebral hemispheres   The two divisions of the CEREBRUM, labeled "left" and "right," that are separated by a deep groove called the longitudinal cerebral fissure. At the base of this fissure lies a thick bundle of nerve fibers called the CORPUS CALLOSUM, which provides a structural and communication link between the two hemispheres.

The left hemisphere controls the right side of the body, and the right hemisphere controls the left, because of a crossing of the nerve fibers in the MEDULLA. Although in many ways the two hemispheres are mirror images of each other, there are important differences.

In most people, areas in the left hemisphere control speech and areas in the right control spatial perceptions.

Two major furrows called the CENTRAL SULCUS and the lateral sulcus divided each cerebral hemisphere into four sections — the FRONTAL, PARIETAL, TEMPORAL, and OCCIPITAL LOBES. The central sulcus also separates the cortical motor area from the cortical sensory area.

Starting from the top of the hemisphere, the upper regions of the motor and sensory areas control the lower parts of the body, and the lower regions of the motor and sensory areas control the upper parts of the body.

Other areas in the cerebral hemispheres have also been identified; the VISUAL CORTEX is found in the occipital lobe, and the AUDITORY CORTEX is found in the temporal lobe.

cerebral hemorrhage   Bleeding within the brain caused by rupture of a blood vessel. See BRAIN HEMORRHAGE.

cerebral palsy (CP)   Also called Little's disease, cerebral palsy is the general term used to describe a group of movement and posture symptoms arising from nervous system damage before birth, during birth, or early in life.

The portion of the nervous system that is injured will determine the symptoms. Groups of symptoms are described as spastic (abnormal stiffness and contraction of groups of muscles), athetotic (involuntary writhing movements), or ataxic (loss of coordination and balance), depending on whether the CEREBRAL CORTEX, BASAL GANGLIA, or CEREBELLUM is the most severely affected.

The degree of disability varies from person to person and can range from simply a slight clumsiness to complete immobility. In addition, children with CP may also experience other nervous system disorders, such as hearing problems or epileptic seizures. While many of these children are also mentally retarded, some are of normal to high intelligence.

Between 2 to 6 out of 1,000 American infants develop cerebral palsy, with only a slight reduction in the number of cases over the past 20 years.

Children who are moderately disabled have a near-normal life expectancy; with special help, most who can move around and communicate effectively grow up to lead relatively independent, normal lives. (See also Appendix A: United Cerebral Palsy Association or National Association of Sports for Cerebral Palsy; see Appendix B: American Academy for Cerebral Palsy and Developmental Medicine.)

Cause   Cerebral palsy can be caused by chromosome abnormalities, inherited metabolic defects, prenatal injury or premature birth, oxygen deficiency or mechanical injury at birth, jaundice, hypoglycemia, or nervous-system infection during the first few months of life.

Most—about 90 percent—of cases occur before or at birth, most commonly due to a lack of oxygen. It's also possible that a mother's infection spreading to the fetus could cause CP. Rarely, babies with severe jaundice develop CP because the bile pigment damages the BASAL GANGLIA (nerve cell clusters in the brain that control movement).

After birth, a child could contract CP via ENCEPHALITIS or MENINGITIS or through a HEAD INJURY.

Symptoms   While severe nervous system damage may be noticeable at birth, it is more usual for symptoms to appear between ages two and four as the child fails to grow and develop normally. Some of the infant's muscles may be floppy; there may also be feeding problems.

In the spastic group, there are three different categories of disability: diplegia, hemiplegia, and quadriplegia. Diplegics have two limbs affected. Hemiplegics experience symptoms only on one side of the body, and the arm is usually worse than the leg. All four limbs of a quadriplegic are severely affected.

About three-quarters of all CP patients are mentally retarded with an IQ below 70; the exceptions occur mostly among those with athetotic CP; many of these patients and some people with diplegic CP are highly intelligent.

Cerebral palsy is not progressive and will not worsen with age, and the conditions of the disease often improve with age and special treatment.

Prevention   Parents of infants at risk (those born prematurely or during difficult births) are encouraged to take their children more frequently for routine checkups; the physician will test for any abnormalities in the baby's muscle tone and reflexes and for delay in reaching developmental milestones.

Treatment   Cerebral palsy is incurable, but there is much that can be done with physical and speech therapy. Physical therapy teaches the child to develop muscular control and maintain balance. Speech therapy can help improve speech; for those children who do not speak, special equipment can help them communicate nonverbally.

cerebral thrombosis The formation of a clot (thrombus) in a brain artery that may cause a STROKE by blocking the artery, cutting off blood and oxygen to the brain.

cerebrospinal fluid A clear fluid found in the four linked brain cavities (VENTRICLES), the central canal in the SPINAL CORD and the space between the brain and spinal cord and the MENINGES (protective covering). The fluid fills the ventricles and flows through special ducts around the brain's outer rim before being reabsorbed by the blood; this surrounding fluid acts as a cushion to protect the brain against shock and makes turning or nodding the head effortless. This fluid also protects the spinal cord. The fluid, which contains sugar (glucose), protein, and salts, can be tested during a LUMBAR PUNCTURE to help diagnose a range of illnesses affecting the brain (such as MENINGITIS).

Excess cerebrospinal fluid that builds up during fetal development or early infancy may cause the skull to grow too large, a condition called HYDROCEPHALUS (or commonly, "water on the brain").

cerebrovascular accident (CVA) Sudden blockage or rupture of a blood vessel within the brain causing a serious local circulation obstruction or bleeding. A block may be caused by a blood clot or a plug of material formed and transported from elsewhere in the body. These problems can lead to STROKE. Several researchers have reported AMNESIA after a blockage in the posterior cerebral artery (a blood vessel that supplies the HIPPO-CAMPUS); less often, CVAs may cause amnesia by damaging the diencephalic structures.

Cause Blockage may be due to a clot formation (thrombosis) or an embolism, and rupture of different blood vessels may cause different patterns of bleeding. About 8 percent of cerebral vascular accidents are due to a SUBARACHNOID HEMORRHAGE, usually affecting a younger age group who are less likely to suffer from widespread cerebral vascular disease. The usual cause of such a hemorrhage is the rupture of a brain ANEURYSM (ballooning of an artery), which bleeds into the SUBARACH-NOID SPACE surrounding the brain. In addition, the ANTERIOR COMMUNICATING ARTERY (located between the FRONTAL LOBES) is often associated with ruptured aneurysms. Other common sites are the middle cerebral artery and the posterior communicating artery. While a hemorrhage may sometimes be caused by a ruptured benign tumor, in about 20 percent of cases no structural cause is known.

Symptoms Shortly after the hemorrhage, symptoms similar to those found in KORSA-KOFF'S SYNDROME may occur, including disorientation, confabulation, and impaired memory. Memory impairment following a subarachnoid hemorrhage may be temporary or permanent. TRANSIENT GLOBAL AMNESIA is almost certainly due to a cerebral vascular cause, with a sudden onset of symptoms in an otherwise normal patient. The episode may begin with a brief clouding of consciousness; the amnesia usually lasts for several hours, ending in complete recovery.

cerebrovascular disease Any disease that affects an artery supplying blood to the brain, such as ATHEROSCLEROSIS (narrowing of the arteries). This type of disease may eventually lead to a CEREBROVASCULAR ACCIDENT (CVA), a sudden block or rupture of a blood vessel commonly resulting in a STROKE.

cerebrum The largest, most highly developed section of the brain (80 percent of the brain), this area is the site of most conscious (voluntary) and intellectual activities. The cerebrum contains centers for sight, sound, smell and touch, intelligence, and memory; if these parts are damaged, the senses they serve may be impaired.

The cerebrum is made up of billions of nerve cells and is divided into two hemispheres, each containing a central cavity (or VENTRICLE) filled with CEREBROSPINAL FLUID. These two hemispheres, outgrowths from the upper part of the BRAINSTEM, are called the right and left CEREBRAL HEMISPHERE. These halves are the part of the brain that is responsible for higher-order thinking and decision making.

The right side of the cerebrum controls the left side of the body, and the left side of the cerebrum controls the right side of the body. For most people (right-handed people and most left-handed ones), the so-called left brain is dominant; this is the hemisphere that focuses on word comprehension, language, speech and numbers. The right brain focuses more on feelings and spatial relationships.

Long ago, the cerebrum functioned as part of the olfactory lobes; over time, it has grown over the rest of the brain, forming a wrinkly top layer. In sheer sophistication and size/body weight comparisons, the human cerebrum is unusual in the animal kingdom (except for certain sea mammals).

The outer layer of the cerebrum is called the CORTEX. Indentations (called *fissures*) divide each cerebral hemisphere into four lobes: the FRONTAL LOBE, PARIETAL LOBE, TEMPORAL LOBE, and OCCIPITAL LOBE. Functions involving memory are thought to take place within the frontal lobe, the parietal lobe, and the temporal lobe.

While scientists have come to a general understanding of the cerebrum's function, the details of its mechanism remains shrouded in mystery, and its complexity remains largely unraveled.

cerebrum, diseases of the   The cerebrum makes up the upper bulk of the brain and can be involved in various neural malformations. It also can be vulnerable to the typical array of brain diseases, including trauma, tumors, infections, demyelinating diseases, neurochemical disorders, and toxins.

chemical brain stimulation   The study of brain function in lab animals by injecting various chemicals directly into the brain or ventricular spaces. The most common studies investigate drugs that stimulate or inhibit NEUROTRANSMITTERS, which are responsible for transfer of information from one NERVE CELL to another.

The chemicals are introduced through very thin stainless-steel tubes implanted into the brain through small holes drilled into the skull. After the animal has recovered from surgery, it is subjected to a variety of behavioral tests that assess the ability to learn new tasks, regulate fluids, etc. In a different type of procedure, glass pipettes are implanted into specific areas of the brain through which drugs are injected; while the animal remains asleep, scientists record the electrical activity of nerve cells and their response to the drugs.

chemoreceptors   A cell (or group of cells) that responds to the presence of specific chemical compounds by triggering an electrical impulse in a sensory nerve. It is the chemoreceptor, for example, that allows us to tell salt from sugar, a fragrance from a stench.

Child Neurology Society   A group of neurologists who have either been certified by the American Board of Psychiatry and Neurology specializing in child neurology; become eligible for the certifying exam; made significant contributions to the field of child neurology; or enrolled in approved child neurology training programs.

The society's goals are to establish a scientific forum for professionals, to define areas of pediatric neurological practices, and to promote interest in the field.

Founded in 1971, the group has 1,000 members and sponsors an annual conference. It publishes the monthly journal *Annals of Neurology* and booklets. For address, see Appendix B.

Children and Adults with Attention Deficit Disorder (ADD) A national support group for parents and professionals with an interest in ATTENTION-DEFICIT DISORDERS, a neurologically based disorder that affects an individuals' behavior and learning.

The association's goals are to maintain a support group for parents of children with ADD, provide a forum for continuing education about ADD, provide resources and information, and assure the best educational opportunities for children with ADD so that their specific difficulties will be recognized and managed. Founded in 1987, the group has 460 local groups and publishes a magazine, newsletter, teacher's guide, slide presentations, booklets, and brochures. For address, see Appendix A.

chlorpromazine (Trade name: Thorazine) A major tranquilizer and antipsychotic drug that is used to treat SCHIZOPHRENIA and mania and to control severe ANXIETY and nausea or vomiting. Chlorpromazine also enhances the effects of painkillers and is used to treat terminally ill patients and those undergoing anesthesia. Chlorpromazine works primarily by blocking dopaminergic receptors.

Side effects Common side effects include dry mouth and drowsiness. Sometimes, it also causes movement abnormalities, such as TARDIVE DYSKINESIA.

choline A basic compound found in plant and animal tissue that is essential to the normal metabolism of fat. This dietary substance is the forerunner of ACETYLCHOLINE (a neurotransmitter). Choline has been implicated as a possible aid to improving memory by increasing the amount of acetylcholine in the brain. Other tests suggest choline may improve thinking ability, muscle control, and the nervous system.

Repeated studies of administering choline to treat the memory problems of ALZHEIMER'S DISEASE patients have resulted in conflicting evidence, although the majority found that giving choline was not helpful. Other studies suggest choline might be useful in heading off some deterioration in the early stages of the disease.

Still other studies have suggested that egg yolk (a dietary source of choline) may be useful to patients suffering from memory problems and seem to show an improvement in alcoholics and drug addicts. The major dietary source of choline is LECITHIN; foods rich in lecithin include eggs (average size), salmon, and lean beef. While some researchers dismiss the idea that eating these foods can significantly improve memory, other scientists note at least that a "normal" level of lecithin in the diet may not be enough as people age.

Phosphatidyl choline is used by the body as part of cell membranes, including those of neurons. NERVE and BRAIN CELLS especially repair and maintain themselves with large quantities of this substance.

In research at the University of Ohio, scientists noted that levels of choline drop as a person ages and that levels are especially low in people with Alzheimer's disease.

choline acetyltransferase (ChAT) An enzyme in the brain that promotes the reaction between CHOLINE and acetyl coenzyme A (an activated form of acetic acid) which produces ACETYLCHOLINE, a NEUROTRANSMITTER involved in many functions including learning and memory as well as the brain's control of skeletal musculature.

cholinergic Refers to those neurons that use ACETYLCHOLINE as a NEUROTRANSMITTER. The term may also refer to a RECEPTOR type.

cholinergic hypothesis of Alzheimer's disease There is a link between the decrease in the activity of the enzyme CHOLINE ACETYLTRANSFERASE (ChAT) in the brain of Alzheimer's patients and memory loss.

ChAT is a crucial ingredient in the chemical process that produces ACETYLCHOLINE, a NEUROTRANSMITTER linked to learning and memory. There has been a link between this change in neurochemical activity and changes in memory loss and disorientation and the physical appearance of Alzheimer brains (especially in the number of plaques).

Researchers have found a marked loss of NERVE CELLS in a part of the base of the brain called the NUCLEUS BASALIS; some patients with classical Alzheimer's disease have been shown to lose as many as 90 percent of these cells. The nucleus basalis is a major site of cholinergic neurons in the brain; its projections reach a number of brain areas associated with learning and memory.

cholinomimetic agents Any non-endogenous compound that activates cholinergic receptors, such as arecoline, nicotine, or muscarine.

chorea Involuntary, jerky movements (especially in the face and limbs) caused by dysfunction deep within the brain. Formerly called St. Vitus' Dance, these unpredictable movements are present in two diseases (HUNTINGTON'S DISEASE and Sydenham's chorea). It may sometimes appear during pregnancy (chorea gravidarum) or as a side effect of some drugs, in CEREBRAL PALSY or in ATHETOSIS.

chronic fatigue syndrome (CFS) A mysterious condition characterized by debilitating tiredness, sometimes derisively referred to as "yuppie flu," that is often associated with an inflammation of the brain. CFS is characterized by tiredness lasting six months or longer, together with irritability, lethargy, and an inability to think clearly. The condi-

tion first received attention in the mid-1980s after reports of about 100 cases appeared in the Lake Tahoe region of California.

Initially, many physicians dismissed CFS as hypochondria or a misdiagnosed depression; it was also called "yuppie flu" because most patients were professionals in their mid-30s (especially women). Because its symptoms were so similar to other diseases, this further complicated attempts to study the condition. Without a solid definition, scientists had problems identifying its cause and seeking a cure.

More recently, studies have begun to link the condition with physiological, rather than psychological, factors. In one recent study, MAGNETIC RESONANCE IMAGING scanned the brains of 259 patients in Lake Tahoe, 183 of whom were afflicted with CFS. In 78 percent of the patients, images showed tiny points of swelling on BRAIN CELLS in the central NERVOUS SYSTEM; the MYELIN SHEATH on some cells was also missing. These swellings did not appear in the same section of the brain for all patients, but researchers did discover a relationship between the region affected and the patient's symptoms. For example, patients who had vision problems also had disturbances in the OCCIPITAL LOBE of the brain—an area that processes vision.

Evidence also suggests that most patients exhibit an active herpes virus 6 (HHV-6), although scientists emphasize this does not mean the virus *causes* the condition. This virus is believed to infect most people in early life without producing any symptoms.

Still other studies suggest that the cause may be linked to a retrovirus in spinal fluid, known as a *spumavirus* or "foamy virus." Moreover, many patients suffer from irregularities in their immune systems and have abnormally low levels of hormones in the brain and endocrine glands.

cigarettes and the brain See SMOKING AND THE BRAIN.

circadian rhythm   A daily activity rhythm that cycles over 24 hours (from the Latin *circa*, "about," and *dies*, "a day"). The best-known human circadian rhythm is the daily sleep/waking cycle. Other circadian rhythms are body temperature, hormone levels, urine production, and levels of cognitive and motor performance.

For hundreds of years, scientists have known that plants underwent daily cycles of leaf and petal movements; more recently, the widespread circadian rhythmicity in animals has been demonstrated.

A person's rhythms are cyclical, rising and falling during certain times of the day and of the week. Although most people experience a period of "peak" efficiency somewhere between 11 A.M. and 4 P.M., every person's internal body clock is different. As the day progresses, a person becomes more involved in activities, but by lunch time, tiredness sets in. The daily biological cycles (body temperature, respiration, and pulse rate) alters the power of attention.

People who go to bed and wake up early learn more readily at the beginning of the day when their attention is best, while those who have a later schedule experience the opposite. Those who work a night shift probably experience different cyclical peak times than those who work a nine-to-five schedule.

What is especially striking is how a living organism will respond differently to a physiological challenge depending on its internal circadian rhythm. For example, the dose of amphetamine that will kill 78 percent of a group of rats at 3 A.M. is lethal for only 7 percent if injected at 6 A.M. or later; identical injections of lidocaine hydrochloride triggers convulsions in only 6 percent of rodents at 3 P.M. but at 9 P.M., 83 percent of rodents experience convulsions. Similarly, allergic reactions to certain antigens tend to be more severe in the evening than during the morning hours.

Importantly, time-related variations in the effectiveness and toxic side effects of drugs is routinely found in human patients.

Years ago, scientists assumed that circadian rhythm was just a direct response to the natural sequence of day and night. However, more recent research has revealed that without such obvious time cues as regularly alternating dark and light, rhythms persist, although the period of time may deviate significantly from 24 hours and differ from one person to another. Researchers now believe that every person has an intrinsic, innate circadian rhythm ordinarily synchronized to 24 hours by recurring stimuli (such as day and night)—but not necessarily bound to those cues.

While most researchers don't believe people "learn" their rhythms, it *has* been shown that early experience with light and dark cycles longer or shorter than 24 hours can have a long-lasting effect on an individual's circadian rhythm.

The limits of a circadian cycle are between 20 and 28 hours; rhythms of slower frequency are called INFRADIAN RHYTHM and those of faster frequency are termed ULTRADIAN RHYTHM.

circulation and the brain   When blood pressure falls to the point where it isn't high enough to pump blood to the brain, especially when a patient stands up, this causes symptoms that can include dizziness, memory loss, and fainting. If the blood does not begin flowing to the brain, the brain tissue will begin to die from lack of oxygen, resulting in coma and death.

clonidine   A drug used to treat high blood pressure that works by reducing nerve impulses from the brain to the heart and circulatory system.

cluster headaches   See HEADACHES.

cocaine and the brain Cocaine, an alkaloid derived from the coca plant (*Erythroxylon coca*), produces its stimulating effects by enhancing the activity of DOPAMINE and NOREPINEPHRINE neurons. (It is dopamine that also plays a key role in the development of SCHIZOPHRENIA and PARKINSON'S DISEASE.) Cocaine works by not only increasing the release of norepinephrine and dopamine, but also by blocking their reuptake. This overuse of the two systems takes its toll on the brain areas that normally rely on these neurotransmitter systems for function—learning and memory areas, and limbic structures. This is why heavy cocaine use leads to emotional and cognitive disorders. The overall effect on the brain and nervous system is to stimulate the part of the LIMBIC SYSTEM known as the NUCLEUS ACCUMBENS, where a large number of dopamine AXONS terminate, producing a feeling of euphoria. Eventually, however, the receptors become desensitized by this process, and it takes more and more cocaine to create the same sensation. Withdrawal can be just as harsh from cocaine as from opiates.

The feeling of alertness experienced by cocaine users is caused by the increasing activity of norepinephrine cells in the higher thought centers of the CEREBRAL CORTEX.

Chronic administration can result in permanent neurological damage, at least among animals; brain damage in humans is still being studied. At its worst, users can experience a frightening psychotic condition known as *cocaine psychosis*, which may appear similar to schizophrenia. It is believed to be related to dopamine. Scientists know that doctors treat schizophrenia by giving drugs that block dopamine receptors; cocaine, which enhances dopamine release, will worsen the condition of schizophrenia. Therefore, a cocaine psychosis may be caused by excessively high dopamine levels in the brain induced by cocaine use.

For reasons little understood, cocaine will cause psychosis selectively; cocaine poisoning is equally unpredictable. An overdose of cocaine can cause convulsions and death by depressing the brain centers that control breathing and heart activity. In these cases, death can occur so quickly that there is no time to treat the overdose. This type of cocaine poisoning was the cause of death in several young athletes, including University of Maryland basketball player Len Bias, the first-round draft choice of the Boston Celtics in 1986.

More than a thousand years ago, South American Indians chewed the leaves of coca plants for the energy boost it gave them. The habit was introduced by Spanish explorers into Europe, where the leaves were used to make beverages. In the United States, the original recipe for Coca-Cola used a coca-leaf extract, but it was eliminated many years ago when the harmful effects of cocaine were discovered.

Cocaine was isolated from the leaves in 1860 by a German chemist, and its use was quickly taken up by Sigmund Freud, who had studied cocaine as a treatment for nervous exhaustion as a young neurologist. In 1884 he published *Uber Coca* in which he stated that a person could enjoy cocaine "without any of the unpleasant aftereffects that follow exhilaration brought about by alcohol." He believed that cocaine could cure many diseases and could also cure narcotic addiction, and he prescribed it for his close friend Ernst von Fleischl-Marxow, who was addicted to morphine. Unfortunately, Fleischl-Marxow became a cocaine addict, suffered toxic psychosis, and died. In spite of this, Freud used cocaine himself for many years, although he did finally begin to write about its newly discovered dangers.

Cocaine was eventually discredited as a medicine except for its use as a local anesthetic that can block pain without putting the patient to sleep. Procaine, a drug derived from cocaine, is still used today in eye surgery and dentistry.

Cognex The brand name for the drug tacrine (tetrahydroamainoacridine, or THA) recently approved for the treatment of ALZHEIMER'S DISEASE. Although tacrine is not a cure for the disease, it is the first drug proved to have some effect on the disease's devastating symptoms and can provide small but meaningful improvement in memory and reasoning ability for some patients suffering from mild to moderate Alzheimer's. It will not help those with very advanced cases. About 40 percent of patients with mild cases who took the drug experienced a brief slowing of progressive memory loss. In addition, research shows improved cognitive abilities in some patients who take the drug. In two of the tacrine tests, patient memory, awareness, and language levels improved, and subjects were better able to handle the activities of daily living.

Cognex blocks the function of enzymes that normally break down acetylcholine, making more of the neurotransmitter available to brain cells. A slow depletion of acetylcholine in the brain is one of the characteristics of Alzheimer's disease. Manufacturer Warner-Lambert Co. of Morris Plains, New Jersey, began to sell the drug in late 1993. The drug coasts about $1,500 a year.

Side effects The most significant side effect, according to Warner-Lambert, is an elevation of liver enzymes that, if untreated, could cause liver damage. This condition was reversed in all cases when therapy was reduced or discontinued. Weekly blood tests are required in order to detect the problem.

colliculus Two pairs of colliculi, the superior and the inferior, protrude from the roof of the MIDBRAIN. The superior colliculus is involved in processing involuntary tracking reflexes of the visual system; the inferior colliculus is a relay area for auditory processing.

coma A state of unresponsive unconsciousness in which the person does not respond to external stimuli (such as a pinprick or a shout) or to inner needs (such as a full bladder). It is caused by damage or a disturbance in the parts of the brain involved in conscious activity or the maintenance of consciousness, including the CEREBRUM, upper parts of the BRAINSTEM, central regions of the brain and the LIMBIC SYSTEM. In particular, coma will result from injury or damage to the RETICULAR FORMATION, the brain structure crucial to maintaining consciousness.

Coma may result from BRAIN DAMAGE such as that caused by brain ABSCESS, BRAIN TUMOR, or INTRACEREBRAL HEMORRHAGE. Coma could also be caused by the accumulation of toxic substances (such as in drug overdoses, acute alcohol intoxication, etc.). All CENTRAL NERVOUS SYSTEM DEPRESSANTS (such as alcohol or BARBITURATES) can lead to coma when taken in overdose, and they are particularly dangerous when taken together. OPIATES (such as heroin or morphine) can also lead to coma. Coma may also result from the interruption of blood flow; inflammatory diseases such as ENCEPHALITIS or MENINGITIS may also cause a coma.

A patient may remain deeply comatose but alive for many years if the brain stem is still functioning. Once brain damage spreads to the lower brain stem laryngeal function (coughing and swallowing), breathing will begin to deteriorate.

Symptoms A coma may occur in various degrees of severity. In mild forms, the patient may respond to stimuli by speaking a few words or moving a body part. In more severe cases, the patient cannot respond in any way. But even deeply comatose patients may continue to breathe, cough, yawn, blink, or exhibit eye movements. These automatic responses indicate that the lower brainstem, which controls these responses, is still functioning.

The depth of coma may be measured by a variety of means, such as assessments of verbal behavior, eye movements, etc.

commissures, cerebral See CEREBRAL COMMISSURES.

commissurotomy Cutting of the CORPUS CALLOSUM and perhaps the other cerebral COMMISSURES (anterior and posterior) as well. See SPLIT-BRAIN RESEARCH.

complementarity The distribution of skills in the cerebral hemispheres so that if language is represented in one hemisphere, some non-language skills will reside in the other.

computerized axial tomography (CAT) scan See CAT SCAN.

concentration See ATTENTION.

concussion Brief unconsciousness after a blow to the head or neck, caused by a disturbance of the neural activity in the brain. An impact to the head creates a sudden movement of the brain within the skull; the outer surface of the cortex actually strikes the inner surface of the skull. This jolt causes aberrant neural activity that can lead to many short- and long-term problems. A concussion produces no evidence of structural damage to the brain, although there may be cuts or bruises on the skin outside the skull. About a third of all those with concussion go on to develop a combination of symptoms called POSTCONCUSSION SYNDROME for some time after the HEAD INJURY. Recent research has suggested that postconcussion syndrome can include significant memory problems, dizziness, and behavior and cognitive changes

that can disturb patients up to a year following the head injury. Despite sometimes significant symptoms, structural damage may not show up on brain scans.

Repeated concussions (such as damage in the boxing ring) can impair concentration and result in slow thinking and slur speech.

Symptoms Common symptoms immediately following a concussion include confusion, memory loss, dizziness, blurred vision, and vomiting. Partial paralysis and shock are also possible. The longer the period of unconsciousness, the more serious and persistent symptoms tend to be. During the 24 hours after the injury, symptoms may include headache, vomiting, increased pulse rate, and anxiety. Symptoms usually begin to disappear within a few days. Any loss of consciousness should be referred to a physician because of the possibility of serious bleeding within the skull that could require emergency surgery. Symptoms of serious damage may be immediately obvious or may not appear for some time.

Treatment A patient who has experienced concussion should be observed in bed for 24 hours and should not drive a car or play sports as blackouts can occur. New symptoms (drowsiness, breathing problems, repeated vomiting, or visual disturbances) should be reported immediately to a physician because they indicate potential damage to the brain or bleeding between the skull and the outer surface of the brain.

Acetaminophen or another painkiller may be prescribed for headache. Aspirin is not generally recommended because it can contribute to bleeding. Rest and relaxation with no activities requiring concentration or vigorous movement will speed recovery within a few days.

congenital brain defects Brain defects present at birth. These defects may be caused by genetic or chromosomal problems and result in a variety of disorders such as DOWN SYNDROME, TAY-SACH'S DISEASE, or CRI DU CHAT SYNDROME (all involving retardation). In addition, brain defects may be structural in nature; these are usually fundamental and untreatable, such as MICROCEPHALY (small head) and ANENCEPHALY (absence of the brain). Others, such as HYDROCEPHALUS (water on the brain) are correctable while the fetus remains in the womb.

Congress of Neurological Surgeons A professional society of neurological surgeons in the United States and 55 other countries who meet annually to discuss the principles and practice of neurological surgery, exchange technical information and experience, and study developments in allied fields. The group also promotes interest of neurological surgeons in their practice and provides placement services.

The congress publishes the annual *Clinical Neurosurgery*; the monthly *Neurosurgery*; the quarterly *Newsletter* and both world and U.S./ Canada directories of members. Founded in 1951, the congress has 2,700 members and sponsors an annual congress. For address, see Appendix B.

consciousness The awareness of the self and of one's surroundings. This awareness depends on a combination of sensations, memories, and experiences. Consciousness relies on the proper function of the CEREBRUM (the main mass of the brain) and the reticular system in the BRAINSTEM.

Some researchers, including Endel Tulving, have postulated that there are three varieties of consciousness: noetic, autonomous and anoetic. Noetic consciousness implies a semantic memory because it involves thinking about objects and events and relationships among them in their absence. Autonomous consciousness is self-knowing; it is related to episodic memory that recognizes events as in the personal past. Anoetic consciousness is

nonknowing, but it is still consciousness because it allows appropriate behavioral responses to aspects of the environment.

Some scientists believe that the perception of consciousness occurs when NERVE CELLS fire at similar frequencies, which imposes a "global unity" on nerve cells in different brain areas.

While a person maintains consciousness, there is still a great deal that goes on without a person's awareness; this is referred to as subconscious activity. According to psychoanalysts, it's the part of the mind through which information passes on its way from the unconscious to the conscious mind. It contains feelings, thoughts or ideas you may be unaware of but that can be recalled.

When consciousness is impaired, the person begins to have problems with attention, concentration, and understanding; memory fails and there is a lack of direction and purpose. As the level of arousal drops, the person may pass into a state of stupor and then COMA. However, despite the common perception of "losing" consciousness, the unconscious state is more of a shift in consciousness that allows the brain to filter incoming information in a different manner.

contrecoup effects French for "opposite blow," this term refers to HEAD INJURY damage to the side of the head opposite the point of impact. For example, a blow to the right side of the head causes the brain to crash into the left side of the inner skull. This is especially likely to occur in the temporal and orbital regions of the brain and may destroy neurons.

corpus callosum A bundle of white matter 4 inches long that contains 300 million myelinated nerve fibers. It is the main bridge between the left and right hemispheres of the brain and carries messages between them.

Some scientists believe that SCHIZOPHRENIA may be associated with abnormalities in the corpus callosum because scans and tests have found a thickened, damaged, or nonfunctioning corpus callosum in some schizophrenic patients.

Other studies of gender differences in brain structure have revealed that a man's corpus callosum is relatively smaller than a woman's. In women, the rear of the corpus callosum is larger than in men; this may explain why women use both sides of their brain for language. The smaller corpus callosum in men may also suggest that the two hemispheres in the male brain may intercommunicate less often. See SPLIT BRAIN RESEARCH.

corpus striatum See STRIATUM.

cortex See CEREBRAL CORTEX.

cortex, limbic See LIMBIC SYSTEM.

corticotropin-releasing factor A chemical secreted by the HYPOTHALAMUS that stimulates the anterior pituitary to produce ADRENOCORTICOTROPIC HORMONE (ACTH). In turn, ACTH stimulates the adrenal cortex to produce glucocorticoids (primarily cortisol), which in turn stimulates the release of AMINO ACIDS. The releasing of corticotropin-releasing factor is an important component of the brain's response to stress.

See STRESS AND THE BRAIN.

Cotugno, Domenico (1736–1822) Italian anatomist who discovered in 1774 that the brain's cavities were not filled with "animal spirit" but with cerebrospinal fluid.

See also BRAIN IN HISTORY.

Council for Learning Disabilities A professional group for those interested in the study of LEARNING DISABILITIES that works to promote the education and general welfare of those who have specific learning disabilities by improving teacher-preparation programs and local special-education programs and re-

solving important research issues. Founded in 1967, the group has 4,500 members and publishes a quarterly *LD Forum* and a quarterly journal. For address, see Appendix B.

cranial nerve, eighth See VESTIBULOCOCHLEAR NERVE.

cranial nerve, eleventh See SPINAL ACCESSORY NERVE.

cranial nerve, fifth See TRIGEMINAL NERVE.

cranial nerve, first See OLFACTORY NERVE.

cranial nerve, fourth See TROCHLEAR NERVE.

cranial nerve, ninth See GLOSSOPHARYNGEAL NERVE.

cranial nerves A series of 12 nerve pairs connecting directly to the brain, emerging through openings in the skull and then dividing into several major branches. All but two of the cranial-nerve pairs connect with nuclei in the BRAINSTEM (the lowest section of the brain). One nerve from each pair serves one side of the body, while the other nerve serves the other side.

The cranial nerves, known by a numbering system invented by the early Greek physician GALEN, include the OLFACTORY NERVE (first cranial nerve); OPTIC NERVE (second cranial nerve); OCULOMOTOR NERVE (third cranial nerve); TROCHLEAR NERVE (fourth cranial nerve); TRIGEMINAL NERVE (fifth cranial nerve); ABDUCENS NERVE (sixth cranial nerve); FACIAL NERVE (seventh cranial nerve); VESTIBULOCOCHLEAR NERVE (eighth cranial nerve); GLOSSOPHARYNGEAL NERVE (ninth cranial nerve); VAGUS NERVE (tenth cranial nerve); SPINAL ACCESSORY NERVE (eleventh cranial nerve); HYPOGLOSSAL NERVE (twelfth cranial nerve).

Each of the cranial nerves plays a part in at least one of the following operations: carrying motor and sensory information to regions of the head and neck; serving as the basic wiring system of the sense of vision, hearing and balance, taste and smell; and transmitting autonomic information to special glands and organs.

Some of the cranial nerves play a variety of roles. For example, the trigeminal nerve wears several hats, carrying sensations from the face, teeth and sinuses to the brain as well as controlling several important muscles, including the strong jaw muscles used for chewing. The facial nerve sends branches to the important facial muscles of expression—those used in smiling, frowning, raising one's eyebrows, etc. The olfactory and optic nerves carry visual and olfactory input from the eyes and nose to the brain for processing. The oculomotor nerve controls eye movements and also helps focus images on the retina. The vagus nerve, in addition to performing sensory and motor functions, sends nerve fibers to the heart, stomach, and intestines to help regulate autonomic activity.

cranial nerve, second See OPTIC NERVE.

cranial nerve, seventh See FACIAL NERVE.

cranial nerve, sixth See ABDUCENT NERVE.

cranial nerve, tenth See VAGUS NERVE.

cranial nerve, third See OCULOMOTOR NERVE.

cranial nerve, twelfth See HYPOGLOSSAL NERVE.

craniopharyngioma A benign, congenital tumor of the PITUITARY GLAND that, if untreated, may cause permanent brain damage due to intracranial pressure. This very rare condition only affects one or two people per million Americans yearly, causing headaches, vomiting, vision problems, stunted growth, and failure to develop sexually.

Treatment The tumors are usually surgically removed; because it is usually in a favorable location, it can often be almost completely excised. Radiation therapy may be indicated if the tumor is not completely removed.

craniosynostosis The early fusion of one or more joints (or sutures) between the skull bones during infancy. A baby with this condition is born without fontanelles (or spaces between the plates of the skull) that allow for growth. For more information, see Appendix A (Society for Children with Craniosynostosis).

Causes Craniosynostosis may appear in an infant with bone disease (such as rickets), multiple birth defects, an abnormally small brain—or in a perfectly healthy infant.

Treatment To prevent brain damage, treatment (surgical splitting of the skull bones) must begin within the first few months of life.

craniotomy Removal of part of the skull during brain surgery. In this procedure, an incision is made into the skin, and using a high-speed drill, a piece of bone is removed from the skull to expose the brain. After the operation, the piece of bone is replaced and the membrane, muscle, and skin are sutured. Patients generally experience a mild headache for a period of time after the operation.

A craniotomy is the most commonly performed surgery for removal of a brain tumor (see TUMOR, BRAIN). *Crani* means "skull," and *otomy* means "cutting into."

cranium The hard shell encasing the brain, made up of eight fused skull bones: the occipital bone, lying at the back of the head; the sphenoid bone, a wedge-shaped bone at the skull base; the parietal bones, forming a wall at the top and sides of the head; the temporal bones forming the "temples" above the ears; the frontal bone forming the forehead; and the ethmoid bone lying behind the nose, which is pierced to take olfactory nerve bundles.

Creutzfeldt-Jakob disease (CJD) A very rare infectious viral disease of the nervous system caused by a transmissible infectious organism, probably a SLOW VIRUS or PRION, that causes a progressive DEMENTIA with seizures. It can usually be distinguished from other dementias by its rapid course—it takes only months from onset of symptoms until death.

It is possible for an infected patient to transmit the disease to monkeys, cats, and guinea pigs, but the disease is not contagious between humans. However, infection has been linked to brain surgery with contaminated instruments or transplantation of an infected cornea. Some cases have been traced to young people treated with contaminated human growth hormone. There are also indications that there may be a genetic link to this condition. It is considered to be more prevalent in Sephardic Jews and in families from Chile and Slovakia.

An accurate diagnosis requires an autopsy.

Symptoms The first symptoms involve a sudden progressive memory loss, bizarre behavior, reasoning problems, visual distortions of objects, HALLUCINATIONS and mental confusion, and a lack of coordination. As the disease progresses (usually very rapidly), mental deterioration becomes pronounced, involuntary movements and muscle jerks appear, and the patient may become blind, develop weakness in the arms or legs, and ultimately lapse into COMA.

CJD patients usually die from infections that proliferate in bedridden, unconscious patients.

Treatment At present, there is no treatment.

cri du chat syndrome Also known as "cry of the cat syndrome" or "5p-syndrome," this is a rare congenital condition characterized by a kittenlike mewing cry caused by a small larynx. The cry usually disappears after the first few weeks, but the syndrome is usually linked with MENTAL RETARDATION, heart problems, unusual facial characteristics (such as widely spaced eyes), small head, and short stature.

The condition is the result of a chromosomal abnormality in which a portion of chromosome 5 is missing in each of the person's cells. There is no treatment, and the child may not survive infancy.

For more information, contact the 5p- Society, a mutual-support, self-help organization for families, that provides information and publishes various materials, including a quarterly newsletter.

For address, see Appendix A.

cryptococcosis A rare infection caused by inhaling a fungus *cryptococcus neoformans* found in soil and pigeon droppings throughout the world that can lead to MENINGITIS, an inflammation of the coverings of the brain. Those most susceptible to cryptococcosis are those with weakened immune systems, such as AIDS patients. Symptoms may include low-grade fever, chest pain, and a cough, but more serious cases resemble bronchitis and lead to meningitis, with symptoms of HEADACHE, stiff neck, fever, drowsiness, blurred vision, mental deterioration, and staggering gait; untreated, it can cause COMA and death.

Cryptococcosis is diagnosed from spinal fluid; if the disease has affected the brain, treatment includes a combination of the antifungal drugs flucytosine and amphotericin B for six weeks. Relapses can occur, however.

CT scan See CAT SCAN.

CVA See CEREBROVASCULAR ACCIDENT.

cysticerocosis Multiple brain cysts produced by the larval form of the pork tapeworm *Taenia solium*. Once the larvae have migrated from the intestine into the blood-stream, they migrate to muscle, eye, and brain, where they are associated with intense inflammation.

Humans become infected by ingesting tapeworm eggs in contaminated food or drinks.

Symptoms Cysticerocosis often causes no symptoms at first. The larvae in muscles causes pain and weakness, but in the brain the symptoms are more serious. The most common symptom that appears is SEIZURES. Other symptoms include mental deterioration, paralysis, giddiness, EPILEPSY, and convulsions, which may be fatal. Imaging studies reveal multiple calcifications and lesions in the brain.

Treatment Broad-spectrum antinematode drugs (such as praziquantel) kill surviving organisms. Surgical removal of cysticerci may be needed to relieve pressure on the brain.

D

da Vinci, Leonardo (1452–1519) Artist and scientist who, in 1505, made the first wax cast of the brain's ventricles using the brain of an ox. Da Vinci shifted the supposed site of sensory analysis in the brain to the second ventricle, where earlier researchers had thought the seat of reason could be found.

decerebrate Absence of a functioning CEREBRUM (cerebral hemisphere), the main control center of the brain. This occurs when the BRAINSTEM (lowest section of the brain) is severed, isolating the cerebrum.

degenerative diseases and the brain There are a whole range of degenerative diseases that can affect the brain, ranging from those that produce only slight problems to those that are rapidly fatal. These diseases include ALZHEIMER'S DISEASE, MULTIPLE SCLEROSIS, PARKINSON'S DISEASE, senile DEMENTIA, MOTOR-NEURON DISEASE, and HUNTINGTON'S DISEASE.

dehydroepiandrosterone (DHEA) One of the four most common steroid hormones in the body, it is produced mainly in the adrenal gland and may play a role in cognition. It is the precursor hormone to testosterone and estrogen. Because nerve degeneration occurs most often when DHEA levels are low, some researchers wonder if DHEA may protect brain cells against ALZHEIMER'S DISEASE and other forms of SENILITY. DHEA has been shown to improve long-term memory in mice.

Because Alzheimer's disease patients have almost half as much DHEA as their same-aged counterparts without the disease, studies have been looking at the possibility of using this drug to enhance their cognitive abilities.

déjà vu The sense of having already experienced an event that is happening at that moment, from the French meaning "already seen." This very common phenomenon has never been fully explained, but some scientists believe that a neurological glitch causes the experience to be registered in the memory before reaching consciousness. Other people believe déjà vu is an unconscious emotional response triggered by similarities between the current event and a past experience. Frequent occurrences of déjà vu may be a symptom of temporal lobe EPILEPSY.

delirium Acute mental confusion caused by a disordered brain function, characterized by disorientation, increased anxiety, failure to understand events, confusion, memory problems, sudden mood swings, illusions, HALLUCINATIONS, extreme excitement, panic, and violence. Symptoms are usually worse at night, either because of disturbed sleep or because the dark and quiet make visual illusions more common. It is an acute reaction to intoxication, disturbance of body chemistry, organic mental disorder, infection, high fever, HEAD INJURY, or trauma. It is most common among the very young and the very old, especially after major surgery or when there is a pre-existing brain disturbance.

Treatment Delirium is usually reversible once the underlying condition is recognized and treated. Patients require calm and clear communication, adequate lighting, appropriate seclusion, and known attendants. It is important to maintain fluids and nutrition; tranquilizers are often necessary to treat restlessness.

delirium tremens (DTs) An acute brain disorder characterized by confusion, trembling, and vivid HALLUCINATIONS, usually occurring in chronic alcoholics who stop drinking. It can be fatal in 10 to 15 percent of untreated cases. The cause of DTs is the withdrawal of alcohol after the brain and other organs have become accustomed to tolerating elevated levels of ethanol.

Symptoms, which usually develop within 24 to 96 hours after drinking stops, include restlessness, agitation, trembling and sleeplessness, rapid heartbeat, fever, sweating, confusion, hallucinations, delusions, paranoia, and convulsions. Symptoms usually subside within three days.

Treatment includes rest, rehydration, and sedation with vitamin injections because some of the features of delirium tremens seem linked with thiamine deficiency.

delta waves Brain wave pattern during deep sleep. In adults, the presence of waves during wakefulness show the presence of BRAIN DAMAGE or BRAIN DISORDERS.

dementia The general decline in all areas of mental ability, including memory, personality, visual skills, spatial relations, and general thinking ability. It may be caused by organic mental disorders (as injury or illness), or it may be a symptom of mental disturbance such as SCHIZOPHRENIA. More than 10 percent of all those over age 65 and 20 percent of those over age 75 have some degree of dementia.

Though there are some "reversible" cases of dementia, caused by HEAD INJURY, pernicious anemia, ENCEPHALITIS, myxedema, SYPHILIS, BRAIN TUMOR, or alcoholism), by far the majority of cases are more permanent, caused by CEREBROVASCULAR DISEASE (including STROKE) and from ALZHEIMER'S DISEASE. While it may be possible to alleviate some dementia by treating high blood pressure or heart disease, gradual deterioration usually occurs. Alzheimer's disease is at present incurable.

Symptoms A person with dementia may forget recent events, may lose touch with immediate surroundings, or may fail to negotiate familiar environments. These problems may become worse very gradually, and the patient may try to cover up the problem. The first obvious signs of dementia may involve emotional outbursts or inappropriate behavior in public (such as urinating outdoors).

As the dementia progresses, the patient may begin to make unreasonable demands or accusations, begin stealing, and even attack others physically. Paranoia, depression, and psychosis may develop as the disease worsens, and personal habits deteriorate. Eventually, demented individuals require total nursing care, including assistance with feeding, toileting, and physical activities.

demyelinating disorders A group of diseases characterized by the breakdown of myelin, the fatty sheath surrounding and insulating nerve fibers that interferes with nerve function. The best-known of these is MULTIPLE SCLEROSIS; others include Schilder's disease and dysmyelination disease. In *multiple sclerosis*, lesions appear in the brain and SPINAL CORD, causing a variety of intermittent neurological symptoms. While the cause of this demyelinating disease is unknown, some researchers believe it may involve a disruption in the body's immune system or by infection from a slow-acting virus. It generally strikes adults in their 30s and 40s, and its symptoms vary: some patients live many years with few symptoms, while others experience frequent attacks. In general, however, each new attack is followed by more severe episodes. The disease is not often immediately fatal; the average duration of life after onset is about 25 years. In the terminal stage, almost every portion of the nervous system is affected.

There is no known treatment that influences the symptoms of multiple sclerosis to any degree.

Schilder's disease, also known as *encephalitis periaxialis diffusa*, is a rapidly progressive sheath-destructive disorder that features widespread demyelination of the NEURONS in the cerebral hemispheres of the brain. This disease occurs more often in children and ends in death within a few years of onset.

Dysmyelination disease is best exemplified by metachromatic leukodystrophy (sulfatide lipoidosis), which results in impaired development of MYELIN in the brain along with a toughening of the brain.

The disorder often appears in the fiber tracts, which should myelinate after birth. The diseased tissues contain granular material that occurs from a defect in the metabolism of fatty substances (sulfatides) appearing in the nerves, pituitary gland, liver, testes, and kidneys and is excreted in the urine.

Symptoms, which appear in infancy, childhood, or early adult life, include convulsive seizures, optic atrophy, paralyses, and DEMENTIA, or emotional abnormalities. The disease ends in death within a few years of onset. There is no satisfactory treatment.

dendrite The branched extension of a NEURON that receives nerve impulses from other nerve cells and carries them toward the cell body.

Denver II A type of developmental screening test that measures four areas of behavior, including gross motor, fine motor, language, and personal-social. It is used for children from infancy through the preschool years. It is not an IQ test.

See also STANFORD-BINET TEST; WECHSLER INTELLIGENCE SCALE FOR CHILDREN REVISED.

deprenyl (Trade names: Eldepryl, Jumex) The treatment of choice for PARKINSON'S DISEASE and also an antidepressant, deprenyl is one of the class of drugs called MONOAMINE OXIDASE (MAO) INHIBITORS; it is currently being studied for the treatment of ALZHEIMER'S DISEASE. The drug has also been said to improve cognition in some patients, improving attention, memory, and reaction times. Newly diagnosed patients who receive deprenyl show much slower progression of their diseases.

Deprenyl is chemically related to AMPHETAMINE and PHENYLETHYLAMINE, a substance found in chocolate, and stimulates the SUBSTANTIA NIGRA, a tiny brain region rich in DOPAMINE-using BRAIN CELLS. (It is the deficiency of dopamine that can result in Parkinson's symptoms.) Degeneration of the NEURONS in the substantia nigra also has been associated with the aging process.

depression and the brain While there are many theories of depression, most experts agree that depression isn't caused by any one specific problem. Instead, it's the result of a collision between genetics, biochemistry, and psychological factors. The physiological basis of depression may be found in neurons in the part of the brain responsible for human emotions centered in the HYPOTHALAMUS, a cherry-sized structure that controls basic functions such as thirst, hunger, sleep, sexual desire, and body temperature.

Each nerve cell in the brain is separated by tiny gaps called synapses; neurons communicate by sending chemical messengers across these gaps to a "RECEPTOR" on the other side. Each neurotransmitter has a special shape that helps it fit exactly into a corresponding receptor like a key into an ignition switch. When the neurotransmitter "key" is inserted into its matching receptor's "ignition," the cell receiving the transmitter may then fire an "action potential," the electrical impulse that travels down the axon, to release its own transmitter to the next neuron. Once the message is sent, the neurotransmitter is either absorbed into the cell or burned up by enzymes patrolling the gaps.

When there are abnormally low levels of certain neurotransmitters, messages can't get across the gaps, and communication in the brain slows down. It appears that depression occurs if there isn't enough of these neurotransmitters circulating in the brain or if the neurotransmitters can't fit into the receptors for some reason.

While there are as many as 100 different kinds of neurotransmitters, NOREPINEPHRINE, DOPAMINE, and SEROTONIN seem to be of particular importance in depression. The pathways for these neurotransmitters reach deep into many of the parts of the brain responsible for functions that are affected in depression—sleep, appetite, mood, and sexual interest.

Scientists aren't sure whether depression is directly related to abnormal levels of these transmitters or whether these neurotransmitters affect yet another neurotransmitter that's even more directly involved in depression. But it is clear that neurotransmitters are related to depression because medications that boost levels of these neurotransmitters also ease depression. Yet, some of the newer antidepressants don't affect the levels of all of these neurotransmitters, while they still relieve depression, and other drugs (such as cocaine) that *do* interfere with neurotransmitter levels *don't* affect depression.

Moreover, antidepressants can raise neurotransmitter levels almost immediately, but depression doesn't improve until weeks after drug therapy has begun.

Depression appears to be far more than a simple problem with the amount of neurotransmitters in the synaptic cleft. It has become clear that it is probably influenced by a profoundly complex interplay of receptor "ignition" responses and the release of the neurotransmitter "keys." It also appears that depression depends not just on the *number* of neurotransmitter "keys," but also the *quality* and *availability* of the receptor "ignitions."

One reason behind the antidepressants' lag time could be that antidepressants may cause a decrease in number of available receptors. When this happens, it could trigger an increase in the production of neurotransmitters. Importantly, these changes don't happen right after antidepressant treatment begins; the changes in the receptors typically can take up to several weeks. This receptor change has been reported in almost all antidepressant drug treatment and also in ELECTROCONVULSIVE THERAPY.

Diagnosis A diagnosis may begin with a brief family history with a medical workup, including tests to rule out low thyroid, mononucleosis, anemia, diabetes, adrenal insufficiency, and hepatitis.

Major depression While symptoms differ from one person to the next, major depression is almost always characterized by general feelings of sadness and a total loss of pleasure in things that once brought joy. There might be sleep and eating problems or a sense of worthlessness, a lack of interest in sex, with apathy or suicidal thoughts.

Like any other illness, there's a definite beginning and an end to major depression, and if it's not treated it may very well recur. Each time major depression strikes again, it tends to last longer and be more debilitating than before.

It's possible to have a major depression and not feel particularly sorrowful, sad, or hurting. Instead, there may be eating problems or problems sleeping, remembering, concentrating, or making decisions. Only a mental-health expert can diagnose a depression that is disguised as some of these symptoms.

Descartes, René (1596–1650) French philosopher, mathematician, and scientist who in 1637 publicized his theory that the soul and the brain were separate. His underlying belief was that the mind is not a product of the brain.

Beginning with his famous phrase, *Cogito, ergo sum* (I think, therefore I am), he described a theory of the mind that was an immaterial substance that engages in a variety of activities, including feeling, thinking, and willing.

See also BRAIN IN HISTORY.

development of the brain The *nervous system* is one of the first recognizable features of a human embryo. Only three weeks after conception, the brain's earliest form—the NEURAL TUBE—appears as a tiny sheet of cells on the back of the embryo, which is then only 3 mm long (a bit thicker than a nickel). The brain begins as a swelling at one end of the neural tube, formed by a ridge of neural tissue that rises and fuses along what will be the fetal back.

Once this occurs, the cells begin to multiply at breakneck speed, creating millions of new cells each day. The brain continues to develop along patterns roughly similar to the way the brain evolved, beginning with the BRAINSTEM. By five weeks, all three main brain regions are recognizable; by seven weeks the brain and SPINAL CORD have emerged. By 10 weeks, the FOREBRAIN has begun to overlap the brainstem, and somewhat later, the CEREBELLUM begins to grow. By 12 weeks, the brain is the size of a large pea.

BRAIN CELLS are especially active during two critical periods of fetal development—between 15 and 20 weeks after conception and again at 25 weeks. The second growth spurt persists slightly less intensively until birth.

During gestation, the brain will grow into a model about two-thirds the size of an adult brain, and is the fastest-growing structure before and shortly after birth than any other part of the body. During pregnancy, NEURONS can grow at a rate of 250,000 a minute, although half die before the baby is born. Scientists suspect this elimination of neural cells may eliminate faulty cells.

This period of brain growth is one of the most sensitive times of fetal development. Damage to developing cells may occur from maternal smoking or drinking, vitamin deficiency, prenatal exposure to chemicals, or excess heat. Illnesses of the mother during pregnancy may also severely affect fetal brain cells; studies suggest that influenza or malnutrition during pregnancy may be associated with the development of SCHIZOPHRENIA in the baby.

At birth, the brain is completely formed with every structure in place, but there is still a great deal of growth to come. Each neuron must make connections to others of its own kind, and all of the cells must be insulated with MYELIN; as the neurons branch and the cells become myelinated, the brain will enlarge and gain weight. These neuronal connections become more and more complex as the child grows. In the CORTEX itself, each cell must make as many as 10,000 connections to enable the child to speak, to perceive, and to develop coherent thought.

This process is far from an isolated exercise; the external environment, genes, and other stimulation affect a cell's connections. It is at this stage that any deprivation, whether emotional or sensory, can distort the brain's healthy growth.

Six months after birth, the child's brain weight has doubled and by age five, the child's brain is nine-tenths its adult weight.

This does not mean that a newborn baby has almost as much brain power as an adult. While its neurons are in place, the vital connections between these cells have not yet been forged.

diazepam (Trade name: Valium) One of the best-known BENZODIAZEPINE tranquilizers. With its muscle relaxant and anticonvulsant properties, diazepam is used to ease tension and anxiety and to treat EPILEPSY and insomnia.

Side effects Drowsiness and lethargy, dizziness and confusion. Alcohol increases the sedative properties of diazepam and should be avoided. Like other drugs in this class, diazepam is habit forming if taken regularly, and tolerance will occur. Patients who have taken diazepam for more than two weeks should not abruptly stop taking this medication but rather should gradually decrease the dose. Otherwise, withdrawal symptoms could include severe anxiety, sweating, or seizures.

diencephalon An anatomical division of the brain that is part of the uppermost part of the BRAINSTEM, that includes the THALAMUS; it connects via the FORNIX to the TEMPORAL LOBES and contains the HYPOTHALAMUS, the PITUITARY GLAND, and the PINEAL GLAND. The diencephalon also may be concerned with memory; it is one of the structures most commonly involved in KORSAKOFF'S SYNDROME. Furthermore, tumors of the third ventricle, a part of the diencephalon, are generally those which cause memory disorders. In fact, AMNESIA following diencephalon damage is quite common.

dimethylaminoethanol (DMAE) This naturally occurring nutrient is found in some types of seafood and in the human brain. Studies suggest this substance may improve memory and learning, elevate mood and increase physical energy, and act as both a mild stimulant and a sleep enhancer. It is believed to improve the brain's production of ACETYLCHOLINE, which plays an important part in memory and maintaining memory ability. Overdoses of DMAE may cause INSOMNIA, HEADACHE, or muscle tension, and while no serious adverse effects have been reported, it may deepen the depression phase in manic-depression patients.

DMAE See DIMETHYLAMINOETHANOL.

dominant hemisphere The tendency for one brain hemisphere to control the processing of information for a particular task. *Dominant hemisphere* is often used to refer to the hemisphere controlling speech.

dopamine A chemical messenger (neurotransmitter) in the brain and a member of the class of Catecholamines (a class of compounds that affects the nervous and cardiovascular systems, metabolic rate, and body temperature). Secreted by NEURONS in the SUBSTANTIA NIGRA, the MIDBRAIN, and the HYPO-

THALAMUS, dopamine is thought to play a role in controlling movements. PARKINSON'S DISEASE, a degenerative condition characterized by muscle rigidity and tremors, is due to loss of cells in the substantia nigra that release dopamine. In fact, drugs that mimic dopamine are used to treat Parkinson's, and drugs that relieve the symptoms of SCHIZOPHRENIA may also cause Parkinsonlike symptoms.

Identified in the late 1950s, this NEUROTRANSMITTER is part of the biosynthetic pathway of the neurotransmitter NOREPINEPHRINE and is believed to help regulate mood; when found in excess amounts in the LIMBIC SYSTEM, it can contribute to the development of schizophrenia.

dopamine hypothesis The theory that SCHIZOPHRENIA is the result (in part) of an excess of dopaminergic transmission in the brain. Schizophrenia can be treated in part by such drugs as CHLORPROMAZINE, a dopaminergic antagonist, which can interfere with dopamine's action.

dopaminergic Those neurons or areas of the CENTRAL NERVOUS SYSTEM that use DOPAMINE as a NEUROTRANSMITTER.

d-phenylalanine This chemical (abbreviated DPA) stops the enzymatic breakdown of ENKEPHALIN.

dreams Dreaming, the sometimes-haunting mental activity that takes place during sleep, is a state of lessened consciousness, lowered metabolism, and limited muscular activity. But scientists don't yet understand how we dream or what the biological function could be. Some believe that dreams represent the right brain talking to itself; others believe dreams are the way the brain discharges nonproductive thoughts; still others insist dreams are the brain's creative method of solving its own problems. Finally, the more purely biological explanation is that the brain is trying to understand random firings of NEURONS during sleep.

Most scientists do suspect that dreams allow mental impressions, feelings, and ideas absorbed during the day to be sorted out; the content of dreams often closely represent the day's preoccupations, although the ideas and memories are distorted by the lack of a conscious, awake mind.

Dreaming is believed to occur only during certain periods (the rapid-eye movement, or REM stage of sleep), which lasts for about 20 minutes four or five times a night. Later in the sleep cycle, one spends more and more time in REM sleep. During this stage, blood flow and brain temperature rise, and there are sudden changes in the heart rate and blood pressure. All this may indicate the brain is restoring itself for further activity. During REM sleep, the brain is actually more active than during waking periods. This is why REM sleep is called PARADOXICAL SLEEP.

While people who are awakened during REM SLEEP report vivid dreams, those who awaken normally may not remember dreaming at all.

REM sleep occurs far more often in young babies and after HEAD INJURY, which may indicate the important role that dreaming plays in promoting brain development and repair. Whether dreams serve important psychological functions is still controversial.

The average person experiences about 300,000 dreams over a lifetime, spending about 20 years of life in sleep.

DTs   See DELIRIUM TREMENS.

dura mater   Also known as pachymeninx, this is the thickest, outermost of the three membranes surrounding and protecting the brain and SPINAL CORD. It includes two layers; the inner dura extends downward between the CEREBRAL HEMISPHERES to form the falx cerebri, forward between the CEREBRUM and CEREBELLUM to form the tentorium. The inner dura is separated from the arachnoid by a thin film of fluid.

dysarthria   A speech problem caused by damage to or disease of the musculature controlling the voice apparatus; unlike APHASIA, patients with dysarthria have no problems with the speech center in the brain. Dysarthritic patients can select and write out words and sentences; they simply cannot form vocal expression.

Dysarthria is a common characteristic of a wide range of DEGENERATIVE DISEASES such as MULTIPLE SCLEROSIS, PARKINSON'S DISEASE and HUNTINGTON'S DISEASE, and occasionally CEREBRAL PALSY. It may be caused by a STROKE, a BRAIN TUMOR, or damage to a particular nerve controlling the structures of speech (larynx, tongue etc.).

Treatment   There is no specific treatment, although medication or surgery may restore the ability to speak by treating the underlying disease. Speech therapy may also be of help.

dysautonomia   A genetic disease of the AUTONOMIC NERVOUS SYSTEM. Also known as Riley-Day syndrome, its symptoms include absence of tears, skin blotching, excess sweating, insensitivity to pain, and excess growth. There seems to be a general defect of the autonomic and sensory nerve fibers. For address, see Appendix A.

See also DYSAUTONOMIA FOUNDATION.

Dysautonomia Foundation   A support group for parents, relatives, friends, and benefactors of children affected with DYSAUTONOMIA. The foundation funds research in the causes and cure of the disease and publishes a semiannual newsletter and an annual journal. Founded in 1954, the group has 5,000 members. For address, see Appendix A.

dyskinesia   Abnormal muscular movements caused by a brain disorder, causing uncontrollable jerking or twitching. The disorder may affect the entire body or just one group of muscles. Types of dyskinesia include CHOREA (jerking movements), athetosis (writhing), choreoathetosis (a combination of jerking and writhing), tics (repetitive movements), TREMORS, or myoclonus (muscle spasms).

dyslexia A specific reading disability characterized by problems in coping with written symbols, despite normal intelligence and vision. This term does not describe other types of reading problems, such as those caused by brain damage or mental retardation.

There have been many suggestions as to the cause of dyslexia, including emotional disturbances, minor visual defects, and failure to train the brain, but more recent research suggests that it arises from an inherited neurological disorder; some 90 percent of dyslexics are male.

Recent research at Harvard University suggests that dyslexia could be a defect in the brain involving the sense of vision. They linked the problem to defects in certain kinds of cells that transmit visual stimuli of low contrast and rapid motion from the eye to the brain.

The key characteristic in dyslexia is that the child has completely normal intelligence; usually, the child has little problem in reading musical notes or numbers. A dyslexic child may see printed words upside down, backward, or otherwise distorted. Letters are often transposed and spelling errors are common. The total inability to read (to interpret written symbols) is called *alexia* or *word blindness*.

See also LEARNING DISABILITIES.

dysmyelination disease A type of MYELIN disease best exemplified by metachromatic leukodystrophy (sulfatide lipoidosis), causing poor development of myelin in the brain along with a toughening of the WHITE MATTER of the CEREBRUM and CEREBELLUM.

The disorder often appears in the fiber tracts which should myelinate after birth. The diseased tissues contain granular material that results from a defect in the metabolism of fatty substances (sulfatides) appearing in the nerves, PITUITARY GLAND, liver, testes, and kidneys and is excreted in the urine.

Symptoms Symptoms, which appear in infancy, childhood, or early adult life, include convulsive seizures, optic atrophy, paralyses, and DEMENTIA or emotional abnormalities. The disease ends in death within a few years of onset.

Treatment There is no satisfactory treatment.

dysphasia A term used to describe a problem with the ability to select words (and/ or to comprehend and read) that is caused by damage to parts of the brain that control speech and comprehension.

See also AGRAPHIA; ALEXIA; APHASIA; APRAXIA.

dystonia Abnormal muscle rigidity resulting in painful muscle spasms, fixed posture, or strange movements. Generalized dystonia usually is caused by neurological disorders, such as PARKINSON'S DISEASE or STROKE, or may be a feature of SCHIZOPHRENIA. It may also be a side effect of ANTIPSYCHOTIC DRUGS.

E

Early Language Milestone Scale (ELMS)
An easily administered screening instrument that provides an indication of delay in expressive and receptive language up to the age of three years.

See also CENTRAL LINGUISTIC AUDITORY MILESTONES SCALE (CLAMS).

eating and the brain What a person eats may have an effect on the brain's performance; when and how much a person eats may have almost as much effect. Research suggests that foods low in protein and high in carbohydrates boost alertness and performance by raising the level of TRYPTOPHAN in the brain.

Other studies have found that eating several small meals or snacks might temporarily sharpen the mind. In one British study, subjects who ate a light lunch of balanced protein and carbohydrates made fewer errors, and those who ate a heavy lunch made more errors on a task requiring close attention. All light snacks are not equal, however; in one Tufts University study, subjects who ate a nutritionally empty snack did worse on tests of memory and attention than did those who ate a caloric snack.

On the other hand, some studies suggest that a big breakfast does not appear to hamper performance, perhaps because of the body's daily rhythms of alertness and fatigue.

echoencephalogram A type of scanning technology that uses ultrasound reflections bounded back from the brain surface to view intracranial abnormality and midline structures.

ECT See ELECTROCONVULSIVE THERAPY.

EEG The abbreviation for ELECTROENCEPHALOGRAM.
See also ELECTROENCEPHALOGRAPHY.

Egas Moniz, António (Caetano de Abreu Freire) (1874–1955) Portuguese neurologist who performed the first LEUCOTOMY (lobotomy) as a radical treatment for certain mental diseases. Egas Moniz was deeply interested in the practice of PSYCHOSURGERY (another term he invented), and he won the 1949 Nobel Prize in physiology or medicine for his leucotomy work. He developed the idea after hearing of experimental lobectomies with chimps. His work inspired American neurologists Walter Freeman and James Watts to perform the first American leucotomies the next year.

Egas Moniz understood that certain mental problems (such as SCHIZOPHRENIA and severe paranoia) involve recurrent thought patterns. He reasoned that aberrant thought patterns might be replaced with more normal ones if he could sever the nerve fibers connecting the PREFRONTAL LOBES that are known to be associated with these psychological responses, and the THALAMUS, as relay center for sensory impulses. The leucotomy, then, severs nerve tracts connecting the frontal association CORTEX with these deeper structures in the brain. Because the procedure carries considerable risk of side effects, Egas Moniz cautioned that the radical procedure should only be attempted if all other treatment options had failed.

The first neurologist at the University of Lisbon, Egas Moniz developed the technique of cerebral ANGIOGRAPHY, a method of visualizing the blood vessels of the brain by injecting radiopaque substances into the CAROTID ARTERY. The technique is helpful in diagnosing intracranial diseases.

Egas Moniz described his procedures in the 1936 textbook on psychosurgery, *Tentative Operatoires dans le Traitement de Certaines Psychoses* (*Experimental Surgery in the Treatment of Certain Psychoses*). In 1955, at the age of 88, he was beaten to death in his office by one of his patients.

electrical activity mapping See ELECTROENCEPHALOGRAM; ELECTROENCEPHALOGRAPHY.

electrical stimulation of the brain Stimulating various areas of the CORTEX produces a range of responses from patients, and stimulation of the TEMPORAL LOBES can elicit meaningful, integrated experiences featuring sound, movement, and color. Stimulating one side of the brain may bring back a certain song or the smell of the sea breeze. Interestingly, stimulating the same point in the brain elicits the same memory most of the time.

electroconvulsive therapy (ECT) and memory An electric shock applied to the body to induce brain seizures while the patient is anesthetized, used primarily as an attempt to treat severe depression. ECT, though controversial, is used widely in psychiatric treatment, most often in cases of severe depression; it can also cause a temporary memory loss. The question of whether ECT affects memory permanently is still debated. Despite its frightening reputation, ECT (formerly known as *shock therapy*) may work for those very serious depressions that just don't respond to any other treatment, especially when there's a risk of suicide. The modern version of ECT is nothing like the sort of mental torture depicted in such movies as *One Flew Over the Cuckoo's Nest*.

Technique The patient is given an anesthetic and a muscle relaxant so that the effects of the shock are basically limited to the brain; two padded electrodes then are applied to the temples. A controlled electric pulse is delivered to the electrodes until the patient experiences a brain seizure; treatment usually consists of 6 to 12 seizures (2 or 3 a week).

After the treatment, the patient usually experiences a period of confusion that is not remembered afterward; there is usually also a brief period of AMNESIA covering the period of time right before the treatment. On regaining consciousness, patients who have received ECT are similar in many ways to those who have experienced posttraumatic amnesia. Typically, patients first regain their personal identity, followed by the knowledge of where they are; orientation in time occurs last of all.

Tests of memory after ECT reveal a substantial memory impairment in addition to a clear anterograde amnesia. However, after a number of treatments, some patients say they experience a more serious memory loss, involving everyday forgetfulness, which usually disappears within a few weeks after treatment. Critics of ECT claim, however, that it produces more substantial effects on memory.

New research suggests that ECT administered to only one side of the brain produces equally beneficial results to the more standard method without any accompanying memory loss.

While many believe the origins of ECT lie in the ancient Roman tradition of applying electric eels to the head as a cure for madness, mild electric shocks had been used since the late 1700s to treat illness. A machine using weak electric currents was used in Middlesex Hospital in England in 1767 to treat a range of illnesses, and London brain surgeon John Birch used his machine to shock the brain of depressed patients.

At about the same time, American inventor and patriot Benjamin Franklin was shocked into unconsciousness—and suffered a RETROGRADE AMNESIA—during one of his electricity experiments; he is said to have recommended electric shock for the treatment of mental illness.

However, the modern practice of electric-shock treatment for the treatment of depression and mental illness is less than 65 years old. In the 1930s, scientists noticed that a number of studies reporting that SCHIZO-PHRENIA and EPILEPSY did not occur in the same patient and wondered if an artificially induced seizure might cure schizophrenia. While the seizures were originally induced through the use of camphor and other drugs, Italian psychiatrist Ugo Cerletti and colleagues explored the possibility of using electric shock to achieve similar results. Cerletti's version was considered an improvement over the drug-induced seizures, which were associated with toxic side effects.

The first patient received ECT to treat schizophrenia on April 15, 1938. Because it was simple and inexpensive, the use of ECT spread, and by the 1950s it was the primary method of treatment for schizophrenia and depression, but the discovery of neuroleptic drugs led to a substantial decline in its use.

Still, the controversy surrounding ECT is likely to continue for some time, and the question of whether ECT affects permanent memory remains unclear. Many studies that have examined long-term experience with ECT and that were controlled for influence of other factors indicate that ECT doesn't have any extensive effect on permanent memory function. All patients show some amount of retrograde amnesia for events immediately before ECT itself.

Some scientists believe that some patients may falsely conclude that their memory is impaired. In one study, scientists found significant differences between patients who reported memory problems and those who didn't. Those who complained tended to believe the ECT hadn't helped their depression, which could mean that their own assessment of memory might be the result of their continuing illness. Three years after treatment, this group insisted their memory problems, which they believed were of an amnesic type, remained—even though there was no objective proof of this. Researchers believe that their initial experience of true amnesia immediately following ECT might have caused them to question whether their memory function had really recovered.

Still, it is true that ECT in elderly depressive patients can worsen their decline in the presence of DEMENTIA, and it is also true that ECT can be abused as a treatment. Even ECT proponents admit there is a chance of adverse reaction to the treatment, although estimates of how great a risk vary.

electroencephalogram (EEG) A recorded tracing of wave patterns of electrical brain activity obtained through electrodes placed on the skull.

The machine that records this activity is known as an *encephalograph*. The pattern of the tracings reflect the state of the patient's brain and the level of consciousness in a characteristic way.

See also ELECTROENCEPHALOGRAPHY.

electroencephalography A diagnostic method for determining the electrical activity of the brain, revealing a person's mental state, possible diseases, and level of anesthesia during surgery. It can also be used to determine BRAIN DEATH. The painless technique has no side effects.

On an ongoing basis—even during sleep—electrical signals are constantly flashing over the brain; these signals can be detected and measured by an encephalograph (EEG). Because the tissues of the body conduct electricity well, metal sensors attached to the skin of the head can detect the signals passing from the brain through the muscles and skin. The signals are amplified and displayed on a monitor or paper chart. These devices show that electrical signals in the brain don't come steadily but are produced in short bursts; the shape of the waves change with the activity level of the brain. The tracings reveal that the electrical activity of the brain varies with the degree of alertness, depending on whether the subject is excited, relaxed, or in a deep sleep. The EEG brain-wave patterns include ALPHA WAVES (the primary pattern of an alert adult with closed eyes); the BETA WAVES (lower, faster activity while a person is concentrating on an outside stimulus); DELTA WAVES (sleep patterns also found in infants; rarely, they are also caused by brain tumors); and THETA WAVES (dominant pattern in children ages two to five and in psychopaths; also produced by frustration). In normal people, there are four types of BRAIN WAVES: alpha, beta, theta and delta waves.

The technique was first tried medically in 1928, although scientists have known since the 1800s that it was possible to record electrical impulses from animal brains. Supplanted today by imaging studies in detecting brain pathology, the EEG is now used primarily to detect abnormal cerebral *function* that can't be otherwise identified. It is therefore best used to evaluate transient states, such as SEIZURES; evolving conditions, such as HERPES SIMPLEX ENCEPHALITIS; global disorders, such as DEMENTIA. Only a few EEG patterns can be used to diagnose a particular disease, but the tracings can be helpful in deciding among several disease alternatives.

In the technique, several small electrodes are attached to the scalp, connected to a device that measures and amplifies the brain's electrical impulses. Brain waves are measured while the patient opens and shuts the eyes, during and after hyperventilation and while looking at a flashing light. Sometimes, measurements are also taken as a patient drifts off to sleep.

electromyography A type of test that involves the continuous recording of the electrical activity of a muscle by inserting electrodes into the muscle fibers. The tracing is displayed on an oscilloscope or chart recorder. It is used to analyze peripheral nerve and muscular disorders and assess progress in recovery from some forms of paralysis.

Some discomfort is to be expected during this test, and patients can be premedicated with codeine or other drugs without altering the test results. The tests can be used to help diagnose MYASTHENIA GRAVIS, MOTOR NEURON DISEASE (AMYOTROPHIC LATERAL SCLEROSIS) and GUILLAIN-BARRE SYNDROME.

embolism, cerebral A blockage of one of the arteries that supplied blood to the brain. A cerebral embolism is one of the most common causes of STROKE. The arteries are blocked by an embolus (blood clot, bubble of air or gas, bacteria, bone marrow, fat, etc.).

Survival depends on the speed with which blood flow is reestablished; if the embolus can be removed, long-term outlook for the patient is good.

Symptoms If the embolus causes a stroke, the symptoms depend on which part of the brain has been affected; it may cause an inability to speak, inability to walk, loss of consciousness, or visual problems.

Treatment Surgery (such as BALLOON ANGIOPLASTY) to open the blocked arteries may be tried; if surgery is not possible, drugs designed to break up blood clots, and anticoagulant drugs (to prevent the formation of clots) may be given.

emotions and the brain Far from being a state of consciousness divorced from the physical brain, a person's emotions are produced by chemicals exquisitely intertwined with the physiological processes of the body so that in the truest sense what affects the body affects the mind and emotions, and vice versa.

The center of emotions in the brain can be found in the LIMBIC SYSTEM where the vast panoply of emotions is regulated through the release of excitatory and inhibitory NEUROTRANSMITTERS: Pleasure may be linked with chemical signals produced by the release of NORADRENALIN, and pain is associated with many neurotransmitters. Mood appears to be linked with SEROTONIN and dopamine.

In response to a variety of stimuli, emotions arise in the limbic system, traveling along neural pathways to the FRONTAL LOBES of the CORTEX, where feelings are monitored and interpreted. These two brain structures next influence the HYPOTHALAMUS, which transmits the messages that trigger appropriate physical responses.

The latest research suggests that different parts of the brain may process emotions differently. Scientists have found that the frontal lobes of the *left* hemisphere display more electrical activity when subjects experience positive emotions such as enthusiasm or happiness, and the frontal lobes of the *right* hemisphere display more electrical activity when the subjects experience negative emotions such as disgust or sadness.

While lower animals are guided by primitive instincts and may experience only rudimentary feelings, most mammals probably do have a richer range of emotional feelings. Evidence of the limbic system's so-called "pleasure center" was discovered in 1953 by scientists at McGill University, when a rat incessantly self-stimulated an area of the brain called the *septum* in the front part of the hypothalamus. Further tests revealed that not just rats, but rabbits, dogs, dolphins, monkeys, and even humans experienced intense pleasure when this part of the brain is stimulated.

The limbic system controls not just pleasure but also a wide variety of emotions with many subtle shades. Separate emotions do not exist in individual, isolated areas of the brain, however; instead, emotional reactions appear to develop from a wide range of neural pathways throughout the limbic system, working together to produce a symphony of human emotion.

encephalitis An often-fatal inflammation of the brain that can cause damage on both sides (especially the MEDIAL TEMPORAL LOBE) and the orbital FRONTAL LOBE. Encephalitis may be caused by several different viruses, but the herpes simplex virus is most commonly the cause. Many times, the MENINGES (membranes that cover and enclose the brain) are also affected.

While an encephalitis attack may be so mild that the patient does not notice anything amiss, more often it is a serious condition.

In addition to the herpes virus, encephalitis may be caused by a virus transmitted to humans by mosquito bites, causing St. Louis encephalitis; other cases may be caused by infection with HIV virus, the organism responsible for AIDS. On rare occasions, the condition may follow viral infections such as measles or mumps.

See also ENCEPHALITIS LETHARGICA.

Symptoms Symptoms often begin with HEADACHE, fever, and prostration that leads to HALLUCINATIONS, confusion, paralysis, disturbed behavior, and problems in speech, memory, and eye movement. The AMNESIA in patients with this disorder is probably caused by the destruction of the HIPPOCAMPUS and AMYGDALA. Some patients may also suffer damage to the front lobes and in extreme cases show symptoms of the Kluver-Bucy syndrome, a condition causing a range of symptoms including amnesia, visual problems, and altered sexual behavior. There may be a gradual loss of consciousness and sometimes COMA; seizures may also occur.

If the meninges area also is inflamed, the neck usually becomes stiff and the eyes are abnormally sensitive to light.

Diagnosis A diagnosis can be determined from symptoms plus results of BRAIN SCANS, and EEG (ELECTROENCEPHALOGRAM), and a LUMBAR PUNCTURE (a sample of SPINAL FLUID). Blood tests may also be necessary.

Treatment   The antiviral drug ACYCLOVIR is an effective treatment for encephalitis caused by the herpes simplex virus. However, there is no treatment for the disease caused by other viruses. Some patients die, and others have brain damage, behavioral problems, and persistent EPILEPSY.

encephalitis lethargica   An epidemic form of ENCEPHALITIS (inflammation of the brain) that has not been seen in major outbreaks since the 1920s. Occasional isolated cases do still occur.

About 40 percent of all patients died during the epidemics; those who survived developed postencephalitic PARKINSONISM, a movement disorder marked by symptoms of tremor, rigidity, and disturbed eye movements.

A few survivors from the post-World War I epidemic were alive in the 1970s when a new antiparkinsonism drug (LEVODOPA) remarkably improved their condition. However, after 50 years of immobility, sufferers were apparently unable to cope with awakening, and they lapsed back into their earlier lethargic state.

Symptoms   Primary symptom is lethargy and drowsiness (hence, the popular name "sleeping sickness") together with symptoms that appear with encephalitis: HEADACHE, fever and prostration, HALLUCINATIONS, confusion, paralysis, disturbed behavior, and problems in speech, memory, and eye movement.

encephalomyelitis   Inflammation of the brain and SPINAL CORD that can permanently damage the NERVOUS SYSTEM. Encephalomyelitis develops as a complication in about one out of every 1,000 cases of measles, usually appearing about three days after the rash. It may also rarely appear after other viral infections, such as chickenpox, rubella (German measles), or infectious mononucleosis or after vaccination against rabies.

About 10 to 20 percent of patients will die; those who recover may experience permanent damage to the nervous system, including MENTAL RETARDATION, EPILEPSY, paralysis, pituitary problems, loss of sensation, or incontinence.

Symptoms   Fever, HEADACHE, drowsiness, confusion, SEIZURES, partial paralysis, or COMA.

Treatment   There is no cure for this disease, but corticosteroid drugs can reduce inflammation, and anticonvulsant drugs can control seizures.

encephalon   The anatomical name of the BRAIN, it is rarely used.

encephalopathy   Any disorder that affects the brain, especially those that lead to chronic degenerative conditions. WERNICKE'S ENCEPHALOPATHY is a degenerative condition caused by a lack of thiamine (B1) and is most often found in alcoholics. Hepatic encephalopathy is a brain disorder caused by toxic substances that accumulate in the blood as a result of liver disease.

encephalopathy, toxic   Serious generalized brain dysfunction, characterized by personality changes, memory problems, and changes in conceptual thinking.

endorphin   One of the brain's natural OPIATES produced by the PITUITARY GLAND and involved in a wide variety of body processes, including pain control and emotions. Endorphins are chemically similar to morphine. In 1973, scientists located a variety of "opiate receptors" in the body where morphine acted, which led to the realization that the body must therefore produce its own opiates. This discovery lead to the identification of protein molecules named *endorphins* (for *endogenous morphines*), produced by the body that also acts at these same opiate receptor sites.

While researchers are still studying the role of endorphins in the body, they have outlined their role in mood, pain mediation, euphoria, stress, and regulating intestinal contractions. Endorphins have also been implicated in the release of hormones from the pituitary gland, such as growth hormone and gonadotropin hormones, which act on the sex organs.

It is believed that both addiction and tolerance to narcotic drugs are caused by the drug's suppression of the body's own endorphins; when the narcotic drug is then stopped, the body's own stores of endorphins is depleted, and withdrawal symptoms appear because the body can't mediate pain as well. It has been proven that acupuncture and possibly some forms of meditation can control pain by stimulating the release of endorphins and enkephalins.

engram   The physical basis of memory, also known as a *memory trace,* this is a unit of information encoded as a pattern of lowered resistance or increased conductance to electrical impulses resulting in an increased readiness to respond to NEUROTRANSMITTERS. The engram is believed to exist in a network of nerve cells as the result of the consolidation of memory. Memories seem to be encoded in the brain's cells, which convert chemical signals to electrical signals and then are converted back to chemical signals again.

Information is carried inside a neuron by electrical pulses, but when the signal reaches the end of the axon, it must be carried across the synaptic gap by chemicals called NEUROTRANSMITTERS. On the other side of the synapse, another dendrite containing RECEPTORS that recognize these transmitting molecules registers the signal. If enough signals are registered, then the second cell fires an action potential. A single neuron can receive signals from thousands of other neurons, and its axon can send signals to thousands more.

When a person experiences a new event such as meeting a new person, an engram is activated in some way, and certain brain cells light up. In order to store this memory of the new person, there must be a way to save the memory—to make new connections between neurons to create a new circuit to serve as a symbol. By reactivating the circuit, the brain can retrieve the memory. The person is recognized when something evokes a neural pattern similar to one already stored in the brain. A picture of the person in a photo album might cause a pattern of neurons to light up that resembled the patterns joined together during the initial experience. However, the brain's circuits are not permanent; circuits break up and form new connections as knowledge is gained.

Engrams also are formed on tasks performed over and over again. To perform the task, the appropriate engram must be activated. The appropriate area of the brain then reads this engram, and the task is performed. Engrams are not constructed easily; the more complex the activity, the more rehearsals it takes to form a reliable engram and most probably a larger number of neurons is involved.

Because all memories aren't stored the same way, not all memories are remembered equally well; some memories have stronger traces. What remains in long-term memory has been used many times, recalled and stored differently with different references so that the trace can be thoroughly integrated.

Every time a memory is retrieved, it appears in a different context and is altered by the new recall. The more time that has elapsed since the memory was first encoded, the greater the chance that the memory trace has been manipulated.

Today, scientists believe that engrams are encoded in the neurons throughout the brain. Like any circuit, electrically stimulating any neuron in an engram circuit could produce the entire memory.

enkephalin   Protein molecules that are produced in the brain, where they act as one type of the body's own (endogenous) OPIATES.

They are believed to produce sedation, affect mood, and stimulate motivation. Originally believed to be the same as ENDORPHINS, they were reclassified when it was determined that they were released from different nerve endings. They are part of the endorphin peptide and, in general, activate the same opioid receptors.

enzyme An organic compound that interacts with other substances to form a new chemical, either by synthesizing or degrading it. Brain function depends on chemical messages transmitted from cell to cell by NEUROTRANSMITTERS which depend on brain enzymes as part of their synthesis and degradation.

The enzyme CHOLINE ACETYLTRANSFERASE is important in the production of ACETYLCHOLINE, a neurotransmitter involved in learning and memory. Scientists have found low levels of this neurotransmitter in the areas of the Alzheimer brain where plaques and tangles are located.

ependymoma A common childhood tumor appearing in the CEREBRAL HEMISPHERES that may be either benign or malignant; it is usually slow-growing. Ependymoma usually cannot be completely removed because of their location on the brain floor or deep in the cerebral hemisphere. This type of tumor may alter the flow of cerebrospinal fluid, causing HYDROCEPHALUS (accumulation of fluid in the brain).

Treatment Radiation therapy, chemotherapy, and a shunt to relieve the excess intracranial pressure that often occurs.

epilepsy Condition of recurrent SEIZURES or temporary alteration in one or more brain functions. Seizures are temporary abnormalities in the brain caused by abnormal electrical activity, resulting in a chaotic type of unregulated discharge. In some cases, a stimulus (such as a flashing or red light) triggers this abnormal electrical activity; in other cases, the seizures occur spontaneously. Sometimes a visual "aura" precedes the seizures.

About 1 in 200 people are affected by epilepsy; in the United States, more than one million people have the condition. The disorder, which often begins in childhood or adolescence, is sometimes outgrown and may not require medication.

An epileptic seizure is either generalized or partial, depending on the part of the brain in which it arises and how widely the seizure spreads.

Hereditary epilepsy that begins in childhood may very likely disappear after adolescence; about one-third of these patients eventually outgrow the condition. Another third experience fewer seizures with drug treatment. The rest experience no change in their condition. Seizure control is more difficult in TEMPORAL LOBE EPILEPSY or if the condition has been caused by serious BRAIN INJURY.

While people with epilepsy can work, their choices of jobs may be limited; there are restrictions against obtaining a driver's license (usually, a person must be symptom-free for several years). Unless the disease is very well controlled, most physicians advise against working in high-risk jobs, such as those involving heavy machinery or heights, and participating in such sports as skiing.

Generalized seizures Generalized seizures result in a loss of consciousness and may arise from wide areas of the brain. There are two types of generalized seizures—GRAND MAL and PETIT MAL SEIZURES. During a *grand mal* seizure, the person loses consciousness and may stiffen, twitch, or jerk. Breathing may stop or become very irregular; afterward, bowel and bladder control may be lost. The person may feel disoriented and confused or may have a HEADACHE and want to sleep. There is usually no memory of the event. Untreated prolonged seizures (called STATUS EPILEPTICUS) may be fatal.

Petit mal (or absence) seizures may involve only a brief loss of consciousness and are found primarily in children. The blank period may last from a few seconds to up to a half minute, during which the person is unaware of his or her surroundings. The person may appear to be daydreaming, and the attack may pass unnoticed. They may occur hundreds of times a day, significantly interfering with schoolwork.

Partial seizures Partial seizures, which may not cause unconsciousness, result from more limited BRAIN DAMAGE. Although partial seizures begin in one small area of the brain, the electrical disturbance may spread, affecting the entire brain and setting off a generalized seizure. *Temporal lobe epilepsy* is an example of a partial type of epileptic seizure; it may result in uncontrollable flashbacks to distant memories.

They are divided into simple (without unconsciousness) or complex seizures. Simple seizures involve an abnormal twitching movement, tingling sensation, or even HALLUCINATION of smell, vision, or taste; they occur without warning and can last for several minutes. Twitching may spread slowly from one part of the body to another on the same side; this is called JACKSONIAN EPILEPSY. These patients are aware during the event and can remember the details.

In a complex seizure, the patient may be dazed and may not respond; there may be involuntary movements (lip smacking, etc.). The patient may not remember anything about the seizure.

Causes Epilepsy can be caused by a wide variety of injuries or diseases that affect the brain, such as birth trauma, head injury, brain infection, tumor, STROKE, drug abuse, or metabolic imbalances. In addition, epilepsy may appear for no known reason; there may also be an inherited predisposition to developing the disease.

Prevention Avoiding extreme fatigue or stress and infectious diseases may all help to avoid seizures. By doing this and taking prescribed medication, epileptics can reduce the frequency of the attacks. Some people discover a distracting technique that can stop a seizure once it begins.

Treatment ANTICONVULSANT DRUGS are the first step in treating epilepsy; in almost all cases they can at least reduce the number of attacks. However, these drugs may have unpleasant side effects (such as drowsiness or impaired concentration). If no seizures occur for two or three years (depending on cause), the physician may recommend reducing or stopping the drugs.

Surgery is only rarely considered if medication does not work and if there is the suggestion that only one area of the brain is responsible (usually the TEMPORAL LOBE). However, temporal-lobe surgery to remove the area that produces the epileptic activity may cause a degree of memory defect. Operations on the dominant temporal lobe often interfere with the ability to learn verbal information by hearing or reading and may last for as long as three years after surgery.

In a series of operations during the mid-1950s, surgeons removed the MEDIAL TEMPORAL LOBE in 10 epileptic patients in order to lessen seizures. While the operations were successful, 8 of the 10 suffered pronounced memory deficits. The most famous of these was known as HM, whose amnesic syndrome is considered to be among the purest ever studied. After the operation, HM was unable to remember anything other than a handful of events since the time of his operation and was described as living in the "eternal present."

The study revealed that AMNESIA was present only in those who had lost both the HIPPOCAMPUS and the AMYGDALA; removal of the amygdala alone did not produce amnesia.

First aid for seizures Most seizures last for only a few minutes. Bystanders should let the attack run its course and not interfere with the patient, beyond checking to make sure the person is in no physical danger and can breathe. Bystanders should not hold the patient down or restrain movements. Any tight clothing around the neck should be loosened, and something soft should be placed underneath the head. The mouth should not be forced open, and objects should not be forced between the teeth.

An ambulance should be called if the seizure continues for more than 5 minutes, if another seizure immediately follows the first or if the person does not regain consciousness a few minutes after the seizure ends.

Epilepsy Concern Service Group National support group for persons with EPILEPSY and concerned friends and relatives. The group starts and maintains self-help groups and operates Long Distance Friends Program whereby individuals may communicate with a member by letter or tape. The group also provides group-leader training and makes an Epilepsy Concern Starter Kit available to those who want to start a group in their community. Founded in 1975, the group publishes a periodic newsletter and a quarterly membership directory. For address, see Appendix A.

See also EPILEPSY FOUNDATION OF AMERICA.

Epilepsy Foundation of America A national voluntary health agency which serves as the focal point for the fight against ELIPESY in the United States. Augmented by 85 affiliates committed to preventing and controlling epilepsy and improving the lives of those who have it, the group provides federal government liaison and supports medical, social, rehabilitational, legal, employment, information, education, and advocacy programs. The foundation sponsors research in the causes, prevention, psychosocial needs, and treatment and provides research and training grants as well as fellowships.

In addition, the foundation offers assistance and counseling for patients and their families through local organizations and a national information and referral service. Annual projects include National Epilepsy Month (November), School Alert (a national educational program for schools), selection of the Epilepsy Poster Child, and a continuing professional and public education and information program. The foundation maintains a library and resource center and provides members with access to mail-order pharmacy programs.

Founded in 1967, the group publishes a quarterly newsletter, a monthly newsletter, pamphlets, and audiovisual material. For address, see Appendix B.

epinephrine Also known as ADRENALINE, this is a naturally occurring hormone and neurotransmitter that has been synthetically manufactured since 1900. It is one of two chemicals (the other is NOREPINEPHRINE) released by the adrenal gland in response to signals from the sympathetic division of the AUTONOMIC NERVOUS SYSTEM. The signals are triggered by exercise, stress, and emotions such as fear.

Epinephrine increases the speed and force of the heart, allowing the heart to do more work. In addition, epinephrine dilates the airways to improve breathing, narrowing blood vessels in the skin and intestine to direct blood flow to the muscles to allow them to cope with exercise.

Epinephrine also seems to be responsible for imprinting memories indelibly in the long-term memory. In fact, people seem to remember better when their bodies are flooded with adrenaline. Additional research also suggests that epinephrine plays an important role in regulating memory storage; it enhances memory for many different kinds of tasks, including those that train animals using rewards as well as punishment. Some scientists suggest that hormones such as epinephrine may act as a "fixative" to lock memories of stimulating or shocking events in the brain. This could allow the brain to discard unimportant information while maintaining the important impressions we experience. It may be that these hormones act directly on the brain, or they may alter brain chemistry that allows another substance to travel to the brain and "fix" the memory.

Unfortunately, because epinephrine has a variety of unpleasant side effects on the heart and other body systems—especially in older patients—more research needs to be completed before epinephrine can be used as some sort of "memory enhancement" drug.

Epinephrine is sometimes injected as an emergency treatment for a heart that has stopped beating and is used to treat anaphylactic shock (a severe allergic reaction) and acute asthma attacks. It can be used during surgery to reduce bleeding, and when combined with a local anesthetic, it prolongs the numbing effect by slowing down the rate at which the anesthetic spreads into adjoining tissue.

Erasistratus of Chios (b. c. 304 B.C.; d. c. 250 B.C.) The Greek anatomist and the founder of physiology who described the brain's main parts, including the MENINGES and VENTRICLES. He studied in Athens, Cos, and Alexandria, dissected the human body, and is alleged to have carried out vivisection on prisoners. He also believed that human intelligence was to be found somewhere in the brain's convolutions.

See also BRAIN IN HISTORY.

estrogen and the brain A growing body of research suggests that the female hormone estrogen may play a protective role against memory loss and ALZHEIMER'S DISEASE and may also improve brain function. In fact, the sharp decrease in estrogen during menopause may be one reason why women are 50 percent more likely to contract Alzheimer's disease at midlife.

While the research has not yet clearly proven the role of estrogen as a brain protector, one study of 2,418 women in southern California showed that those who took estrogen supplements after menopause were 40 percent less likely to have Alzheimer's. In this study, the higher the dose of estrogen, the lower the risk of Alzheimer's. In other studies of women over age 65, women who had taken estrogen supplements continuously since menopause had significantly higher scores of verbal memory than other women.

Other studies at Columbia University suggest that estrogen may also improve brain function, boosting the level of the important brain chemical called NERVE GROWTH FACTOR (NGF) and stimulating the growth of AXONS and DENDRITES (the long projections from NERVE CELLS that allow nerves to communicate with each other).

In fact, the brain is a major target for estrogen and has plenty of estrogen receptors, especially in regions associated with learning and memory (the basal FOREBRAIN, CEREBRAL CORTEX, and HIPPOCAMPUS)—the areas most affected by Alzheimer's. Other studies at Rockefeller University note that (at least in rats) the number of SYNAPSES (points at which nerves communicate) fluctuate during reproductive cycles. When estrogen levels are high, there are more synapses (especially in the memory centers); when estrogen levels are low, the synapses disappear.

While extensive research has also found that estrogen significantly reduces the risk of heart disease and osteoporosis, it is far from a harmless wonder drug. Estrogen supplements taken during menopause have been linked to increased risk of breast cancer.

evoked response A painless recording of electrical brain activity in response to a single, specific stimulus. This technique, which was first demonstrated in 1947, is a refined version of ELECTROENCEPHALOGRAPHY, in which the brain's activity can be analyzed to assess the function of various sensory systems. Evoked potential can reveal problems caused by tumors, inflammation, and some diseases and is used to confirm the diagnosis of MULTIPLE SCLEROSIS. The test is usually used in concert with other tests of the NERVOUS SYSTEM, such as EEGS or CAT SCANS.

The testing of each sensory system (eyes, ears, touch, etc.) takes about 30 minutes. A set of electrodes is attached to a portion of the scalp (depending on which sensory system is being tested). The patterns produced by the brain are fed to a computer, which can produce a printout of the activity after a specific period of stimulation. The amount of time between the stimulus and the response can be analyzed by the computer, which separates the information from background brain activity.

exercise and the brain   Aerobic exercise can improve cognitive function, perhaps because of the increased oxygen to the brain or a rise in GLUCOSE metabolism.

Studies at the University of Pennsylvania show that a person who exercises consistently over a period of years will not show the same mental decline as someone who doesn't exercise. In tests of rapid decision making (such as how quickly a person could slam on the brakes if a child jumped in front of his or her car), researchers found that older men who had exercised were better at quick decision making than older men who hadn't. It is known that those who exercise for a long period have healthier hearts, lungs, and muscles; now scientists suspect that exercise might also slow the decline in CENTRAL NERVOUS-SYSTEM processing as well. Even walking around the block has been shown to be beneficial.

There's now solid evidence that regular aerobic exercise (such as running, biking, or swimming) can ease some more moderate cases of depression by raising the level of certain brain chemicals responsible for mood—some of the same brain chemicals that are affected by antidepressants. Even a brisk midday walk for 10 or 20 minutes can help. To be most effective, a person should exercise regularly at least three times a week (five or more is better) for at least a half-hour each time. Exercise has not been shown to be effective for severe depression.

extradural hemorrhage   Bleeding into the space between the external surface of the DURA (the outer layer of the protective cover of the brain) and the inner surface of the skull. A BRAIN SCAN can confirm the diagnosis.

Cause   This type of hemorrhage is usually caused by a skull fracture that ruptures the artery running over the surface of the dura. The person may briefly lose consciousness and then appear to recover. This leads to a collection of clotted blood (HEMATOMA) that rapidly enlarges, increasing pressure within the skull.

Symptoms   The main cause of symptoms occurring a few hours to days later is pressure within the skull, leading to a HEADACHE, drowsiness, vomiting, SEIZURES, and paralysis on one side of the body opposite the hemorrhage. The patient may lapse into a COMA and eventually die.

Treatment   CRANIOTOMY (drilling burr holes in the skull) and clipping the ruptured blood vessel. If the problem is diagnosed before serious symptoms occur, the patient's chances of recovery are excellent. This is why it is so important to seek medical care after even moderate blows to the head.

extrapyramidal system   A network of nerve pathways that link nerve nuclei in the surface of the CEREBRUM (main brain mass), the BASAL GANGLIA deep within the brain, and some of the BRAINSTEM. It is a collective term for those structures involved in the central nervous control of motor function other than the pyramidal tracts and their connections.

Damage of any part of this system may interfere with voluntary movements or muscle tone and induce involuntary movements such as jerks or writhing movements.

These disturbances are found in PARKINSON'S DISEASE, HUNTINGTON'S DISEASE, and some forms of CEREBRAL PALSY. The movements (called TARDIVE DYSKINESIA) can also appear as a side effect of taking some drugs, including the phenothiazines (used in treating some psychiatric disorders).

F

facial nerve Also known as the seventh cranial nerve; with both sensory and motor aspects, this nerve is responsible for facial expressions and taste.

See also CRANIAL NERVES.

fainting A loss of consciousness caused by a temporary lack of oxygen to the brain. Known by the medical term *syncope*, fainting may be preceded by dizziness, nausea, or a feeling of extreme weakness.

Usually, an attack may be caused by extreme pain, fear, or stress, resulting from an overstimulation of the vagus nerve, which helps control breathing and circulation. A person could faint from prolonged coughing or by straining to defecate or to urinate or to blow a wind instrument. Another cause could be remaining in a stuffy environment with not enough oxygen.

In addition, standing still (or standing erect) for long periods of time may cause fainting due to blood pooling in the leg veins, cutting down on the amount available for the heart to pump to the brain. This is common in the elderly, those who have diabetes mellitus, and those taking drugs to treat high blood pressure.

Fainting could also be a symptom of STOKES-ADAMS SYNDROME, in which the blood flow to the brain is temporarily reduced because of an irregular heart beat, usually associated with the interruption of electrical impulses of the heart.

In some people, fainting may be associated with VERTEBROBASILAR INSUFFICIENCY, a temporary problem in speaking or a weakness in the limbs caused by an obstruction to the blood flow in vessels passing through the neck to the brain. (This is one form of TRANSIENT ISCHEMIC ATTACK.)

Treatment A fainting episode fades away as soon as a normal blood flow to the brain is restored. This usually happens as soon as the person hits the ground because the head is then placed at the same level as the heart. To head off another attack, the patient should not stand for 10 or 15 minutes after regaining consciousness.

If a person does not regain consciousness within a minute or two after fainting, medical help should be obtained immediately. Repeated attacks should be checked out by a physician.

Prevention When a person senses that he or she is about to faint, the attack may be prevented by sitting with the head between the knees or lying flat with the legs raised.

Fallopio, Gabriel (1523–1562) An illustrious Italian anatomist who contributed to our early knowledge of the ear and the reproductive organs. He discovered several major nerves of the head and face and described the semicircular canals of the inner ear that are responsible for maintaining body equilibrium.

Fallopio was an anatomy professor at the University of Ferrara, the University of Pisa, and at Padua. He made most of his observations of the human body during dissection of cadavers and wrote about his findings in *Observationes anatomicae*, published in 1561.

Family Survival Project for Brain-Damaged Adults This nonprofit organization helps those who care for adult victims of chronic brain disorders.

Famous Faces Test A test of a person's ability to recall events and significant people from the past, designed by Nelson Butters, M.D., a Boston specialist in the evaluation and treatment of memory-impaired patients. The test consists of a series of photographs of famous people from the 1950s to the present.

A person without memory problems should be able to identify 80 percent of the faces, such as those of Ronald Reagan, Dwight Eisenhower, Marilyn Monroe, etc.

fatal familial insomnia An extremely rare progressive SLEEP DISORDER (there are just nine known families with the disease in the world) caused by PRIONS. In affected families, the condition appears out of nowhere and affects succeeding generations.

The latest case was discovered in the spring of 1994 by Pierluigi Gambetti of Case Western Reserve University School of Medicine in Cleveland.

fear and aggression Feelings of fear and aggression trigger strong stimulation of the sympathetic nerves of the AUTONOMIC NERVOUS SYSTEM—a reaction commonly known as the FIGHT-OR-FLIGHT RESPONSE. The emotions of fear and aggression appear to be linked, at least to some degree, by the HYPOTHALAMUS and LIMBIC SYSTEM.

When this area is stimulated in cats in the laboratory, the animals respond with a dramatic representation of fear or anger: hissing, arched back, raised fur, and extended claws. When the neural connections between the CEREBRAL CORTEX and the hypothalamus are severed, the cats exhibited even more intensely aggressive behavior.

Moreover, damage to limbic structures deep within the brain can result in a variety of emotional and behavioral changes, including docility, calming of emotions, and submission.

Federation for Children with Special Needs A coalition of parents' organizations (acting on behalf of children and adults with developmental disabilities) that provides information on special education laws and resources and tells how to obtain related services. The federation operates Collaboration Among Parents and Health Professionals Project to increase and encourage parent involvement in the health care of children with disabilities or chronic illnesses. Other projects include Parent Training and Information Project (which provides workshops in basic rights, parent consultations and training, and an information service) and Technical Assistance for Parents Project and also provides assistance to parent training and information programs in the U.S. Coordinates National Network of Parents Center. Although membership is concentrated in the New England area, activities are conducted on a national level. Founded in 1974, the federation publishes the triennial *Coalition Quarterly* and a newsletter five times a year. For address, see Appendix A.

See also CENTER FOR FAMILY SUPPORT; JARC; MENTAL RETARDATION ASSOCIATION OF AMERICA; NATIONAL ASSOCIATION OF DEVELOPMENTAL DISABILITIES COUNCILS; NATIONAL DOWN SYNDROME CONGRESS; NATIONAL DOWN SYNDROME SOCIETY; PARENTS OF CHILDREN WITH DOWN SYNDROME; PILOT PARENTS; VOICE OF THE RETARDED; YOUNG ADULT INSTITUTE AND WORKSHOP.

fetal alcohol syndrome (FAS) A condition in which a mother's excessive drinking during pregnancy produces a specific range of physical and mental characteristics in the developing fetus. First recognized in the early 1970s, the syndrome is now considered to be one of the most common causes of MENTAL RETARDATION.

About 5,000 American babies per year are born with FAS, and a great number of others are both with "fetal alcohol effects" that include several, but not all, of the typical features of FAS.

No one knows for sure how much drinking is dangerous; in part, it depends on how a woman's body metabolizes alcohol. Some women consume very large amounts of alcohol without harm to their babies, while other women who drink only very small amounts have babies with the syndrome.

In particular, *sudden heavy drinking*—such as at just one celebration—may be the most harmful of all, according to some research, especially if the drinking occurs at a crucial time of fetal development.

For these reasons, women are advised to stop drinking altogether while they are pregnant and—if they breast-feed—until their babies are weaned.

Symptoms Abnormally small head and brain, growth deficiency, deformities of face, joints, and limbs, brain and SPINAL CORD defects, varying degrees of malfunctions in major organs (especially the heart), small wide-set eyes, short upturned nose, flat cheeks. Babies with this syndrome tend to weigh less at birth and fail to catch up later; they often suffer with HYPERACTIVITY, short attention span, poor coordination, nervousness, and behavioral problems.

Cause Exactly how alcohol produces these devastating brain defects and other problems is not clearly understood. Scientists do know that alcohol consumed by the mother crosses the placenta, and while a baby's organs are still developing, they can't break down alcohol as quickly as an adult can. As a result, the alcohol in the baby's bloodstream remains high for a much longer time.

fetal brain development While in the womb, the brain is the largest organ of the fetus's body; by the fifth month, it is almost the same size as the trunk. This early growth spurt of the brain is a result of the multiplication of cells, not their enlargement. Cells divide or multiply at different times in different parts of the brain.

The two hemispheres of the FOREBRAIN are the first to experience a spurt in NERVE-CELL growth, which happens between the third and fourth month of pregnancy, peaking at 26 weeks. At this stage, 250,000 nerve cells are being created every minute. Most of the NEURONS, however, are formed during the second trimester; at birth, the infant's brain weighs one pound and contains about 100 billion neurons—just about the same number as in the adult brain.

GLIAL CELLS are also growing at a rapid rate in the brain, starting in the fifth month in the womb. This glial-cell division peaks at birth and begins to decline within three months, although glial cells still grow until the child is two or three.

By the 10th week of pregnancy, electrical activity in certain areas of the brain can be detected, especially in areas concerned with waking and sleeping. By the 12th to 16th week the brain can direct the fetus's hands and face to move, and by two-and-a-half months, the fetus can swallow amniotic fluid. By seven-and-a-half months, the fetal brain can direct the opening of eyes and sucking of fingers.

Nutrition and fetal development The mother's nutrition is critical to fetal brain development because a lack of proper nutrients can interfere with the rate of fetal cell division, resulting in a permanent reduction in the number of brain cells. Severe malnutrition during fetal development primarily affects neurons, whereas malnutrition during the early postnatal period affects glial cells.

Even if the mother suffers a nutrient deficiency for a short time, the rate of cell division in the fetal brain will increase again but not always normally. The complex programming of brain growth and development requires that development take place in certain steps; interference during any of the steps may cause harm that is irreversible once its "developmental window" has passed. This will then interfere with all stages of growth that come after it. Therefore, the earlier the period of nutritional interference, the more serious the subsequent developmental problems.

fetal hydantoin syndrome A group of birth defects, including small head (MICRO-CEPHALY) in babies of women with EPILEPSY who have taken antiseizure medication derived from the chemical hydantoin. Other symptoms include MENTAL RETARDATION, growth problems, and abnormalities of nails and fingers.

field dependence When making a perceptual judgment, the tendency to be influenced by surrounding information.

fight-or-flight response The almost instantaneous reaction of the brain to sudden fear that triggers a cascading chain of physiological reactions to prepare the body either to fight or flee from a perceived threat. This physical response triggers the sympathetic division of the AUTONOMIC NERVOUS SYSTEM to become activated, a situation that is common to all animals in reaction to threat.

The response usually begins with a visual signal that the brain interprets as a threat. This triggers fear or anger in one part of the brain, which induces the HYPOTHALAMUS to send an urgent message to the PITUITARY GLAND's anterior lobe to release the stress hormone ADRENOCORTICOTROPHIC HORMONE (ACTH) into the blood. ACTH enters the adrenal glands located on top of the kidneys, producing more stress-associated hormones (EPINEPHRINE and NOREPINEPHRINE). Due to this increase in systemic epinephrine and norepinephrine, drastic changes affect the body's blood supply; as the heart races, blood vessels supplying the skin and digestive system constrict, draining color from the skin. This shunts blood to the vital musculature where it is needed. The chest expands, widening bronchial tubes and increasing respiration rate; muscles tense; pupils dilate; the mouth grows dry; and the body sweats.

These physiological changes also occur during ANXIETY and its disorders.

fipexide This centrally active drug has been shown in some studies to enhance the release of DOPAMINE, the NEUROTRANSMITTER related to

fine motor coordination, motivation, emotions, and the immune function. In one double-blind study of 40 elderly patients with severe cognitive problems, fipexide improved cognition and performance, short-term memory, and attention. Average improvement in cognition was estimated to be 60 percent.

Fissure of Sylvius The groove that separates the TEMPORAL LOBE of the brain from the FRONTAL and PARIETAL LOBES.

fissures, cerebral See SULCI.

Flourens, Marie-Jean-Pierre (1794–1867) French physiologist who was the first to demonstrate the general function of the major portions of the vertebrate brain, who proved that the brain's respiratory center lies low in the BRAINSTEM, and who pioneered the idea of nervous coordination. In 1814, Flourens began a series of experiments to discover physiological changes in pigeons after he removed certain portions of their brains. He published these findings in *Recherches expérimentales sur les propriétés et les fonctions du système nerveux dans les animaux vertébrés* (*Experimental Studies on the Properties and Functions of the Nervous System in Vertebrate Animals*).

Flourens discovered that the absence of the CEREBRAL HEMISPHERES at the front of the brain destroys the sense of perception but not of equilibrium. He also discovered that removing the CEREBELLUM at the base of the brain destroys the sense of equilibrium and that removing the MEDULLA OBLONGATA at the back of the brain is fatal.

As a result of these experiments, he concluded that the cerebral hemispheres are the seat of higher cognitive abilities, that the cerebellum regulates movement, and that the medulla controls breathing and other vital functions. Flourens also learned how the semicircular canals of the inner ear regulate equilibrium and coordination.

See also BRAIN IN HISTORY.

fluent aphasia   See WERNICKE'S APHASIA.

fluid balance   See THIRST.

fluid imbalances and the brain   Too much or too little water will disturb brain function by changing the osmotic balance of electrolytes (potassium, sodium chloride, calcium, and magnesium) crucial to brain function. Especially during hot weather, aging patients are particularly at risk for electrolyte-induced brain problems.

folic acid   A B vitamin essential to the production of red blood cells by the bone marrow, this vitamin plays a particularly important role in the development of the fetal NERVOUS SYSTEM and formation of fetal red blood cells. Its lack during pregnancy has been linked to NEURAL TUBE DEFECTS. (Neural tube defects are a devastating birth disorder that takes place when the spinal column fails to close early in pregnancy; the condition can cause a baby to be born with part of its brain missing.)

Because of the link between folic acid and neural tube defects, an advisory committee to the Food and Drug Administration (FDA) has recommended that food (especially flour) be fortified with folic acid to prevent these birth defects. An estimated 2,500 babies were born in the United States each year with this condition, and the FDA panel estimates that this number could be cut in half if women consumed the suggested daily allowance of folic acid (0.4 mg). The average women ingests only 0.2 mg. of the substance each day; the vitamin is found in green leafy vegetables, dried beans, liver, citrus juices, nuts, avocadoes, and cereals.

Other scientists suggest that low levels of folic acid are closely tied to psychiatric symptoms in the elderly; one study has found that elderly patients with mental disorders (especially DEMENTIA) were three times more apt to have low folic acid than others their age.

Among healthy aged people, those with low folic-acid intake scored lower on memory and abstract-thinking ability. Studies have also found that low daily doses of folic-acid supplements lifted mood and relieved depression.

In other studies, scientists found that a pregnant woman's diet full of fruits and vegetables may dramatically reduce the risk of the child's subsequent development of NEUROECTODERMAL TUMORS in the part of the brain that controls coordination.

forebrain   The largest and most expansive part of the brain, also known as the prosencephalon, this part of the brain is made up of two subdivisions: the telencephalon (endbrain) and the DIENCEPHALON (interbrain). Structures in the telencephalon account for about 75 percent of the weight of the entire CENTRAL NERVOUS SYSTEM and include the CEREBRAL HEMISPHERES connected by a mass of crossing fibers in the CORPUS CALLOSUM and preoptic area. The surface of the hemispheres is a layer of tissue called the CEREBRAL CORTEX, which is divided into subregions according to creases along the brain's surface (also known as SULCI). The largest subregions are the four lobes in each hemisphere (FRONTAL, PARIETAL, TEMPORAL, and OCCIPITAL).

The cerebral hemispheres are attached to the diencephalon by large bundles of fibers called the *corona radiata*. The major parts of the diencephalon include the THALAMUS, the subthalamus, the HYPOTHALAMUS, and the epithalamus (containing the pineal body).

fornix   A circular arrangement of fibers connecting the hippocampus to the hypothalamus and connecting the two hippocampi.

Fragile X Foundation   A support organization concerned with FRAGILE X SYNDROME and other forms of X-linked MENTAL RETARDATION. The group seeks to educate and provide information about diagnosis and treatment.

The foundation also encourages research and publishes materials including a quarterly newsletter and a brochure. For address, see Appendix A.

See also FRAGILE X SUPPORT.

Fragile X Support   A national support organization concerned with FRAGILE X SYNDROME, the group helps families in enhancing the lives of children with the condition, provides information, and publishes brochures. For address, see Appendix A.

See also FRAGILE X FOUNDATION.

fragile X syndrome   An X-linked congenital condition caused by a chromosomal abnormality in which a male's X chromosome is malformed; some evidence links the syndrome with AUTISM or LEARNING DISABILITIES.

Many children with fragile X are MENTALLY RETARDED (as often are their mothers), but many people with the syndrome have normal mental capacity. In fact, fragile X is the most common cause of mental retardation in males after DOWN SYNDROME. Although males are mainly affected, women are able to carry the genetic defect that is responsible for the disorder and pass it on to some of their sons, who are affected, and some of their daughters, who in turn become carriers of the defect. Approximately one in 1,500 men are affected and one in 1,000 women are carriers. About one-third of female carriers show some degree of intellectual problems.

See also FRAGILE X FOUNDATION; FRAGILE X SUPPORT.

Symptoms   In addition to mental retardation, the syndrome is characterized by large testicles, protruding long ears, and a pronounced nose, chin, and forehead; those affected tend to be tall and physically strong. The syndrome affects every 2,000 to 3,000 births; a child of a mother who carries the fragile X chromosome has a one chance in two of inheriting the disorder.

Treatment   There is no treatment.

free radicals   A highly charged, potentially destructive molecule (most commonly, a species of oxygen) that is generated naturally by breathing and by the body's response to stress. While free radicals are destructive, they have a positive role to play in the body as well. Generated by the immune system, they fend off microbes and help the digestive system break down food. In the brain, it can interact with lipids, harming the brain.

While a certain amount of free radicals is necessary to maintain proper body function, high levels are toxic. Each day, the body generates thousands upon thousands of free radicals in response to ultraviolet (UV) light, smoke, and pollution. Once activated, they tear through the membrane that protects the body's cells, causing inflammation and cell breakdown.

Friedreich's ataxia   A hereditary degenerative disease of the CEREBELLUM and spinocerebellar tracts, this disorder is characterized by the development of ATAXIA of the trunk and extremities, absence of deep reflexes, loss of sensations in the arms and legs, clubfeet, and curvature of the spine (scoliosis). The late stages of this disease may involve atrophied muscles and degeneration of the optic nerve. In mild forms, patients may be able to live a normal life, but most cases are slowly progressive to complete incapacity by age 20. Death is usually caused by infections or degeneration of the heart muscle.

Friedreich's Ataxia Group in America   A support group that aids patients with FRIEDREICH'S ATAXIA and their families, provides information to the public and to health professionals, supports research, and publishes a newsletter. For address, see Appendix A.

Friends of Brain Tumor Research   A national organization that encourages formation of mutual-support, self-help groups of those concerned with BRAIN TUMOR. The group also publishes various materials, including a quarterly newsletter and a resource guide. For address, see Appendix A.

frontal aphasia See BROCA'S APHASIA.

frontal lobe The area just in front of the central fissure; one of the roles of the frontal lobe is concerned with intellectual functioning, including thought processes, behavior, and memory.

frontal lobotomy See LOBOTOMY; LEUCOTOMY.

fundus Cortical valleys of brain tissue that lie beneath the outer layer of the brain that, according to new research, may help coordinate problem solving and other complex types of thinking.

The new research, using PET SCANS, suggests that more-demanding and complex cognitive functions rely on cortical fundal activity to a higher degree than do less-demanding processes. The research found that these cortical valleys showed the most activity during especially complex problem-solving and memory tasks, and yet these areas make up only about 8 percent of the entire CORTEX.

Because fundal cells handle short-range communications in the brain, some scientists suggest that these NEURONS may also function as a central point where related lines of information converge to make complex thinking possible.

fusiform gyrus A band of tissue that runs lengthwise along the base of each side of the brain. Recent research suggests that parts of the fusiform gyrus show distinctive electrical responses to patterns of letters; one part of the fusiform gyrus responds comparably to all types of letter strings but not to illustrations or visual patterns. Another part is activated only during presentations of actual words.

The two parts of the fusiform gyrus play a part in the brain's visual system that specializes in word recognition some researchers believe. While the first site in this part of the brain perceives separate letters in an array and in meaningful arrangements of those letters, the second appears to form visual meanings of words or to helps retrieve memories of word meanings based on emotional qualities of a word or on its context in a sentence.

This whole process of word recognition takes about a fifth of a second to complete.

See also READING.

G

GABA The abbreviation for *gamma-amino-butyric acid*, this is an AMINO-ACID NEUROTRANS-MITTER released by nerve terminals in the brain and SPINAL CORD. GABA is known as an inhibitory neurotransmitter, for its action is to inhibit the electrical activity of the neuron it is released upon. GABAergic systems shape the activity of other transmitter systems through the inhibition or reduction in firing rate of target neurons. BENZODIAZEPINE drugs boost the activity of GABA, and anticonvulsant drugs decrease its activity. It is believed that it helps control anxiety.

Some research indicates that patients with HUNTINGTON'S DISEASE may have too few GABA-producing NERVE CELLS in the areas that coordinate movement. Huntington's is associated with involuntary movement and mental problems.

Galen (A.D. 129–199) The great Greek physician of the second century A.D. who established some basic (albeit slightly garbled) theories of the brain and body that were practiced for the next 1,500 years. He was born the son of a gifted architect in the city where the healing shrine of the god Asclepius was located. At the medical school that was connected with the shrine, Galen observed many of the treatments for a variety of diseases and eventually became chief physician for the gladiators in 157. Galen based his anatomy on the dissection of lower animals such as the African monkey. His important contributions included the discovery of seven pairs of CRANIAL NERVES and the discovery that the brain controls the voice.

Gall, Franz Joseph (1758–1828) German anatomist and physiologist who dissected the brain, established the basis of modern neurology, and was the first to ascribe particular functions to various areas of the brain. Gall is also the cofounder of PHRENOLOGY, the practice of assessing a person's intellect and personality from shape of the skull. He was also the first to identify the GRAY MATTER of the brain with NEURONS and the WHITE MATTER with GANGLIA (conducting tissue).

Gall was convinced that mental functions were to be found in specific areas of the brain (localization); these theories were proved correct when French physician Pierre-Paul Broca (see BROCA, PIERRE-PAUL) demonstrated the speech center of the brain in 1861. Unfortunately, he enlarged on these theories to assume that the surface of the skull reflected the development of the various brain regions lying underneath. It was later found that the thickness of the skull varies and so does not reflect the underlying brain.

gamma-aminobutyric acid (GABA) See GABA.

ganglia Groups of peripheral neuron cell bodies in which nerve signals are processed.

gender differences in the brain Although the sex of every fetus is genetically determined at the moment of conception, sexual anatomy begins to appear during the sixth to eighth week. In addition to affecting sexual organs, testicular hormones guide the development of the brain, leading to gender differences in the HYPOTHALAMUS and other areas. Moreover, exposure to the androgen testosterone before and immediately after birth seems to change the way the NERVOUS SYSTEM responds to hormones after puberty.

More and more studies are suggesting that sex-linked hormones may indeed help shape some behavioral and cognitive differences between men and women, although it's hard to figure out which are learned and which are due to hormonal influences. While it is always difficult to separate the role of the environment from innate differences, some studies suggest that girls tend to show more parenting-rehearsal behavior, while boys respond more to things that deal with human interaction.

While some gender differences in the brain appear to be the result of sex hormones, other are simply structural in nature—it's clear that male brains tend to be bigger and heavier than female brains. Of course, this does not mean that intellectual capacity is likewise more advanced in males.

This is because the brain operates through electrical and chemical processing, not through the *physical* storage of facts; therefore, the actual size of the brain should have no bearing on intellect. Beyond that statement, the issue of male-female brain differences is extremely controversial. There are other structural differences in the brain between men and women as well, although it is not clear what these may mean. First of all, females tend to have a left cortical dominance while males usually have a right cortical dominance. This is why, scientists believe, women appear to be predisposed toward better verbal abilities; they usually speak earlier and more clearly, learn languages more easily, and can repeat tongue twisters better. They also have better fine-motor control (and therefore tend to have better penmanship). On the other hand, men typically are inclined to outperform women in spatial functions, such as negotiating a maze.

The CORPUS CALLOSUM (fiber network joining the left and right hemispheres) is proportionately much larger in a female brain than in a male brain. For hundreds of years, doctors noted that women seemed to recover more quickly and more completely from BRAIN INJURIES than did men. More recently, scientists have discovered that this is possible because the bridge that joins the two hemispheres is more closely connected in women, allowing one side of the brain to better compensate for damage to the other. Moreover, brain hemispheres in both men and women become more and more specialized with each year of life from birth until puberty; after this, the corpus callosum becomes thinner and thinner. Because women generally reach puberty first, their brains tend to be less specialized than men and therefore are able to recover more quickly from BRAIN DAMAGE. Men are also far more likely to suffer from DYSLEXIA, stuttering, AUTISM, and HYPERACTIVITY.

This thicker "bridge" between the two hemispheres might also explain the mystery of "women's intuition," according to Dr. Jerre Levy of the University of Chicago. Dr. Levy suggests that this close connection between the two hemispheres in women makes it easier for them to integrate the details and subtleties of a situation.

Of course, scientists emphasize that the skill differences between men and women due to brain configuration are only slight. In fact, they emphasize that only a small part of the difference between men and women in any one skill is due to the structure and chemical makeup of their brains. The rest— probably as much as 80 percent—of the differences reflect a person's expectations, encouragement, education, and environment.

genetic disorders of the brain There are a number of genetic disorders that can affect the brain and its function. These include inherited chromosomal abnormalities resulting in mental retardation (such as TAY SACHS DISEASE or DOWN SYNDROME), degeneration of brain tissue (such as HUNTINGTON'S DISEASE) and structural problems, such as ANENCEPHALY (absence of the brain), MICROCEPHALY (very small head), or HYDROCEPHALUS (water on the brain).

genetic influence on the brain The debate between nature and nurture—what is inherited and what is a product of our environment—is an ongoing scientific argument. Nowhere is this more clear than in the study of the brain and its influence on individual thought, personality, and behavior.

However, by studying twins separated at birth and reared apart, it is possible to make some conclusions about what is inherited and what is controlled from outside. Among other traits, scientists have found that

- Leadership ability (about 60 percent of a person's ability) is inherited.
- Aggression, neatness, social closeness, and intellectual achievement depends primarily on upbringing (only a 33 to 48 percent is contributed by inheritance).
- Shyness is strongly linked to heredity; fears and phobias are also primarily inherited.

Even in the most clearly inherited traits, however, the brain influences behavior subtly by influencing what environments a person will seek; this in turn determines behavior. For example, someone born to lead may never have the opportunity to do so—at least in a positive way—if born to a life of poverty and isolation.

Gilles de la Tourette's syndrome See TOURETTE'S SYNDROME.

ginkgo biloba This extract from the oldest known species of tree (also known as a *maidenhair tree*) is drunk as a tea and seems to increase the flow of nutrients and oxygen to the brain. As it increases circulation, it also boosts the production of ADENOSINE TRIPHOSPHATE (ATP) and streamlines the brain's ability to metabolize GLUCOSE. It also appears to prevent platelet clumping in arteries and serves as a powerful ANTIOXIDANT.

The tree dates back 300 million years and is the only living representative of the order Ginkgoales. Called a *living fossil* because it does not exist in the wild, it has been planted since ancient times in Chinese and Japanese temple gardens and is now widely used throughout the world as an ornamental tree.

It also has been used for millennia in China as a valuable medicine, and it is still used today throughout Europe for the same purpose. Among its many alleged benefits, leaves from this tree are said to improve short-term memory loss, and some people believe it is of some benefit to ALZHEIMER'S DISEASE patients. While some studies have found ginkgo to improve cognitive function in Alzheimer's disease patients, another study could not substantiate such a link.

Research suggests that ginkgo leaves are most effective for those with reduced blood flow to the brain. While most research has been done with a ginkgo-biloba extract (with a 24-percent flavonoid concentration), many products on the market are not as strong. Ginkgo-biloba leaf and extracts are available in vitamin and health-food stores.

glia cells See GLIAL CELLS.

glial cells One of the types of cells composing the brain that protect, support and feed NEURONS, outnumbering them 10 to 1—the brain contains more than 100 trillion glial cells. Some of the glial cells seem to act as a sort of bed for NEURONS. Unlike neurons, glial cells don't generate electrical impulses, but they do play an important supportive role in maintaining efficiency along the brain's nerve network. They help to form a covering to protect the large neurons in the SPINAL CORD; MYELIN is placed around the axons of some neurons by a particular type of glial cell, and AXONS covered by this myelin sheath conduct impulses up to 12 times faster than those without it. The areas of the brain that contain myelin-covered axons are called the WHITE MATTER because the myelinated axons look white. In addition, some glial cells may get rid of dead neurons.

glioblastoma A fast-growing, highly malignant type of BRAIN TUMOR. Glioblastoma multiforme is a type of GLIOMA, a tumor arising from the GLIAL CELLS within the brain. Most glioblastomas develop within the CEREBRUM (the main mass of the brain). This type of brain tumor occurs in 10 out of a million people in the United States each year.

The most common primary brain tumor of adults and the third most common of preteens, it occurs most often in those between ages 48 and 60, affecting twice as many men as women and whites more often than nonwhites.

It is a rapidly spreading tumor with tentacles that invade nearby tissue, resembling a butterfly pattern of distribution throughout the WHITE MATTER of both CEREBRAL HEMISPHERES. The spread of this tumor outside the brain and SPINAL CORD is rare.

While glioblastomas may occur in any part of the cerebral hemispheres, they are most common in the FRONTAL, TEMPORAL, and PARIETAL LOBES.

Cause Its cause is unknown, and although there have been cases of this type of tumor appearing in the same family, research has not yet proven a hereditary link. Some research has suggested a possible link to a type of rare virus. Males with type A blood appear to be at higher risk, as are children who swallow lead or BARBITURATES; occupational chemical factors have also been associated with this type of tumor, such as those employed in rubber-manufacturing industries or who are exposed to vinyl chloride or pesticide sprays.

However, some factors have been excluded as a possible cause, including birth control pills, smoking, alcohol use, prior HEAD INJURY or exposure to dental X RAYS.

Symptoms Because the tumor can grow so quickly, doubling its size every seven to eight days, the primary symptom is related to the compression of brain tissue by the tumor. Because the skull can't enlarge to accommodate the increased pressure, it causes an "all-over" HEADACHE that is worse in the morn-

ing, together with vomiting (though not usually nausea). Other symptoms may include weak muscles, sensory disturbances, speech problems, SEIZURES, visual disturbances, and impaired mental processes.

Diagnosis Checking for a suspected brain tumor involves a fairly standard procedure, including a basic neurological exam testing eye movement and pupil reaction, observation of walking pattern, repeat rapid alternating movements, heel-to-toe walking, heel-to-shin movements, balance with feet together and eyes closed, sensation by pin prick, and smelling. Other tests may evaluate concrete and abstract thinking.

This may be followed by a set of plain skull X rays together with some combination of scanning procedures. In order to locate the tumor and determine its extent, physicians may use ANGIOGRAPHY together with CT SCANNING, MAGNETIC RESONANCE IMAGING (MRI), ELECTROENCEPHALOGRAMS (EEG), RADIONUCLIDE BRAIN SCAN (RN), or POSITRON EMISSION TOMOGRAPHY (PET).

Treatment The tumor is surgically removed when possible, but too often this type of tumor is inaccessible or too extensive to be removed. In this case, survival rates are not high; less than 20 percent of these patients survive one year. When a tumor cannot be totally removed, as much of the growth as possible will be cut out to relieve pressure on the brain, followed by chemotherapy or radiation therapy. Corticosteroid drugs can be used to reduce tissue swelling around the tumor.

Laser microsurgery may be able to remove (by vaporization) some tissue past the tumor border in order to try to remove microscopic tumor infiltrates without damaging normal tissue too much. However, glioblastomas can never be totally removed because cells too small for the surgeon to see are present in the surrounding area. With luck, aggressive surgery can reduce the number of tumor cells so that chemotherapy or radiation therapy can be more effective. If the tumor recurs, a second or even third surgery may be performed.

Radiation is the second most common treatment for brain tumors after surgery, usually administered soon after surgery. The cells of many malignant brain tumors are readily killed by radiation, which is why this type of treatment is almost always recommended. (One possible exception is the treatment of very young children, whose developing brains may be injured by the radiation). Most tumors do shrink from the effects of radiation, although it may take some time for swelling and dead cells to diminish so that the true size of the growth can be seen.

After radiation has reduced the number of tumor cells, chemotherapy is given to try to destroy any that remain. Chemotherapy may also be given at the same time as radiation.

Other possible treatments include brachytherapy (also called interstitial radiation or "seeding") in which radioactive pellets are implanted directly into the tumor during surgery. Brachytherapy is used primarily in recurrences when the tumor is confined to one side of the brain and measures less than six centimeters (about the size of a golf ball).

Other research is investigating the use of different types of radiation (such as neutrons), intraoperative radiation, etc. Immunotherapy is also being studied, using drugs such as interferon, levamisole, interleukin-2, and thymosine in conjunction with chemotherapy or radiation therapy in the hopes of stimulating the body's own immune system.

There are also a whole range of new drugs being tested, plus better methods of drug delivery.

Prognosis Long-term survival with this type of tumor is not very good. With surgery alone, median survival is 17 weeks; with radiation, 37.5 weeks; and with chemotherapy, 50 to 60 weeks. Chemotherapy increases the number of long-term survivors (those who live more than a year) from 4 percent to 20 percent; a few patients do survive for five years or more.

The ASSOCIATION FOR BRAIN TUMOR RESEARCH maintains a current list of specialists in the glioblastoma field, who will agree to review medical records for a consultation fee.

glioma A general name for a variety of brain tumors (see TUMOR, BRAIN) arising from the supportive tissue (GLIAL CELLS) within the brain. (See also ASTROCYTOMA, OLIGODENDROGLIOMA, EPENDYMOMA, and GLIOBLASTOMA.) About 60 percent of all primary brain tumors (tumors originating within the brain) are gliomas; there are about two to four new cases per 100,000 people each year in the United States.

Symptoms Compression of brain tissue by the tumor may cause weak muscles, sensory disturbances, speech problems, and epileptic seizures. Pressure can also cause HEADACHES, vomiting, visual disturbances, and impaired mental processes.

Diagnosis In order to locate the tumor and determine its extent, physicians use ANGIOGRAPHY together with various types of BRAIN SCANS: CT SCANNING, MAGNETIC RESONANCE IMAGING (MRI), and X-RAY studies.

Treatment The tumor is surgically removed when possible, but too often it is inaccessible or too extensive to be removed. In this case, survival rates are not high; less than 20 percent of these patients survive one year. When a tumor cannot be totally removed, as much of the growth as possible will be cut out to relieve pressure on the brain, followed by chemotherapy or radiation therapy. Corticosteroid drugs can be used to reduce tissue swelling around the tumor.

Radiation is the second most common treatment for brain tumors after surgery, usually administered a few weeks after surgery. The cells of many malignant brain tumors are readily killed by radiation, which is why this type of treatment is almost always recommended. (One possible exception is the treatment of very young children, whose developing brains may be injured by the radiation). Most tumors do shrink from the effects of radiation, although it may take some time for swelling and dead cells to diminish to the true size of the growth can be seen.

glioma of the optic nerve A type of GLIOMA commonly found in children causing blindness in one eye because of the pressure on the optic nerve; sometimes, the tumor extends to the third ventricle of the brain.

Treatment The usual treatment is radiation therapy because this type of glioma is sensitive to radiation. However, if the tumor extends into the third ventricle, the chances for survival are not good.

glossopharyngeal nerve Also known as the ninth cranial nerve, this mixed nerve is mainly responsible for taste and throat sensations.

See also CRANIAL NERVES.

glucose A simple sugar (dextrose) that is the primary source of energy for the brain. Because glucose is not stored within the brain, a continuous supply is essential. If the brain is deprived of glucose for 10 to 15 minutes, irreversible brain damage can occur.

Free glucose is not found in many types of food (except for grapes), but it is a part of both sucrose and starch, both of which break down and form glucose after digestion. Glucose is stored in the body in the form of glycogen; its concentration in the blood is maintained by a variety of hormones (especially insulin and glucagon).

If the blood-glucose concentration falls below a certain level, neurological symptoms of low blood sugar (hypoglycemia) may occur. These symptoms include dizziness, apprehension, and fainting; in severe cases, COMA and death may follow. On the other hand, if there is too much glucose in the blood, hyperglycemia (the primary symptom of diabetes) may result.

glucose utilization scan See PET SCAN.

glutamate An amino acid found in every cell in the body, it is also used in the nervous system as a "fast excitatory" neurotransmitter. Glutamate is important in the proper function of the HIPPOCAMPUS, among other brain areas, and an imbalance will cause epileptic seizures, memory disorders, or both.

Glutamate is the best known of a group of excitatory amino acids that plays an important part in initiating and transmitting signals in the brain. Almost half of the brain's neurons use glutamate as a primary transmitter.

Normally, glutamate is bound tightly in the cells, and only tiny amounts are allowed into the spaces between brain cells at any one time. But new research suggests that abnormal glutamate activity may *also* be responsible for BRAIN DAMAGE following lack of oxygen from injury, STROKE, or SEIZURE. When the brain is deprived of oxygen and some of the cells that store glutamate shut down, glutamate comes flooding out of the cells; in such high levels, it kills brain cells—just five minutes of excess glutamate is enough to kill cells.

grand mal seizure The most severe type of EPILEPSY in which a person cries out and falls to the floor unconscious, jerking uncontrollably from muscle contractions. The seizure may last for a few minutes, and unconsciousness may last for some time afterward. The person may not remember anything about the seizure upon awakening. Sometimes, people experience warning symptoms before a *grand mal* attack.

gray matter Parts of the brain and SPINAL CORD that include mostly closely packed, interconnected nuclei of NERVE CELL bodies (instead of the AXONS that make up WHITE MATTER). Gray matter in the brain is primarily found in the outer layers of the CEREBRUM (the main mass of the brain) and in some deeper areas of the brain. Gray matter also makes up the inner core of the spinal cord.

growth hormone A hormone that promotes growth of the long bones and increases protein synthesis, both produced and stored in the anterior PITUITARY GLAND. The release of growth hormone is controlled by the growth hormone releasing factor and the hormone somatostatin. The release of too much growth hormone can result in gigantism before puberty, and acromegaly (increase in hands, feet, and face) in adults. Lack of this hormone in children can produce dwarfism.

Guardians of Hydrocephalus Research Foundation National support group for hydrocephalics and their families, health-care professionals, and others who seeks to find the cause and cure of HYDROCEPHALUS, the buildup of cerebrospinal fluid in the brain activity. The foundation provides information, conducts fund-raising projects, and maintains an evaluation center that provides comprehensive patient services.

The group also plans to conduct research and educational programs and to operate computerized services. Founded in 1977, the group has 5,000 members and publishes an annual journal and various brochures. For address, see Appendix A.

Guillain-Barre syndrome A rare disease of peripheral nerves characterized by numb, weak arms and legs. The condition usually appears 10 to 20 days after a respiratory infection that triggers an allergic response in the peripheral nerves, inflaming and destroying the MYELIN nerve sheath. The condition is also known as acute polyneuritis or ascending paralysis.

In 1976, an epidemic occurred in the United States following mass vaccination against swine flu, but further evaluation showed the vaccination did not cause the flurry of cases. Two-thirds of cases occur after a viral infection that may be a form of herpes (such as Epstein-Barr virus), or it may follow flu, a cold, or other minor infection. The syndrome may also appear with conditions such as Hodgkin's disease.

Occasionally, Guillain-Barre is associated with medical procedures and 5 to 10 percent occur after operations.

A severe attack of Guillain-Barre is a medical emergency and may require a stay in intensive care; a few patients need artificial ventilation during the illness. Generally, recovery begins after a few months, and most people recover completely without specific treatment, although there is permanent weakness in about 10 percent of cases. Others may suffer from repeated attacks of the disease. The mortality rate is 3 to 4 percent.

See also GUILLAIN-BARRE SYNDROME FOUNDATION INTERNATIONAL.

Symptoms A few days to a week or so after infection, or one to four weeks after an operation, symptoms appear, including tingling sensations in fingers and toes and general muscle weakness. A sensation of weakness can spread from legs to arms and face; in severe cases, weakness turns into paralysis and may affect respiratory muscles. Muscles controlling eye or facial movements, speaking, chewing, or swallowing may also be affected. About 3,500 cases occur every year in the United States and Canada.

Diagnosis Tests (such as ELECTROMYOGRAPHY), analysis of cerebrospinal fluid extracted by LUMBAR PUNCTURE (spinal tap) and physical exam.

Treatment Patients are treated in the hospital with supportive care; mechanical ventilation may be necessary. Some patients benefit from plasmapheresis (removal of plasma and damaging antibodies from the blood) during the first few weeks of a severe attack; this may improve the chance for a full recovery. Once the condition has stabilized, rehabilitation will include whirlpool baths to relieve pain and retrain movements, physical therapy, and training with adaptive devices.

Guillain-Barre Syndrome Foundation International A national support group for individuals concerned with GUILLAIN-BARRE SYNDROME, a rare paralyzing disorder of the peripheral nerves. The foundation provides information about the disease and support groups; fosters research on the cause, prevention, and treatment of the syndrome; encourages financial support for research; and develops support groups across the country. The foundation also arranges for recovered or recovering patients to visit patients in acute care and rehabilitation hospitals, helps patients deal with disabilities, and maintains a steering committee of physicians, some of whom have had the disorder. Founded in 1980, the group has 15,000 members and publishes various informational brochures. For address, see Appendix A.

H

habituation The process by which a NERVE CELL adapts to an initially novel stimulus and decreases its response to that stimulus after repeated presentation.

Haller, Albrecht von (1708–1777) Swiss biologist and the father of experimental physiology who showed that the sensation of touch depends on nerves and that nerves activate muscles. Von Haller also traced nerves from the body's limbs to the brain's CEREBRAL CORTEX. While serving as professor of medicine at the University of Göttingen, he wrote the eight-volume landmark in medical history: *Elementa Physiologiae Corporis Humani* (*Physiological Elements of the Human Body*).

See also BRAIN IN HISTORY.

hallucination Seeing, hearing, touching, smelling, or tasting something that does not actually exist.

hallucinogens A class of drugs that cause HALLUCINATIONS by interfering with the normal chemical balance of the brain, mimicking the naturally occurring OPIATES in the brain that affect the LIMBIC SYSTEM.

There are four main groups of hallucinogens, each containing drugs derived from plants: the *indole alkaloid derivatives* (including LSD, harmatine, ibogaine, and psilocybin); *piperidine derivatives* (atropine, belladonna, and scopolamine); *pheylethylamines* (amphetamines and mescaline) and *cannabinols* (cannabis, or marijuana).

Most hallucinogens, including LSD, stimulate the SYMPATHETIC NERVOUS SYSTEM, boosting pulse rate and blood pressure resulting in sweating and palpitations. Others (such as the cannabinols) reduce stomach acid secretion and have a calming effect on the brain.

Hallucinogens also have an intense effect on the brain's LIMBIC SYSTEM, influencing mood and emotions and suppressing centers controlling memory and higher functions such as judgment. This combination of limbic system effects (which can cause violent mood swings) together with loss of judgment can be dangerous.

Particular effects depend on the type of drug and the dose; some emphasize feelings while others influence fantasies. Effects may also depend in part on the user's personality, and those unused to drugs may experience ANXIETY, depression, or nausea. Those who have used drugs often report euphoria and irrational thoughts or mystical experiences that may be confused with a higher state of consciousness. While not normally addictive, hallucinogens may trigger a psychological dependence.

handedness A person's preference for using the right or the left hand; 90 percent of healthy adults use the right hand for writing, and most (66 percent) favor the right hand for most other activities requiring coordination. The rest are either left handed or ambidextrous (able to use either hand). Handedness has no correlation to gender, and if the brain becomes damaged before age 12, it is possible to switch handedness.

Handedness is related to the two hemispheres of the brain, each of which controls movement and sensation in the opposite side of the body. The dominant hemisphere in right-handed people is always the left one, but oddly enough, this is true for left-handers as well, although a few have dominant right hemispheres. Some display no dominance at all. Scientists suspect that some language disorders such as DYSLEXIA and stuttering are more common in left-handed people and may be related to a problem in developing cerebral dominance.

Scientists believe that a tendency toward the right or the left hand is inherited, although it is possible to "force" a left-handed child to use the right hand. In early centuries, a left-handed person was considered to be unlucky at best and evil at worst (indeed, the word *sinister* comes from the Latin word for "left"). While this is no longer true today, so many people are right handed that the pressure to conform is very high, especially in cultures that reserve the left hand for cleaning the anal area after defecating.

It is not clear whether handedness is related to special abilities, and while the left brain is related to verbal ability and local reasoning and the right to emotional and spatial ability, there is no evidence that more artists are left handed or more writers are right handed. In fact, about 60 percent of left-handed people, like right-handers, process speech in the left hemisphere, while the other 40 percent use both sides of the brain. This is one indication that each of the brain's hemispheres has the potential for processing any function. It often takes advantage of this potential following BRAIN INJURY from trauma or STROKE. A few scientists suspect that the CEREBRUM evolved into two almost identical parts to provide a sort of "back-up" brain in case of accidents.

The right brain does seem to be critically involved in appreciating and interpreting spatial relationships and visualizing complex three-dimensional shapes, in addition to recognizing faces.

Harvey, William (1578–1657) The British physician who discovered the secret of blood circulation and who also believed that sensory nerves took sensations to the brain and that motor nerves worked muscles. A graduate of the University of Padua medical school, he was a member of the Royal College of Physicians. The physician extraordinary to James I of England, he was one of the doctors in attendance at the death of the king in 1625. He was also appointed personal physician to Charles I.

See also BRAIN IN HISTORY.

headaches Pain in the head, front of the face, or back of the head that can range from mild to extremely severe. One of the most common medical complaints, each year headaches affect as many as 24 million Americans seriously enough for them to miss work. While most headaches don't represent a life-threatening condition, they can significantly interfere with the activities of daily living. Headaches that *may* represent a more serious medical problem are those that appear suddenly, that are extremely severe, or that change in pattern or severity of pain.

The many different causes for headache are diagnosed according to how they occur, plus their severity, onset, and location. There are many types of headaches that scientists divided into three categories: tension headaches, vascular headaches, and headaches caused by trauma or disease.

Tension headaches These most-common headaches are set off by severe muscle contractions caused by stress or exertion. People who are so anxious that they grind their teeth or hunch their shoulders may find that the strain can travel to the nerves in the brain, producing constant pain. Many people report this pain as a kind of tight band around the forehead, affecting both sides of the head. Tension headaches occur most often in the front of the head, although they may also appear at the top or the back. Eyestrain caused by coping with a great amount of paperwork can cause a tension headache that builds up during the day.

Tension headaches respond very well to over-the-counter drugs such as aspirin, ibuprofen, or acetaminophen or by massaging the tense muscle groups responsible for the pain. Those who often get tension headaches

TYPES OF HEADACHES

Symptoms	Type	Cause
Pain on both sides of head	Tension headache	Muscle contraction
Agonizing pain on one side of head; nausea or vomiting	Migraine	Stress, hunger, fatigue, addiction withdrawal, sensory overload, hormone fluctuation
Less pain than migraine; stuffy sinus	Cluster	Same as migraine
Dull head pain	Hypertensive	High blood pressure
Head pain	Toxic	Food or chemicals, allergies
Pain with weakness, loss of balance, numbing	Injury/disease	Infection, anemia, trauma, neurological problems

should consider taking stress breaks throughout the day.

Vascular headaches Vascular headaches can be divided into four subcategories. The first is the *migraine*, the most delibitating of all headaches, which causes a profound throbbing pain that is often accompanied by nausea and vomiting. Researchers thought that migraines were caused by abnormally dilated blood vessels in the head, but more recently they have found the pain is caused by electrochemical activity in the brain that is usually caused by stress, hunger, fatigue, sensory overload, hormone fluctuations, or addiction withdrawal. Some people with migraines see spots, auras, flashes, or blank spots right before a migraine strikes. Migraines are almost always limited to one side of the head. People who place a great deal of stress on themselves are more likely to suffer with treatment-resistant migraines.

Migraines are treated by prescription drugs that affect the brain's chemistry, such as ergotamine, methysegide, and verapamil. Migraines also respond to antidepressants (especially the new SELECTIVE SEROTONIN REUPTAKE INHIBITORS such as Prozac), not because the patient is depressed but because the drugs normalize the brain's level of SEROTONIN, which is believed to be askew in migraine patients.

Cluster headaches are milder cousins of the migraine that do not announce their onset with visual disturbances, don't cause nausea, and don't last very long. They usually occur in two or three episodes in one day, lasting between 10 minutes to a few hours each time. Unlike migraines, cluster headaches include the sensation of a stuffy sinus. Cause and treatment are the same as for migraines.

Cluster headaches are treated by the same type of prescription drugs used to treat migraines—drugs that affect the brain's chemistry, such as ergotamine, methysegide, and verapamil.

Toxic headaches are caused by chemical fumes (such as CARBON MONOXIDE) or by chemicals in food (such as chocolate, cheese, or citrus fruits). They also may be caused by allergies or weather changes. Medical tests can determine whether a person's headache is of toxic origin.

Hypertensive headaches are caused by high blood pressure, characterized by a dull pain that is easily relieved by bed rest.

Headaches caused by trauma/disease This type of headache can be the most difficult to diagnose. The headaches may be caused by a wide range of problems, including sinus infections or infection in the blood or lymph system; a neurological problem in the brain, eyes, ears, teeth, face, or spine; anemia; or trauma caused by blows, tumors, or blood clots. They may be particularly severe or accompanied by numbness, balance problems, or weakness.

head injury Even the mildest bump on the head is capable of damaging the brain; research suggests that 60 percent of patients who sustain a mild BRAIN INJURY continue to have a range of symptoms called POSTCONCUSSION SYNDROME as long as six months after the injury. These symptoms can result in a puzzling interplay of behavioral, cognitive, and emotional complaints that can be difficult to diagnose. Although research is still limited, studies have found that symptoms following even the mildest head injury can linger, causing ongoing discomfort and destroying personal lives.

The fact that head injury can have effects throughout the body has been known for at least the past 3,000 years; the Edwin Smith Surgical Papyrus written between 2,500 and 3,000 years ago contains information about 48 cases in which eight people describe head injuries that affect other parts of the body.

Symptoms Symptoms following head injury may be due both from the direct physical damage to the brain and also to secondary factors, such as lack of oxygen, swelling, and vascular disturbance. A penetrating injury may also cause a brain infection. The kind of injury the brain receives in a closed head injury is determined by the type of accident; whether or not the head was unrestrained upon impact; and the direction, force, and velocity of the blow. If the head is resting upon impact, the maximum damage will be found at the impact site; a moving head will cause a "contrecoup" injury where the damage will be on the side opposite the point of impact.

Both kinds of injuries can cause swirling movements throughout the brain, tearing nerve fibers and causing widespread vascular damage. There may be bleeding in the CEREBRUM or SUBARACHNOID SPACE leading to HEMATOMAS. Swelling may raise intracranial pressure and may block oxygen to the brain.

After a head injury, there may be a period of impaired consciousness followed by a period of confusion and impaired memory with confusion, disorientation, and impairment in the ability to store and retrieve new information. For some reason, the physical and emotional shock of the accident interrupts the transfer of all information that happened to be in the short-term memory just before the accident; this is why some people can remember information several days before and after the accident, but not information right before the accident occurred.

There may be a temporary AMNESIA following head injury that often begins with memory loss over a period of weeks, months, or years prior to the injury, diminishing as recovery proceeds. Permanent amnesia, however, may extend for just a few seconds or minutes before the accident; in very severe head injuries, however, the permanent amnesia may also cover weeks or months before the accident.

A small minority are plagued by symptoms, including HEADACHE, dizziness, confusion, and memory loss which may continue for months.

A 1981 study of 424 patients diagnosed with mild head injury showed that many had recurrent problems with deviant behavior, headaches, dizziness, and cognitive problems; only 17 percent were symptom-free three months after the accident. A later study reached the same conclusions.

Diagnosis Until recently, diagnostic tools were not sensitive enough to detect the subtle structural changes that can occur and sometimes persist after mild head injury. Typically, CT SCANS have yielded negative results from this group of patients. But studies involving MAGNETIC RESONANCE IMAGING (MRI) and brain electrophysiology indicate that contusions and diffuse injuries associated with mild head injury are likely to affect those parts of the brain that relate to memory, concentration, information processing, and problem solving.

While CT scans are widely available in emergency rooms to help in the diagnosis of neural hematomas, many experts believe these scans may not pick up the subtle damage following a mild head injury. Magnetic resonance imaging is more sensitive in diagnosing many brain lesions, and it may be more sensitive in detecting the diffuse shearing and contusions.

In many patients, neither scan can detect the microscopic damage that occurs when fibers are stretched in a mild, diffuse injury. In this type of injury, the AXONS lose some of their covering and become less efficient. This mild injury to the WHITE MATTER reduces the quality of communication between different parts of the brain. A quantitative EEG plays signals from the brain into a computer, where they are digitized and stored. This type of EEG can measure the time delay between two regions of the cortex and the amount of time it takes for information to be transmitted from one region to another.

PET (POSITRON EMISSION TOMOGRAPHY), which evaluates cerebral blood flow and brain metabolism, may help diagnose mild head injury. SINGLE PHOTON EMISSION COMPUTED TOMOGRAPHY (SPECT) is less expensive than PET and might provide data on cerebral blood flow after mild head injury.

Evoked potential tests are not generally used in patients with less serious mild head injury because they aren't sensitive enough to document physiologic abnormalities unless testing is done within a day or two of injury.

Neuropsychological testing may clarify results when scans and neurologic exams are unclear.

Treatment Only a small percentage of patients with mild head injury are hospitalized overnight, and instructions they receive upon leaving the emergency room usually do not address behavioral, cognitive, and emo-tional symptoms that can occur after such an injury.

Patients who do experience symptoms are advised to seek out the care of a specialist; unless a family physician is thoroughly familiar with medical literature in this newly emerging area, experts warn that there is a great chance that patient complaints will be ignored. Patients with continuing symptoms after a mild head injury are advised to call a local head-injury foundation that can refer patients to the best nearby practitioner.

hearing The sense of hearing occurs when the ears convert sounds into electrochemical signals that travel to the brain's TEMPORAL LOBES (the "hearing centers") where sounds are interpreted.

Sound waves travel through the outer ear tunnel to the eardrum, the gateway to the middle ear. Sound waves vibrate the eardrum, which in turn vibrates a sequence of tiny movable bones (the hammer, anvil, and stirrup [or malleus, incus, and stapes]). Sound vibrations also reach the inner ear via the skull bones. As the vibrating stapes plunges in and out of the oval window leading to the inner ear, waves are sent through fluid-filled membrane chambers including the cochlea of the inner ear. In turn, this stimulates the organ of Corti, a tunnel surrounded by rods with thousands of sensitive hairs attached to nerve fibers. When the hairs vibrate, the nerves send signals corresponding to the pitch and volume of the sound, through the ACOUSTIC NERVE (or eighth cranial nerve) to the BRAINSTEM.

In the brainstem, nerve fibers from both sides of the head cross, taking signals up through the CEREBRAL HEMISPHERES to the tops of the temporal lobes to be analyzed. This way, signals from each ear reach both temporal lobes, which means if one lobe is damaged, the patient will not necessarily be functionally deaf in one ear.

Signals arriving from both ears help pinpoint the location of sound. Humans are capable of detecting sound waves with frequencies ranging from a low of 20 cycles per second to a high of 20,000 cycles per second.

Any sound loud enough to cause physical pain is capable of damaging a person's hearing; in addition, some diseases or drugs can cause deafness. *Central hearing loss* is caused by damage or impairment of the nerves of the CENTRAL NERVOUS SYSTEM, either in the pathways to the brain or the brain itself. This type of hearing loss may result from congenital brain abnormalities, tumors, or lesions in the central nervous system, STROKES, or some types of medications.

hemangioblastoma   A rare type of tumor of the brain of SPINAL CORD (also known as Lindau's tumor) that consists of blood-vessel cells usually developing in the form of cysts in the CEREBELLUM or the MENINGES. The tumors are usually found in children and young adults.

In von Hippel-Lindau disease, hemangioblastomas (especially in the cerebellum) are associated with renal and pancreatic cysts, tumors in the retina, cancer of the kidney cells, and red birthmarks.

Symptoms   HEADACHE, vomiting, incoordination, and aberrant nystagmus (rapid involuntary eye movements).

Treatment   The tumor is slow growing and is normally clearly differentiated from the surrounding brain tissue; it can usually be removed surgically. In most cases, this surgery completely cures the condition.

hematoma   A collection of clotted blood caused by bleeding from a ruptured blood vessel that may occur anywhere in the body; however, it is most serious when it presses on the brain (such as an extradural hematoma or a subdural hematoma). Hematomas are usually caused by an injury that ruptures a blood vessel under the skull; they may be fatal unless treated promptly.

hemiballismus   The irregular, uncontrollable movements of an arm or a leg on one side of the body caused by disease in the BASAL GANGLIA. The movements are unpredictable, and they may be so severe that they injure the person or other people.

hemispatial neglect   The tendency for a patient with BRAIN DAMAGE (usually to the right side of the brain) to ignore one side of space; the side ignored is almost always the left side.

hemispherectomy   The surgical removal of half of the human brain as a way to treat severe SEIZURES that do not respond to any other treatment. The procedure is most successful when performed in childhood because the growing brain is capable of taking over many of the functions of the missing lobe. Many children who have had the operation show surprisingly intact cognitive function.

Once the CORTEX is removed, the skull fills with CEREBROSPINAL FLUID to take up the empty space.

When the operation was first performed in the 1940s, few patients survived. However, by the mid-1980s advances in BRAIN SCANS and new methods to stop bleeding made the procedure far safer, although it still carries a risk of COMA or death. Today, several dozen hemispherectomies are performed on children in the United States each year, as a treatment for Rasmussen's ENCEPHALITIS and certain forms of EPILEPSY (those that destroy the cortex but don't cross over from one hemisphere to the other).

It is possible to survive such a profound insult to the brain because surgeons are careful not to remove areas that control basic bodily functions, such as the DIENCEPHALON (controlling emotion and body function), the CEREBELLUM (which coordinates movement), or the BRAINSTEM (overseeing breathing, heart rate, etc.).

hemispheres of the brain See CEREBRAL HEMISPHERES.

hemisphericity The tendency for one hemisphere of the brain to be dominant, no matter what the task.

hemorrhage, brain Bleeding within the brain caused by rupture of a blood vessel.

See also EXTRADURAL HEMORRHAGE; INTRACEREBRAL HEMORRHAGE; SUBDURAL HEMORRHAGE.

Hereditary Disease Foundation A professional organization that supports research into the cause, prevention, diagnosis, and treatment of genetic disease, especially HUNTINGTON'S DISEASE. The group believes that methods and strategies developed in Huntington's research will be applicable to other hereditary diseases. The foundation gathers and disseminates information and maintains a tissue bank for research purposes. It also maintains grant programs to support scientific projects in major medical and basic science labs throughout the United States and offers grants and postdoctoral fellowships. In addition, it sponsors a series of interdisciplinary workshops to stimulate new ideas and approaches to understanding hereditary problems. Founded in 1970, the group holds an annual meeting during the second week of January. For address, see Appendix A.

heroin and the brain Researchers in the 1970s discovered that OPIATES like heroin are effective because the brain contains built-in opiate receptors whose selective activation by opiates kills pain. Researchers realized the only reason the brain had such an opiate system must be that the brain was capable of producing its own opiates—which they subsequently discovered and named ENDORPHINS.

Endorphins may be released during powerful emotions, during childbirth, during pleasurable activities, or during exercise.

But when a person adds external opiates to the brain, the body's own production of the endorphins drops. The body requires more and more to achieve the same degree of pleasure, and the withdrawal pains worsen; finally, withdrawal can cause intense physical pain, HALLUCINATIONS, and even death.

See also SUBSTANCE ABUSE.

Herophilus of Chalcedon (335 B.C.–280) The father of anatomy, Herophilus was an Alexandrian physician who performed public dissections of human cadavers.

Herophilus practiced medicine during one of the brief periods in Greek medical history when it was acceptable to dissect humans and spent his time studying the VENTRICLES of the brain. As early as 300 B.C., Herophilus believed that the brain was the central part of the NERVOUS SYSTEM and associated nerves with movement and sensation. He traced the sinuses of the DURA MATTER (the tough membrane covering the brain) to their junction, where he classified the nerve trunks as either motor or sensory.

A proponent of Hippocrates' doctrine of medicine (based on balancing the four humors of the body—blood, phlegm, choler, and melancholy), he also emphasized the importance of medications, diet, and exercise. He wrote at least nine books, including discussions of anatomy and the cause of sudden death, all of which were lost in the destruction of the library of Alexandria in 272 A.D.

See also BRAIN IN HISTORY.

hindbrain One of the three major sections of the brain, also known as the *rhombencephalon*, part of which exits into the SPINAL CORD at the base of the skull. The hindbrain is made up of the metencephalon (including the PONS and CEREBELLUM) and the myelencephalon (the MEDULLA OBLONGATA). The pons and medulla oblongata transmit all signals between the spinal cord and the higher parts of the brain and contain clusters of cranial nerve nuclei that connect the nerves going to and from the face and head; it also governs automatic functions such as heart rate and breathing. Because of the shape and position of the pons and medulla at the brain base, they are referred to as the BRAINSTEM, although this term usually also includes structures in the MID-BRAIN and lower DIENCEPHALON.

hippocampus A structure located beneath the TEMPORAL LOBE that may be the site of learning ability. This ridge, a part of the LIMBIC SYSTEM, is named for its curving shape, which reminded ancient scientists of a seahorse. One of the earliest structures of the brain, the paired structure found on each side of the brain links nerve fibers involved in touch, vision, sound, and smell with the limbic system.

The hippocampus receives NERVE-CELL input from the CORTEX and appears to consolidate information for storage as permanent memory in another brain region (probably also the cortex). It appears to be particularly important in learning and remembering spatial information. The hippocampus is related to memory because of its response to repetitive stimulation; its SYNAPSES change according to previous experience, which may form the structural basis of memory itself. But because research shows that a person with a damaged hippocampus can still retain long-term memory, it is not likely that this part of the brain is the primary storehouse for this type of memory.

A damaged hippocampus interferes with the ability to form new memory, but only the conscious memory or recall of facts and events is lost. The ability to learn both mental and physical skills remains intact, nor is there damage to the memory used in immediate recall (that is, matters to which a person is paying current attention).

In addition, the hippocampus does not play a vital role in storing older memories but is profoundly important in the short-term memory of contextual information (such as the series of clues a person would recall when trying to find a parked car in a crowded lot). It is also important in converting new sensory information into a form that can be preserved elsewhere in the brain.

Other research into the action of the hippocampus has found that people use different areas of their brains to perform different types of memory tasks. Using PET SCAN (POSITRON EMISSION TOMOGRAPHY), researchers monitored changes in blood flow in the volunteers' brains as they provided endings to words flashed before them. Areas of increased blood flow revealed the brain regions used during the various tasks.

When subjects drew upon memories of previous lists to complete the fragment "mot-," the right hippocampus showed an increased blood supply. This means that subjects were using this part of the brain to remember the word, even though researchers had always attributed such verbal processing to the left brain. If the subjects did not search their brains for a word they had already seen and instead gave the first word that came to them, blood flow did *not* increase to either side of the hippocampus.

Sometimes, subjects spontaneously recalled words from the lists even if they didn't remember having seen the words before. Psychologists call this phenomenon *priming*, and it prompted increased blood flow to the visual cortex.

Still other studies found that monkeys that learned to recognize objects 16, 12, 8, 4, and 2 weeks before surgery damaged their hippocampus forgot what they had learned 2 to 4 weeks before the damage, but they recalled early learning better. Normal monkeys remembered more recent learning better than older memories.

Both the NEUROTRANSMITTER GLUTAMATE and the inhibitor neurotransmitter GABA (GAMMA AMINOBUTYRIC ACID) are important in the proper function of the hippocampus; an imbalance in either of these transmitters will cause epileptic seizures, memory disorders, or both. (Patients with EPILEPSY usually demonstrate memory problems as well.)

The most common cause of damage to the hippocampus is ANOXIA (loss of oxygen) to the brain during a difficult birth and delivery; most patients with idiopathic epilepsy suffered from anoxia at birth which damaged the hippocampus. One reason why memories may be so vulnerable to the loss of oxygen is that hippocampus cells are the quickest to die when oxygen to the brain is cut off.

Hippocrates (460 B.C.–377) The fourth-century B.C. Greek physician popularly known as the *father of medicine*. In his writings, Hippocrates noted that madness is the result of too much "moistness" in the brain. This belief was based on the then-popular belief that human health was based on the four "humors" (earth, fire, air, and water).

Interestingly, the idea of an excess moistness appears to be curiously accurate in the case of schizophrenic patients; recent research suggests that SCHIZOPHRENIA patients have larger fluid-bearing VENTRICLES than normal patients.

hologramic brain The theory that any part of the brain contains the entire mind, just as any part of a hologram holds the entire image.

hormones Chemicals made of protein produced and released by a gland, they circulate through the bloodstream until they reach target cells, which they stimulate into activity. Hormones control the rate and the way that various reactions in the body happen. The PITUITARY secretes nine hormones into the blood which control targeted tissues.

hot tubs Women who use hot tubs or saunas during early pregnancy nearly tripled their chances of giving birth to babies with SPINA BIFIDA or BRAIN DEFECTS, according to research. One study, which surveyed 22,762 women, was designed to explore other issues relating to childbirth and did not include detailed questions about hot tubs and saunas. Nevertheless, the findings showed that women who used a hot tub during the first two months of pregnancy were 2.8 times more likely to bear a child with birth defects than were women with no exposure to heat. The study found no such effect for electric blankets. (Saunas and hot tubs already carried warnings against using during pregnancy.)

These findings support what has already been known about the detrimental effects of heat on animal pregnancy.

hunger An uncomfortable feeling caused by the need for food (unlike APPETITE, which is a pleasant sensation felt when expecting a meal).

Hunger occurs when the stomach is empty and blood GLUCOSE (the primary sugar that the body uses for food) is low. Special sugar receptors in the HYPOTHALAMUS monitor the blood levels of glucose; when these levels drop, sugar receptors stimulate eating by causing the stomach to contract. When pronounced, these contractions produce hunger pains.

In the past, NEUROLOGISTS thought feelings of hunger and fullness were controlled by just two areas in the hypothalamus called the *feeding center* and the *satiety center,* but today we know that a person's hunger is affected by many different brain regions; at least 25 NEUROPEPTIDES all over the brain affect food intake.

Recently, researchers at Rockefeller University in New York City discovered that two chemicals in the brain are responsible for causing some types of food cravings: neuropeptide Y causes carbohydrate cravings in rats, and galanin seems to underlie a desire for fatty foods. The more of these chemicals the body produces, the stronger the drive to eat those particular foods. Hormones and the amount of glucose used by cells moderate the amount of neuropeptide Y production. Scientists hope that once the neurochemical signals for hunger are better understood, doctors may be able to deal with appetites for fats and sugars.

Huntington's disease An inherited disorder that causes abnormal involuntary movements (CHOREA) and progressive mental impairment, including memory loss. It is caused by the degeneration of the CAUDATE NUCLEUS in the BASAL GANGLIA (paired NERVE-CELL cluters in the brain) and of the frontal association NEOCORTEX.

The genetic marker for Huntington's disease has been identified on chromosome 4, and researchers are working on locating the gene itself.

The origins of this brain atrophy are unknown, but some scientists believe the damage may be caused by a buildup of natural chemicals that flood the bundles of NEURONS within the FOREBRAIN, killing them and causing the progressive memory loss, angry rages, and muscle spasms that mark the disease.

The two main chemicals believed responsible for the nerve-cell degeneration are quinolinic acid and GLUTAMATE. These two play essential roles in normal concentrations (quinolinic acid is a breakdown product of TRYPTOPHAN and glutamate is a NEUROTRANSMITTER and metabolic agent). But too much of either chemical kills certain cells, and both bind to the receptor site for a chemical called NMDA. Researchers have found that the brains of Huntington's disease patients had 93 percent fewer NMDA RECEPTORS, indicating that the cells with those receptors had died. In two other studies, researchers found decreased number of receptors for five other chemicals in the brains of Huntington's patients.

Symptoms Symptoms usually appear between the ages of 35 and 50, although in rare cases they appear during childhood. This is a genetic disorder with an autosomal pattern of inheritance; each child of an affected parent has a 50 percent chance of developing the condition. Huntington's is found in about five out of every 100,000 Americans.

The jerky movements usually affect the face, arms, and trunk, causing random grimaces, twitches, and general clumsiness. These changes usually occur first, followed in several years by dementia beginning with personality and behavior changes, irritability, problems making decisions, memory loss, and apathy. Language tends to remain normal for a much longer period than it does in other cortical dementias. Psychotic disorders may also become apparent, including both manic-depressive psychosis and schizophreniclike HALLUCINATIONS.

Diagnosis/treatment Today, offspring of affected parents can take a test to discover, with 95 percent accuracy, whether they have inherited the abnormal gene responsible for the condition.

There is no known cure for Huntington's disease, but drugs like CHLORPROMAZINE can lessen the jerky movements. Most people with Huntington's disease live for about 15 years after the onset of symptoms, although some have lived as long as 30 years.

Researchers suggest that some cells may be more vulnerable to damage from glutamate and quinolinic acid because they contain more NMDA receptors. It is hoped that finding a way to block those receptors might slow the disease; however, selective NMDA-block has not been effective. Although there is no treatment available to stop the progression of the disease, the movement disorders and psychiatric symptoms can be controlled by drugs.

Huntington's Disease Society of America A national support group for individuals and volunteers concerned with HUNTINGTON'S DISEASE (HD), an inherited and terminal neurological condition causing progressive brain and nerve deterioration. The society provides information on the disease, offers referrals to physicians and support groups, and answers questions on presymptomatic testing. The society hopes to identify HD families, promote and support basic and clinical research into the cause and cure of HD, maintain patient-services programs, and coordinate with various community services to help families meet social, economic, and emotional problems. The society is working to change the attitude of the working community toward the HD patient, to enhance the HD patient's lifestyle, and to promote better health care and treatment, both in the community and in facilities.

The society has launched a nationwide campaign in support of federal and state legislation establishing clinics, genetic counseling and screening centers, and diagnostic and treatment centers for HD patients and those suffering from other chronic debilitating diseases. The group actively cooperates with researchers in ongoing studies, cosponsors and supports workshops and symposia, provides grants to researchers, and sponsors brain donor programs.

Crisis intervention and other support services are available, and the group also maintains a lending library of audiovisual materials and general and scientific displays. Founded in 1986, the group has 37,000 members and publishes a variety of books and pamphlets. For address, see Appendix A.

See also HEREDITARY DISEASE FOUNDATION.

Hydergine This extract of ergot, a fungus that grows on rye, is a widely used treatment for all forms of SENILITY in the United States. Proponents believe that hydergine may improve learning, memory, recall, and intelligence; inhibit FREE RADICALS; enhance BRAIN-CELL metabolism; and increase blood supply and oxygen to the brain. Some scientists believe that the drug may mimic the effect of NERVE-GROWTH FACTOR, a substance that stimulates DENDRITE growth in the brain.

Hydergine was the first drug that showed promise in use against ALZHEIMER'S DISEASE; by 1979, at least 20 double-blind studies had produced statistically significant improvements in behavior and psychological tests of demented patients.

hydrocephalus Also known as "water on the brain," this is an excess of CEREBROSPINAL FLUID within the skull (usually under increased pressure). This condition is often associated with other abnormalities present at birth, especially SPINA BIFIDA.

The condition is diagnosed with CAT SCANS or MRI, which show the location and nature of an obstruction.

Untreated, the condition will progress to extreme drowsiness, severe BRAIN DAMAGE, and SEIZURES, which may be fatal within a few weeks.

See also NATIONAL HYDROCEPHALUS FOUNDATION; GUARDIANS OF HYDROCEPHALUS RESEARCH FOUNDATION.

Causes Hydrocephalus is caused by the excessive formation of cerebrospinal fluid, by a circulation block of this fluid, or both. It may be present at birth, or it may develop following severe HEAD INJURY, brain hemorrhage, infection (such as MENINGITIS) or a brain tumor (see TUMORS, BRAIN).

Symptoms If present at birth, the symptom is an enlarged head that continues to grow at an excessively fast rate because the skull bones are not rigid and expand to accommodate the fluid. Other features include leg rigidity, EPILEPSY, irritability, lethargy, vomiting, and absence of REFLEXES.

If the condition occurs in late childhood or in adulthood, the skull cannot swell, and the symptoms will be caused by a rising pressure within the skull; this is characterized by HEADACHE, vomiting, loss of coordination, and deteriorating mental function.

Treatment Usually, excess fluid will be drained away by a shunt from the brain to another part of the body (such as the lining of the abdomen), where it will be absorbed. The shunt (or tube) is inserted into the brain through a hole in the skull; sometimes, the shunt will be left in place indefinitely.

In older children and adults, treatment may be for underlying cause only.

hyperactivity A behavior pattern in which a person is constantly moving around and making rapid, often disorganized, motions. A general term, *hyperactivity* is used loosely to refer to a wide range of behaviors and is considered to be part of a wider complex of behaviors called ATTENTION DEFICIT HYPERACTIVITY DISORDER (ADHD).

Hyperactivity may affect as many as 5 to 10 percent of children in the United States and is four to five times more common in boys.

It is important to realize that some symptoms of hyperactivity are present at some time in almost all children and that overactivity in itself does not indicate hyperactivity. But when other causes are ruled out and the intense behavior continues past age four—and appears significantly different from other children's behavior—it may be reasonable to think of the child as hyperactive.

In many cases, hyperactivity fades away in adolescence, while others experience a transmutation of symptoms into sluggishness, depression, and moodiness. Occasionally, all symptoms of hyperactivity continue into adulthood.

Cause Some research suggests that hyperactive children may have a subtle form of brain damage. Scientists also know that there appears to be a genetic component to the problem and that hyperactive children appear to be more likely to have hyperactive fathers. Children who have MENTAL RETARDATION, CEREBRAL PALSY, or TEMPORAL-LOBE EPILEPSY are also more likely to be hyperactive.

Because stimulant drugs appear to ease the symptoms of hyperactivity, this suggests that the condition may be caused by an underaroused MIDBRAIN, which is unable to control movements or activity. Stimulant drugs appear to work by inducing this area of the brain to suppress extra activity.

Scientists have found that adults suffering from hyperactivity since childhood display markedly reduced metabolism in brain regions regulating motor activity and attention. It is suspected that stimulants increase metabolism in this area.

Symptoms Continual overactivity which often worsens in group situations; it may not appear during a physical exam in the doctor's office. There appears to be a lessened need to sleep, with impulsive and reckless behavior. Hyperactive children are often irritable, emotionally immature, and aggressive; they have a shortened attention span and do not conform to orderly routines.

Hyperactivity may lead to antisocial behavior and learning problems, although IQ is usually normal. It is unclear whether the behavior is part of the disorder or is simply a result of the child's poor attention span.

Treatment Stimulant drugs such as amphetamine or Ritalin appear to be effective. Behavior therapy and counseling of child and parents also may be helpful.

More controversial are special diets that exclude certain additives, artificial colorings, preservatives, etc.

hyperbilirubinemia See KERNICTERUS.

hyperkinetic syndrome (hyperkinesis) Another term for HYPERACTIVITY, now generally called ATTENTION DEFICIT HYPERACTIVITY DISORDER (ADHD).

hyperzine A A chemical found in a type of tea brewed with club moss (*Huperzia serrata*) brewed by Chinese folk doctors, now being investigated as a possible treatment for ALZHEIMER'S DISEASE. A natural compound in the tea inhibits acetylcholinesterase, the enzyme that breaks down ACETYLCHOLINE, a key chemical messenger in the brain involved in awareness and memory. Like the drug TA-CRINE (approved for the treatment of Alzheimer's disease), when also used, hyperzine A prevents acetylcholinesterase from breaking down acetylcholine, thus raising levels of acetylcholine in the brain. The chemical has not yet been approved for use.

hypnosis A trancelike psychological state of altered awareness characterized by extreme suggestibility and certain physiological attributes. Hypnosis was once believed to be a form of sleep, but an EEG tracing during hypnosis does not show normal BRAIN-WAVE patterns typical of sleep. A hypnotized person functions at a level of awareness other than the ordinary conscious state, characterized by receptiveness and responsiveness in which inner experiences are given as much significance as external reality. While hypnotized, a person can think, act, and behave as well or better than during ordinary awareness, probably because of heightened attention. It is not possible to hypnotize someone who does not want to be hypnotized.

hypoglossal nerve The twelfth cranial nerve, this "undertongue" nerve transmits motor signals from the brain to the tongue; poking out the tongue and using the tongue to talk both involve this nerve.

See also CRANIAL NERVES.

hypoglycemia A deficiency of glucose in the blood, causing weakness, confusion, and sweating. Because BRAIN CELLS require an adequate amount of sugar to maintain metabolic activity, a drop in the blood-sugar level can lead to brain-function problems. Insulin (a hormone secreted by the pancreas) helps maintain normal levels of blood sugar; too little insulin and the level will rise; too much and the level will fall. Diabetics are at particular risk for brain problems resulting from low blood sugar; excess amounts of insulin can cause blood sugar to plummet, triggering a seizure.

Even a slight decrease in blood sugar, however, can alter brain function and trigger memory problems in almost anyone. It's not just diabetics who can get too much insulin—stress or nerves can activate the production of this hormone, as can eating too much sugar. One way to avoid this is to eat another food (such as peanut butter) during high-sugar meals; this helps slow the stomach's emptying and helps the body absorb sugar.

See also GLUCOSE.

hypothalamus The cherry-sized part of the brain involved in pleasure, body temperature, and sleep is situated behind the eyes and beneath the THALAMUS. The hypothalamus controls the SYMPATHETIC NERVOUS SYSTEM (part of the AUTONOMIC NERVOUS SYSTEM, which controls body organs) and is responsible for the FIGHT-OR-FLIGHT mechanism.

Other groups of nerve cells within the hypothalamus control body temperature; some are sensitive to heat and some to cold so that when the blood flowing to the brain fluctuates in temperature, the hypothalamus induces temperature-regulating mechanisms such as shivering or sweating.

The hypothalamus receives information from sense organs about the GLUCOSE level in the blood and the body's water levels, stimulating the urge to eat or drink. The hypothalamus also regulates sleep, sexual behavior, and mood and emotions.

The hypothalamus also coordinates nervous control of the endocrine systems, connecting neuronally to the PITUITARY GLAND via the hypophyseal tract, thereby controlling hormonal secretions from the gland. In this way, the hypothalamus can convert nerve signals into hormonal signals.

Because of its many responsibilities, damage to this part of the brain can have wide-ranging consequences. Impaired hypothalamic function can result in hormonal disorders, malfunctioning temperature regulation, and increased or decreased appetite for sleep, food, and sex. Disorders involving the hypothalamus are usually linked to a brain hemorrhage or a pituitary tumor. In addition, LAURENCE-MOON-BIEDL SYNDROME is believed to be associated with a malfunctioning hypothalamus.

hypothyroidism Severe hypothyroidism (underactivity of the thyroid gland) can cause depression and DEMENTIA because of a drop in metabolic activity in the brain; borderline hypothyroidism can cause memory disturbance, poor concentration, and mental confusion. Patients with a severe lack of thyroid hormone may appear to be drugged, exhausted, and weak, exhibiting a slow heart rate, dry flaky skin, hair loss, a husky voice, thickened skin, weight gain, and goiter. The severity of the symptoms depends on the degree of thyroid deficiency.

Hypothyroidism can be detected by taking the temperature immediately upon awakening while still in bed; temperature below 97.8° F. may indicate hypothyroidism. It can also be diagnosed by measuring the level of thyroid hormones in the blood.

Treatment includes replacement therapy with the thyroid hormone thyroxine for life. Once replacement therapy has begun, most or all of the symptoms with this disorder can be reversed.

hypoxia Lack of oxygen to the cells of the brain, which may be caused by the interference or block of blood or the oxygen it carries. Hypoxia may occur during drowning, childbirth, or choking. Hypoxia during birth is one of the primary causes of CEREBRAL PALSY and may be related to LEARNING DISABILITIES.

I

idebenone A molecule found in the heart, idebenone plays an important role in the production of ADENOSINE TRIPHOSPHATE (ATP).

imaging techniques There are a wide range of techniques that have been developed to allow physicians to look at the living brain, including the oldest (X-RAYS) to computer-augmented techniques such as CAT SCANS, MAGNETIC RESONANCE IMAGING (MRI), ULTRASOUND SCANNING, PET SCANS, etc.

While X rays are still be used to view the skull following trauma, this method is less effective in visualizing the soft tissues of the brain. Instead, CAT and MRI scans are particularly valuable in diagnosing disorders of the brain, whereas PET scans have been extremely helpful in visualizing brain activity.

immune system A collection of cells and proteins that protect the body from harm from bacteria, viruses, and fungi. The AUTONOMIC NERVOUS SYSTEM has primary responsibility for controlling the body's immune system, which fights infections by producing antibodies or immunoglobulins (protective proteins).

More and more researchers are coming to believe that there may be a link between people's vulnerability to infectious disease and their state of mind. The term *psychoneuroimmunology*—from *psycho* (the mind), *neuro* (nerve cells or the nervous system), and *immuno* (the immune system)—is the study of how one's beliefs and emotions influence one's brain chemistry and state of health. Coined by Dr. Robert Ader of the University of Rochester in 1975, psychoneuroimmunology is a controversial discipline that may hold promise if researchers can discover how the mind, the brain, and the immune system communicate.

A range of studies have linked depression, separation and loss, and stress with poorer health. It could be, some researchers suggest, that prolonged stress impairs the function of the immune system, and when the immune system is depressed, infection can take hold.

Both the brain and the immune system communicate through chemical signals. Moreover, studies have found that the HYPOTHALAMUS not only transmits emotional signals but also regulates the immune system.

Research by NEUROPSYCHOLOGIST Candace Pert at the National Institute of Mental Health has shown that infection-fighting white cells, like BRAIN CELLS, can both send or receive a wide variety of messages and can make and release hormones. Moreover, her work has also shown that the thymus and the spleen—two of the main structures used by the immune system—are connected by an especially intricate network of nerve cells to and from the brain.

indomethacin An anti-inflammatory drug used to treat arthritis that may be helpful in treating ALZHEIMER'S DISEASE.

infection Bacteria, fungi, or viruses can attack the brain or other parts of the CENTRAL NERVOUS SYSTEM and can cause considerable damage, although the body's immune system can usually successfully fight off these challenges. These infections may include ENCEPHALITIS, RABIES, MENINGITIS, POLIOENCEPHALITIS, and POLIOMYELITIS.

An infectious agent may pervade the entire nervous system, and others may attack selective regions of the brain. Organisms may also directly infect the brain following head trauma or from an infected ear or sinus. The blood may carry other infections to the brain or by following the nerves.

Infections may also physically affect the brain, causing pus, inflamed blood vessels, excess fluid, and inflammation.

Symptoms Infections in the head tend to produce inflammation, nausea, photophobia, fatigue, confusion, vomiting, fever, convulsions, and partial paralysis. Infections in the meninges may produce a stiff neck. Rabies may produce fear of water and maniacal behavior.

Treatment Depends on the infectious cause of the disease. Antibiotics may cure bacterial meningitis, but there is no cure for the encephalitis virus or rabies.

inflammation of the brain See ENCEPHALITIS; INFECTION; MENINGITIS.

infradian rhythm Rhythms that occur over a period of time longer than a day, from the Latin *infra* ("below"), because their length is "below" a day. The monthly cycle of ovulation and menstruation is a good example of infradian rhythms in humans. These longer-than-normal rhythms are more difficult to study than daily (circadian) rhythms. Many animals exhibit seasonal swings in hormone levels by certain behavioral events, but in humans there is less outward appearance of small changes in hormonal levels.

The mechanism that controls the infradian reproductive cycle in humans isn't well understood, although there seems to be a relationship between circadian rhythms of body temperature and the infradian reproductive cycle. (An increase in body temperature at awakening of 0.4°F. or more above the average temperature of the five preceding days indicates that ovulation is taking place.)

intelligence The ability to understand ideas and their relationships and to reason about them. An extremely complex function of the brain, intelligence consists of the capacity for general knowledge, memory, learning, attention, comprehension, judgment, abstract thinking, language, orientation, perception, and association.

Scientists have tried to quantify intelligence and developmental level by a number of tests with many different psychological methods. The most common include the WECHSLER ADULT INTELLIGENCE SCALE REVISED (WAIS-R), the WECHSLER INTELLIGENCE SCALE FOR CHILDREN REVISED (WISC-R), the STANFORD-BINET (fourth edition), the DENVER II and the EARLY LANGUAGE MILESTONE SCALE (ELM), and the CENTRAL LINGUISTIC AUDITORY MILESTONES SCALE (CLAMS).

Interestingly, while more and more scientists disagree about the notion of general intelligence, scientists at the University of California at Irvine have shown that intelligent brains appear to solve problems by conserving rather than expending energy. In the studies, PET SCANS chart the rate at which the brain burns GLUCOSE; as subjects puzzle out mental tests, the scans track the level of cerebral activity. Studies with volunteers scoring high on IQ tests show reduced energy use in areas of the brain uniquely activated by tests; other tests with these subjects record sharp drops in overall brain activity after one or two months of daily practice in a video game.

However, glucose efficiency appears to provide only a partial picture of the intelligent brain. Highly intelligent subjects showed a jump in brain activity when moving from an easy version of a task to a difficult version. On the other hand, moving from the difficult version to an easier memory task resulted in a drop in brain activity.

International Academy for Child Brain Development A group of professionals from a variety of disciplines including physicians, psychologists, and anthropologists who are interested in the physical and psychological processes involved in child brain development. The group seeks to gain recognition of the study of child brain development and a discipline in itself and establish criteria for the certification of child brain developmentalists. It conducts research, offers courses in child brain development and bestows awards.

Founded in 1985, the group sponsors an annual convention in Philadelphia during the last week of November and publishes a periodic *Journal for Child Brain Development*. For address, see Appendix B.

International Association of the Study of Pain   A professional association for healthcare professionals interested in pain research and therapy. The group encourages research on pain mechanisms and syndromes, seeks to improve the well-being of patients with acute and chronic pain, and promotes education and training in the field. The organization also informs the public and develops an international databank, adoption of a uniform classification and, definition regarding pain and pain syndromes and creates a uniform records system on information relating to pain mechanisms. Founded in 1974, the group has 6,000 members and publishes a bimonthly newsletter, a monthly journal, and various other publications. For address, see Appendix B.

See also AMERICAN PAIN SOCIETY.

International Federation of Clinical Neurophysiology   A national ELECTROENCE-PHALOGRAPHY/neurophysiology society whose purpose is to ensure the highest standards of EEG are reached in all countries, encourages research, and promotes effective international collaboration.

Founded in 1949, the group has 46 members and sponsors a quadrennial world congress and periodic conferences in specialized areas. It publishes the monthly journal *Electroencephalography and Clinical Neurophysiology*; the bimonthly journal *EMG and Motor Control*; the bimonthly journal *Evoked Potentials*; and the *Handbook of EEG and Clinical Neurophysiology*. For address, see Appendix B.

International Joseph Disease Foundation   A national support group for geneticists, neurologists, and patients and their families that offers diagnostic services and treatment at free clinics for those with JOSEPH DISEASE, a neurological genetic disorder of the motor system. The foundation provides genetic counseling to those concerned with inheriting the disorder or passing it on to future generations and locates families throughout the world affected by the disease. The foundation also educates the medical profession and the public on Joseph disease in an effort to promote more accurate diagnoses and better treatment. For address, see Appendix A.

International League Against Epilepsy   A group of national organizations united to encourage scientific research on EPILEPSY and to promote optimal treatment and rehabilitation of patients. The league fosters the development of and cooperation among associations with common interests. Founded in 1909, the group has 46 members and publishes a bimonthly journal.

International Neural Network Society   A professional group for those interested in theoretical and computational understanding of the brain. The group promotes research into behavioral processes and models of the brain and encourages development of computing applications that use neural modeling concepts.

Founded in 1978, the group has 4,000 members and sponsors an annual world congress. The society publishes the quarterly newsletter *Above Threshold*; the bimonthly *Neural Networks*; and *The Directory of Government Funding*. For address, see Appendix B.

International Rett Syndrome Association   A support group for parents of children with RETT SYNDROME, professionals, and others interested in RETT Syndrome, a disorder affecting females who seem normal until between 7 to 18 months of age when autisticlike withdrawal sets in. Although this symptom eases in time, higher brain functions continue to deteriorate, leading to severe retardation.

The association provides support to parents, encourages research, collects and disseminates information, helps identify Rett syndrome patients, and conducts activities aimed at the prevention, treatment, and eventual eradication of the condition.

Founded in 1985, the association has 1,500 members and publishes a quarterly newsletter and various informational brochures. For address, see Appendix A.

International Tremor Foundation A national support group for those suffering from tremors, their families and friends, and health-care workers. TREMOR is a common symptom of neurologic disease and may be caused by trauma, tumor, STROKE, or degenerative disease.

The foundation promotes research and development of clinical care programs and provides patient information and referrals. The group publishes a quarterly newsletter and sponsors educational meetings. For address, see Appendix A.

interneuron Small intercommunicating neurons that connect major pathways. Neither purely sensory nor purely motor, interneurons are local nerve cells whose processes are confined within a small, restricted area. The largest number of interneurons are found in the CEREBRAL CORTEX. When a baby is born, the interneurons are not connected; as a result of experience, learning, and repetition, the interneurons weave synaptic links with countless programmed pathways in other parts of the brain.

intracerebral hemorrhage Bleeding *within the brain* from a ruptured blood vessel, one of the three main incidents that can cause a

STROKE. Each year, this type of hemorrhage strikes one out of every 2,500 Americans—usually older people with untreated high blood pressure or ATHEROSCLEROSIS (fatty deposits causing narrowed arteries).

Unlike most SUBDURAL and EXTRADURAL HEMORRHAGES in which bleeding occurs between the surface of the brain and the skull, an intracerebral hemorrhage can occur spontaneously, without any injury to the head. The blood seeps outward from the rupture, forming a round or oval mass that may grow to a few inches in diameter, disrupting brain tissue as the blood volume increases. Usually the rupture is found in the CEREBRUM (main mass of the brain), although it may occur in other brain structures, such as the BRAINSTEM or CEREBELLUM.

Only about 25 percent of patients survive, especially if the hemorrhage is large. However, if the patient survives, recurrent bleeding from the same site does not usually occur.

Symptoms Sudden HEADACHE, weakness, confusion, loss of consciousness. Over a period of minutes or hours, other symptoms resulting from disturbed brain tissue include speech problems, paralysis, or one-sided weakness.

Treatment Surgery is not usually possible because of the difficulty of reaching the rupture. Treatment usually involves life support and attempts to reduce blood pressure.

intracranial pressure (ICP) A measure of pressure depending on the amount of brain tissue, intracranial blood volume, and CEREBROSPINAL FLUID within the skull. Normally, a person's ICP fluctuates depending on the position of the body and the head, but it is usually considered to be less than or equal to 15 mm/Hg.

The volume and pressure of the brain tissue, blood, and cerebrospinal fluid is usually considered to be in a state of equilibrium. Because the skull does not allow much room for expansion, an increase in any of these three will alter the volume of the other two. Normally, the brain undergoes constant minor changes in blood volume and cerebrospinal fluid during changes in posture, blood pressure, internal pressure due to coughing, sneezing, or straining or fluctuations in arterial blood-gas levels.

Moreover, a range of brain problems (including STROKE, HEAD INJURY, inflammation, BRAIN TUMOR, or intracranial surgery) change the relationship between the volume and pressure within the skull. An increase in ICP may reduce cerebral blood flow, which is usually accompanied by a slow, bounding pulse and breathing problems. Such changes in blood pressure, pulse, and breathing give important clues to the existence of an increased ICP. Eventually, a consistently high ICP can cut off blood flow. Exquisitely sensitive to lack of blood flow, the BRAIN CELLS will die if the flow is cut off for more than three to five minutes.

Elevated ICP is most often associated with head injury, but it can also occur as a side effect of a range of other conditions, including brain tumors, SUBARACHNOID HEMORRHAGE, and toxic and viral brain inflammations.

In the initial phase of increased pressure, the brain and its components can adjust their volume to allow for the expanding volume, but after a certain point the brain simply can't continue to compensate for the high pressure. At this point, the patient may show changes in consciousness, with slowed heartbeat and breathing changes. The earliest sign of increasing ICP is lethargy, with slowed speech and a lag in responding to verbal directions. The patient may become more and more sleepy or exhibit sudden changes in condition (such as shifting from quiet to restlessness). As the pressure continues to increase, the patient may begin to react only to very loud or exaggerated stimuli, indicating a probably serious problem in brain

circulation and the onset of COMA. As the condition worsens, the patient's arms and legs become flaccid and reflexes disappear.

Profound coma with pupils fixed and dilated and impaired breathing usually leads to death.

Treatment Immediate action is necessary to reduce the size of the brain by reducing swelling, decreasing the volume of cerebrospinal fluid, or lowering blood volume. This can be done by administering corticosteroids and osmotic diuretics, reducing the restricting fluids, draining cerebrospinal fluid, controlling fever, and reducing metabolic demands.

Iowa Test of Basic Skills A set of group-administered, paper-and-pencil tests that measures basic academic skills in grades K through 9. The tests cover vocabulary, reading, language, spelling, capitalization, punctuation, usage, work and study skills, visual materials, reference materials, concepts in mathematics, problem solving and computation, listening, word analysis, science, and social studies. For older students (grades 9 to 12), the Iowa Tests of Educational Development may be used, which focus on more sophisticated material and skills. Any of these tests may be scored either by hand or by computer. The "Iowas" are used to identify strengths and weaknesses in basic skills, to evaluate classroom instruction, and to monitor a student's progress from year to year.

IQ tests A group of tests of varying reliability that purport to assess an individual's general intelligence and developmental level. It is difficult to reproduce results using any of the IQ tests (especially among young people), and all fail to correct for the known effects of cultural and educational background, interest, motivation, and effort. In addition, some mental disorders (especially SCHIZOPHRENIA and DEPRESSION) may appear to lower IQ scores. Whether this occurs because these disorders actually lower intelligence or because the disorders impair motivation is not known.

Still, IQ tests are the only way of estimating intelligence, and they can be useful, providing their limitations are taken into consideration. The most common tests include the WECHSLER ADULT INTELLIGENCE SCALE REVISED (WAIS-R), the WECHSLER INTELLIGENCE SCALE FOR CHILDREN REVISED (WISC-R), the STANFORD-BINET (fourth edition), the DENVER II and the EARLY LANGUAGE MILESTONE SCALE (ELM) and the CENTRAL LINGUISTIC AUDITORY MILESTONES SCALE (CLAMS).

J

jet lag Interruption of the body's sleep-wake cycles causing fatigue and mental confusion as a result of flying across different time zones. The human body is regulated by a biological clock that sets the pace for everyday rhythms of sleep, activity, temperature, cortisol, and melatonin release on a 24-hour cycle (called the CIRCADIAN RHYTHM). When an air traveler flies across several time zones, the person's day—as timed by an external clock—is longer or shorter than 24 hours, depending on the direction of the flight.

Most of the traveler's circadian rhythms are not able to adjust, causing jet lag when the flight is over. People with jet lag have the urge to sleep during the day, feel awake at night, are generally tired, and have problems with physical and mental activity. Memory may also be affected.

Jet lag tends to be worse when flying eastward, which shortens the traveler's day; it is also more likely to affect people over age 30 who normally follow a specific daily routine.

Prevention/treatment The capacity for the human hormone MELATONIN to modulate the circadian rhythm has led to its use in the treatment of sleep disorders associated with jet lag. In one study of 17 subjects during a period of two weeks following a flight from London to San Francisco, melatonin significantly reduced the negative feelings of jet lag and significantly increased alertness. Those who received melatonin also reported they fell asleep much more easily and slept better than they otherwise would have expected. Melatonin is available without prescription in most health-food stores.

It's also possible to somewhat modify the symptoms of jet lag by staying away from heavy meals and drinking plenty of nonalcoholic fluids during the flight. In addition, people who expect to be flying east should try to go to bed earlier than usual for a few days before the flight; people flying west should do the opposite. If possible, travelers should try to arrive in the new time zone in the early evening and go to bed early.

Your body may take a few days to readjust after traveling to a new time zone—about a half-day to a day for each time zone crossed. This adjustment can be eased by taking a stopover on a long journey and by resting after the flight.

Jewish Association for Retarded Citizens (JARC) A Jewish association providing residential care and support services to developmentally disabled adults; the group operates 16 group homes that provide access to Jewish services, maintains kosher kitchens, and observes Jewish holidays. Although the group primarily services individuals in the Detroit area, JARC has a national membership. The group is affiliated with the ASSOCIATION FOR RETARDED CITIZENS. Founded in 1969, the group publishes brochures and a bimonthly newsletter.

See also CENTER FOR FAMILY SUPPORT; FEDERATION FOR CHILDREN WITH SPECIAL NEEDS; MENTAL RETARDATION ASSOCIATION OF AMERICA; NATIONAL ASSOCIATION OF DEVELOPMENTAL DISABILITIES COUNCILS; NATIONAL DOWN SYNDROME CONGRESS; NATIONAL DOWN SYNDROME SOCIETY; PARENTS OF CHILDREN WITH DOWN SYNDROME; PILOT PARENTS; VOICE OF THE RETARDED; YOUNG ADULT INSTITUTE AND WORKSHOP.

Jordan Left-Right Reversal Test A paper-and-pencil test for children aged 5 to 12 to measure the frequency of transpositions (reversals of letters, numbers, or upside down) among groups of numbers and letters and to identify words with similar errors. Children with perceptual errors often miss the real transpositions while identifying others. The test may be given to individuals or groups and is scored by hand. Scores are sometimes used as a kind of developmental screening test or diagnostic assessment for children believed to have learning disabilities.

Joseph Disease A neurological genetic disorder of the motor system which affects all races and many ethnic groups and which is often misdiagnosed as MULTIPLE SCLEROSIS, PARKINSON'S DISEASE, or spino-cerebellar degeneration. For address of INTERNATIONAL JOSEPH DISEASE FOUNDATION, see Appendix A.

See also INTERNATIONAL JOSEPH DISEASE FOUNDATION.

jugular vein One of three veins on each side of the neck that carry deoxygenated blood from the head to the heart. The largest of the three is the internal jugular, which arises at the base of the skull, travels down the neck alongside the CAROTID ARTERIES and passes behind the collarbone, where it joins the subclavian vein—the large vein draining blood from the arms. Because the jugular lies deep in the structures of the neck, it is rarely injured.

K

kernicterus A rare disorder caused by the buildup of bilirubin (bile pigments) from destruction of the blood cells as part of hemolytic disease in the newborn. The bilirubin buildup damages the BASAL GANGLIA deep within the brain, leading to kernicterus. Untreated kernicterus causes BRAIN DAMAGE and MENTAL RETARDATION in newborns (especially premature infants).

Without treatment, the infant will probably die by the end of the first week of life; those who survive may be deaf and may suffer from uncontrollable writhing movements and spasticity (muscle stiffness). This may be followed by mental retardation, bizarre eye movements, speech problems, and SEIZURES.

Symptoms Jaundice in the first few days of life, together with listlessness and arched back and neck.

Treatment Prompt treatment of jaundice (by resting under special lights or temporary weaning from mother's milk) will completely prevent kernicterus. There is no cure for the brain damage that arises from untreated kernicterus.

ketoconazole (Brand name: Nizoral) An antifungal drug used to treat severe fungal infections of the brain (as well as other organs). To avoid nausea, this drug should be taken with food. Other possible adverse effects include rash and (rarely) liver damage. Taking this drug with alcohol increases the chance of liver damage; taking with tobacco products decreases the drug's effect. The drug may also trigger an increased sensitivity to light.

Kohs Block Design Test A type of intelligence test for children or adults with a mental age of 3 to 19 years, especially handicapped people with defects of language or hearing, disadvantaged children, or those who are not native English speakers. In the test, the person is given a variety of colored blocks with which to copy designs shown on a series of cards. The person is tested not only on success in copying the design, but also in attention, adaptive behavior, and self-criticism. This test may be included in other tests, such as the Merrill-Palmer Scales of Mental Development.

Korsakoff, Sergey Sergeyevich (1854–1900) A Russian psychiatrist who may have been the first to recognize that amnesia does not necessarily have to be associated with dementia. Korsakoff noted a severe but specific amnesia for recent and current events among alcoholics with no problems in intelligence or judgment. This observation, now called the KORSAKOFF'S SYNDROME, is found in a number of brain disorders in addition to problems resulting from alcoholism and appears to be caused by damage in a relatively localized part of the brain.

See also KORSAKOFF'S SYNDROME; WERNICKE-KORSAKOFF SYNDROME.

Korsakoff's syndrome Also known as *Korsakoff's psychosis*, this condition is believed to be caused by the interaction of chronic alcohol abuse and a thiamine deficiency brought on by poor diet typical of chronic alcoholics. Korsakoff's syndrome is found in a number of brain disorders besides alcoholism and appears to be caused by damage to a relatively localized part of the brain.

Symptoms Korsakoff's syndrome includes severe AMNESIA, apathy, and disorientation. Recent memory is affected, and a patient may only be conscious of each moment as it passes without storing any new memories at all. No matter how volatile the patient might have been before the onset of the disorder, afterward these patients tend to be extremely passive.

While Korsakoff disease seems similar to other types of amnesic disorders, patients with Korsakoff's have normal consciousness and perception. Korsakoff patients also differ from each other in the nature and extent of their cognitive deficits.

Gross recent memory defects are the primary sign of Korsakoff's; sometimes impairment is so profound that a person is only conscious of each moment as it passes without storing any new memories at all. While this most severe form of Korsakoff's is rare, many Korsakoff's patients only have the ability to store memories for a brief period of time.

In addition, most subjects experience a retrograde amnesia ranging from a week to as much as 20 years prior to onset of the condition, with the exception of clumps of isolated memories. Many patients are not oriented in place or time, often believe they are younger than they are, often lie and deny they have memory problems; otherwise, they usually exhibit normal personality.

Korsakoff's syndrome may appear only in an acute phase, but it may also be a chronic problem; even when patients do improve, there are often lingering recent memory problems.

See also WERNICKE-KORSAKOFF SYNDROME.

kuru A rare, progressive, and fatal brain infection that occurs in some natives of the New Guinea highlands, caused by a virus spread by cannibalism. The disease is caused by a slow virus with an incubation period of up to 30 years.

Because of certain similarities to HIV (human immunodeficiency virus), which causes AIDS, scientists have become more interested in studying kuru. In particular, HIV and kuru share many of the same characteristic brain changes. There is no treatment.

Symptoms Progressive movement disorders and eventually DEMENTIA.

L

language Most linguistic processing takes place in the dominant HEMISPHERE OF THE BRAIN (usually the left hemisphere, although in a few people the right hemisphere is dominant). The two most important areas for language in the dominant hemisphere are BROCA'S AREA and WERNICKE'S AREA. Broca's area is found in the rear of the FRONTAL LOBE near the face and tongue portions of the MOTOR CORTEX, and Wernicke's area is located in the TEMPORAL LOBE. These two areas are linked by a bundle of nerve fibers called the *arcuate fasciculus* and also are connected to the visual, auditory, and motor areas.

Spoken language travels to the AUDITORY CORTEX, where nerve fibers carry those sounds that have been translated into electric pulses to Wernicke's area, where they are consciously recognized as words. In much the same way, visual information about the shapes and combinations of letters pass from the eye through the VISUAL CORTEX and VISUAL ASSOCIATION AREAS to Wernicke's area, where the information is interpreted as words. In WERNICKE'S APHASIA, the patient cannot comprehend spoken or written language because of a problem in this area, although the person may still *produce* language.

Language *production* takes place in Broca's area, which signals the appropriate portions of the motor cortex (such as the hand muscles for writing) to produce language. BROCA'S APHASIA is therefore not a disorder of comprehension, but of articulation—the person understands written and spoken language but can't speak or write normally.

When the various language areas are used together, it becomes possible, for example, to read a prepared text to an audience. In this case, the written words would first travel to Wernicke's area via the visual cortex, and these impulses would then travel to Broca's area and on to the motor cortex for articula-

tion. In cases of a conduction aphasia caused by disruption of the arcuate fasciculus, the link between language comprehension in Wernicke's area and language production in Broca's area malfunctions. Patients with this condition will have trouble reading aloud or repeating phrases they have heard.

While one hemisphere is dominant for language, this doesn't mean that the other hemisphere has nothing whatsoever to do with the process. Scientists have discovered areas in the opposite (usually right) hemisphere that are analogous to language centers in the left and that appear to be responsible for imbuing communication with emotion. This is where the normal intonation and rhythm of human language are coordinated. The right-side equivalent of Wernicke's area interprets this important aspect of speech. Other right-brain functions in language include the analysis of facial expression and responding to the emotional content music. In APROSODIA, damage to these right-brain regions result in a curiously flat, emotionless speech or problems in appreciating the emotional qualities of speech or gestures.

language areas Language functions within the brain are situated in the dominant cerebral hemisphere, especially in the BROCA'S and WERNICKE'S AREAS. Damage in these areas is the most common cause of APHASIA.

lateral geniculate bodies The region of the brain into which the optic nerve first feeds its signal.

lateralization The functional asymmetry of the two individual cerebral HEMISPHERES OF THE BRAIN, despite the fact that both halves typically work as a coordinated unit.

While many scientists traditionally refer to the left hemisphere as dominant, in fact both halves have important roles to play in brain function. The most typical example of lateralization is a person's HANDEDNESS—whether the person favors the right or left hand, which is often related to the lateralization of other functions. For example, people who are right-handed almost always have primary speech function in the left hemisphere, which controls the right hand; while this is also true for most left-handers, they are more likely to have speech function primarily in the right or distributed equally in both hemispheres.

Interest in lateralization and handedness began in the mid-1800s when French physician Paul Broca (see BROCA, PAUL) discovered that patients with serious speech problems had lesions in the left frontal lobe.

Laurence-Moon-Biedl syndrome A very rare inherited disorder characterized by MENTAL RETARDATION, obesity, retinitis pigmentosa, abnormal number of fingers or toes, or absence of secondary sexual characteristics. It is believed that the syndrome is caused by a problem with the HYPOTHALAMUS (the area of the brain that helps regulate hormone balance).

Treatment There is no treatment.

L-dopa See LEVODOPA.

lead poisoning and the brain Contrary to public opinion, lead poisoning is not just an inner-city problem. Lead poisoning can be found anywhere there are old buildings, old paint, lead pipes—even in vegetable gardens that receive lead-contaminated runoff. Alarmingly, fully *one out of six American children* is considered to be lead poisoned, and lead poisoning can have serious effects on the brain.

Chronic exposure can lead to a "motor neuropathy" that looks identical to AMYOTROPHIC LATERAL SCLEROSIS; acute exposure features disturbances of higher brain function, DELIRIUM, mania, SEIZURES, and blindness.

Lead poisoning is unfortunately one of the most common and preventable childhood health problems today, infecting more than 6 million preschool children and another 400,000 pregnant women. Even very small exposures can produce subtle but dangerous health effects. In 1991, the Centers for Disease Control lowered the amount of lead it considers dangerous in children from 25 microliters to 10 micrograms per deciliter of blood (mcg/dl).

Lead, as most heavy metals, is a NEUROTOXIN, which means that it will impair both physical and mental function and development. For many years, people assumed that children would have to ingest large amounts of lead before being harmed. Today, most experts believe even small exposures (the amount released by raising and lowering a window painted with lead paint in the presence of a child) can result in subtle developmental and intellectual delays.

Youngsters ingest lead by licking or eating flakes of old paint containing lead or by drinking water flowing through pipes contaminated with lead, solder, or brass fittings. Babies who drink reconstituted formula made with water flowing through lead pipes can ingest an alarming percentage of tainted water.

Lead poisoning in children is particularly serious because it doesn't take much to harm a child—and the potential damage to the child's developing neurological system is serious. Lead poisoning causes the most damage to the brain, nerves, red blood cells, and digestive system. The molecular basis for lead's toxic effects on the brain seems to be that lead interferes with the GABA-ergic neurotransmission. A cumulative poison, it remains in the kidneys for seven years and in the bones for more than 30 years.

Symptoms Unfortunately, there may be no symptoms of lead poisoning for a very long time, until the damage has already been done. Because lead's effects vary from one

---

HOW TO REDUCE A CHILD'S LEAD EXPOSURE

- To reduce lead paint and dust temporarily, clean floors, windowsills, and window wells at least twice a week with a trisodium phosphate detergent, available at hardware stores. Sponges used for this purpose should not be used for anything else.
- Move cribs and playpens away from chipped or peeling paint, mantels, windowsills, and doors. Replace or strip baby furniture that may be decorated with lead paint.
- Wash the child's hands, face, bottle nipples, and toys often.
- Children and pregnant women should not be in the area while lead paint is being removed.
- Don't buy large-size canned foods and juices; lead-soldered seams can leach into food; avoid imported brands.
- Feed children plenty of calcium, iron, and protein, with plenty of milk, breads, low-fat foods, and green leafy vegetables (these foods diminish lead's effects in the body).
- Limit the amount of dirt tracked in the home.
- Avoid storing acidic food (such as orange juice and tomatoes) in ceramic or crystal containers, which may contain lead glaze.
- Lead levels in the home water supply should not exceed 15 parts per billion; for high levels, consider a water-treatment device to remove lead from tap water.
- Never boil water to eliminate lead; boiling only concentrates lead.
- Allow water to run on cold for a few minutes before using; never cook with hot water from the tap (especially when making baby food) because lead leaches more quickly into hot water.
- If your soil tests high in lead, cover with clean soil and seed or sod.

---

child to another, it is almost impossible to predict how an individual child will fare. The body absorbs about 10 to 15 percent of the ingested metal; the rest is slowly excreted. Most of the absorbed lead is stored in the child's bones, with smaller amounts deposited in bone marrow, brain tissue, and red blood cells. If the lead poisoning continues, it will accumulate to toxic levels. Lead is excreted very slowly from the body, so it builds up in tissues and bones and may not even produce detectable physical effects, although it can still cause mental impairment. If they do appear, early symptoms include listlessness, irritability, loss of appetite and weight, constipation, and a bluish line in the gums, followed by clumsiness, vomiting and stomach cramps, and a general "wasting away."

If untreated, the toxic lead levels in a child's body can lead to serious cognitive complications, including MENTAL RETARDATION. Babies exposed to high levels of lead before birth reveal impaired attention span, hearing, language ability, and intelligence. After birth, the affected infants may recover, but only if they are no longer exposed to lead. If lead exposure continues, their cognitive performance will continue to be affected for at least the first five years of life.

In addition, some researchers suggest that there may be an association between exposure to lead and pre- and postnatal hyperactivity, behavior disorders, and attention deficit disorder.

While lead poisoning is almost always a chronic problem, it is possible—albeit extremely rare—to suffer from an acute case of lead poisoning when a large amount of lead is taken in by the body over a short period of time. This is generally found among adult drinkers of bootleg whiskey. Acute poisoning symptoms include metallic taste in the mouth, abdominal pain, vomiting, diarrhea, collapse, and COMA. Large amounts directly affect the nervous system and cause HEAD- ACHE, convulsions, coma, and sometimes death.

Treatment According to the Centers for Disease Control, unless widespread screening has revealed no lead problems, parents should have their baby tested at 12 months of age and again at two years, *even without symptoms*. This is because symptoms may be subtle or nonexistent.

Lead screening includes a simple blood test, which can determine the level of lead in the blood. A new noninvasive test using X-RAY fluorescence that assesses lead levels in the bones may soon be approved.

A child with elevated blood lead levels or enough absorbed lead in the body to show symptoms will probably require hospitalization. Treatment usually includes the administration of medicines (calling chelating agents) to help the body rid itself of lead. In mild cases, the chelating agent penicillamine may be used alone; otherwise, it may be used in combination with edetate calcium disodium and dimercaprol. Chelation therapy has its risks, however, and must be properly monitored to avoid kidney damage. In acute cases, gastric lavage (stomach pumping) may be necessary.

Lead prevention The most effective way to protect children from lead poisoning is to prevent lead from building up in blood, tissues, and bones. While many products contain lead, it is most often associated with paint; until about 40 years ago, *all* house paint contained some. Lead was added to paint because it helped the paint dry more quickly and gave it a shiny, hard finish. In fact, the more lead in a can of paint, the better and more expensive the product—some paints were as much as 50 percent lead.

By the late 1970s, the government began to regulate the amount of lead in paint, but nothing was done about the lead-filled paint already on the walls in millions of older homes and schools throughout the United States. It is this lead-based paint that causes most of the lead poisoning in children. More than three-fourths of American homes built

LEAD POISONING GUIDE
The following recommendations have been provided by the U.S. Centers for Disease Control:

Lead levels	Complications	Treatment
0–9 mcg/dl	None	Annual checks until age 6
10–14 mcg/dl	Borderline (possible test inaccuracy); risk for mild developmental delays even without symptoms	Nutrition, housecleaning changes will bring level down
15–19 mcg/dl	Risk for IQ decrease; no symptoms usually noticed	Test for iron deficiency; nutrition, housekeeping changes will lower level
20–44 mcg/dl	Risk of IQ impairment increases; usually no symptoms	Complete medical evaluation; eliminate lead; drug treatment possible
45–69 mcg/dl	Colic, anemia, learning disabilities	Remove from home until lead is removed; drug treatment
70 mcg/dl	Vomiting, anemia, critical illness	Immediate hospitalization; lead removal

mcg/dl = micrograms per deciliter of blood

before 1980 (that's 57 million dwellings) still contain lead paint, and 14 million housing units have high levels of lead in dust or chipping paint—3.8 million of them housing young children. If a house was built before 1950, it's almost guaranteed that its paint contains the toxic substance; if it was built between 1950 and 1978, there is a 50 percent chance of lead paint.

The average blood level of lead in the general population has been gradually dropping during the past 20 years since lead was eliminated from gasoline—but an estimated 7 million tons of lead remain in the soil.

During renovation of an older home, experts should ascertain whether or not there is a lead problem and, if so, how to handle the situation. Because children who live near factories that melt metal may also have a lead-poisoning problem, it's important for parents who live near these factories to find out if lead is being released from the stacks by checking the EPA's Toxics Release Inventory, available at public libraries (or call 1-800-532-0202).

learning A general term for a category of changes whereby behavior or information is acquired or modified; learning begins as soon as a baby is born.

The learning process is believed to rely on the creation of new pathways from the synaptic connections established among the vast network of NEURONS in the brain. A SYNAPSE is where one neuron contacts another.

As people learn, scientists believe, their synapses undergo functional changes. For example, if someone is learning to play the violin, the neural signals from their brain to the muscles they're using travel through existing pathways. But the person's movements are slow and uncoordinated while they are learning. With more practice, the same signals are passed more and more often. These neural pathways begin to change; more connections are made; the pathways are becoming more efficient. As new, faster, more coordinated pathways develop, the budding musician can eventually move fingers and hands more quickly and precisely. Eventually, the person can play accurately without looking at the position of the hands on the instrument.

In autopsies of children, scientists found that new babies have fewer connections between their neurons, but the number quickly increases as children age, indicating that the child has learned more about the world.

The ability to learn is vulnerable to injury to those areas of the brain that process learning. For instance, Alzheimer's disease causes a depletion of ACETYLCHOLINE, a neurotransmitter used by the brain for, among other functions, the processing of learning and memory. This depletion of acetylcholine causes problems in learning and memory.

See also DYSLEXIA; LEARNING DISABILITIES.

learning disabilities A general term for a wide variety of educational problems that involve difficulties in reading, listening, speaking, writing, interpreting, understanding, or remembering. They are not caused by other handicaps (such as MENTAL RETARDATION), poor instructional methods, or cultural or language unfamiliarity. In general, learning disabilities involve problems in four areas: input, integration, memory, and output.

Children with *input problems* have difficulties in the process of receiving and registering information in the brain; they often have problems hearing or seeing accurately, although their eyes and ears are normal. They may have problems decoding (extracting meaning from symbols), such as written or spoken words or numbers. The may confuse letters or numbers because of reversals (transpositions) and therefore may be confused by directions. This type of input problem may also affect eye-hand coordination in addition to visual or motor skills.

Those with *integration* problems have difficulty with the process of putting information together in a meaningful way and understanding it. Because of this, people with LD may have problems getting words, letters, or ideas in the correct order.

Memory problems in LD may involve difficulties in the storage or retrieval of information in the brain. People with LD may have short-term memory problems so that they have trouble remembering directions long enough in order to carry them out. It may be that other problems with *input* and *integration* may scramble the information in the brain. People with LD may also have long-term memory problems (such as in remembering their address).

Problems with *output* in LD can involve difficulties in the process of carrying out commands given by the brain (such as writing or speaking), performing gross motor skills (such as jumping), or fine motor skills (such as writing). In addition, people with LD may have problems encoding information and may often misuse or struggle for words.

Youngsters with LD often have other problems, including short attention span and HYPERACTIVITY (as in ATTENTION DEFICIT HYPERACTIVE DISORDER), social-skills problem, distractibility, or general frustration.

Cause While the cause of learning disabilities is still unclear, it appears to be triggered by some disorder in the brain. This may be linked to injuries at birth or in early childhood, prematurity, serious illness in infancy or early childhood, inherited traits, or gender (boys are five times more likely than girls to have LD). Learning disabilities affecting children exposed to lead, some medications, cocaine, and alcohol are the most common environmentally related neurological disorders.

Warning signs There are a group of warning signs for learning disabilities, according to the ASSOCIATION FOR CHILDREN AND ADULTS WITH LEARNING DISABILITIES:

- *spoken language* – delays or disorders in listening and speech
- *written language* – problems in reading, writing, or spelling
- *arithmetic* – problems in understanding basic mathematical concepts
- *reasoning* – problems in organizing thoughts

See also APHASIA; COUNCIL FOR LEARNING DISABILITIES; LEARNING DISABILITIES ASSOCIATION OF AMERICA; NATIONAL CENTER FOR LEARNING DISABILITIES; ORTON DYSLEXIA SOCIETY.

Learning Disabilities Association of America A national support group for parents of children with LEARNING DISABILITIES and for interested professionals. The group works to advance the education and general well being of children with adequate intelligence who have learning disabilities arising from perceptual, conceptual, or subtle coordination problems, sometimes accompanied by behavior problems. The group provides information to the public and helps state and local groups carry out direct services to parents and children via schools, camps, recreation programs, parent education, information services, and publication of books and pamphlets. Founded in 1964, the group has 60,000 members and publishes the bimonthly *LDA Newsbriefs* and a semiannual journal. For address, see Appendix A.

See also COUNCIL FOR LEARNING DISABILITIES; NATIONAL CENTER FOR LEARNING DISABILITIES.

lecithin Called "nature's nerve food," this is the major dietary source of CHOLINE, the brain chemical implicated as a possible aid to improving memory. Repeated studies of administering lecithin to treat the memory problems of ALZHEIMER'S DISEASE patients have resulted in conflicting evidence, although the majority found it was not helpful. Other studies suggest it might be useful in heading off some deterioration in the early stages of the disease.

Although it is available in supplemental form, many researchers do not believe lecithin can offer significant memory improvement. Still, according to the U.S. Food and Drug Administration, lecithin is not toxic and has no side effects. It is found in the cells of all animals and plants and helps build the insulation around nerves called the MYELIN SHEATH.

left brain–right brain The popular idea that the left side of the brain is the home of logical thought and the right brain controls intuition. While this concept has grown astronomically popular during the past 20 years, the separation of abilities between left and right brains is not nearly so straightforward in actuality. It is true that the left cortical hemisphere does tend to be responsible for such analytical functions as understanding language, speech, computing, and judgment. The right cortical hemisphere tends to be involved with more imaginative tasks, such as recognizing faces, visualizing images, and reconstructing songs. But both hemispheres are much more alike than they are different, and almost every mental process a person undertakes actually requires the cooperation of *both* hemispheres.

It was not until the 1960s that Dr. Roger Sperry published his research on the functional differences between the brain's two hemispheres based on his studies of epileptics whose hemispheres had been surgically severed.

leucotomy A surgical procedure invented in 1935 in which nerve tracts connecting the frontal association CORTEX with deeper structures are severed. The term is derived from the Greek words meaning "white" and "to

cut," alluding to the fact that the white fibers connecting the FRONTAL LOBE to the rest of the brain are cut. The first United States leucotomy was performed in 1935 in Washington, D.C., by American neurologists Walter Freeman and James Watts. Because the term *leucotomy* referred specifically to severing specific fibers, *lobotomy* was preferred as a more general term for any psychosurgical procedure involving the cutting of the lobe's nerve fibers.

While a leucotomy was a type of major brain surgery in which the skull was opened, Freeman developed a less severe "transorbital lobotomy" using an ice-picklike instrument through the eye socket to pierce the brain; a few quick jabs damaged enough brain tissue to tranquilize the patient. For his first patients, Freeman used an ice pick from his own kitchen. The development of this lobotomy technique was an attempt to treat severe mental illness, but it led to the mass BRAIN DAMAGE of thousands of institutionalized psychiatric patients in the 1940s and 1950s, causing harmful personality changes. Lobotomy is now used only as a last resort.

levodopa Also known as L-dopa, this drug is used in the treatment of PARKINSON'S DISEASE, a neurological disorder caused by a deficiency of the neurotransmitter DOPAMINE in the brain. L-dopa is absorbed into the brain where it is converted into dopamine. It's usually given together with an enzyme such as carbidopa, in order to boost the amount of L-dopa available to the brain by reducing the amount that is first broken down by the liver. This allows for a lower dose of L-dopa, which can reduce the risk of adverse effects.

These adverse effects may include nausea and vomiting, nervousness, and agitation. Prolonged use of L-dopa can worsen these side effects.

Unfortunately, L-dopa does not work in the long run and there is still no real treatment for Parkinson's.

limbic system A network of ring-shaped structures in the center of the brain's NEO-CORTEX perched on top of the BRAINSTEM, associated with control of emotion and behavior—especially motivation, gratification, memory, and thought. It is also responsible for controlling body temperature, blood pressure, and blood sugar.

But it is the complexity of emotions, as mediated by the limbic system, together with a sophistication of sensory and motor systems, that lead to the profoundly complex behavior that is uniquely human. While much is still to be learned, scientists do know that the limbic system and the HYPOTHALAMUS are deeply interconnected with emotional feelings and with certain types of basic primitive behaviors such as eating, drinking, and sexual activity.

The limbic system (and the hypothalamus) developed early in evolution, which is not surprising considering that this area governs such basic survival necessities as fear, aggression, hunger, and sexual desire. The neural function and connectedness of the limbic system are fundamentally similar in all mammals. This extensive system includes a range of substructures including the HIPPOCAMPUS, cingulate gyrus, and AMYGDALA. Because it contains the mechanisms that make an organism warm blooded, it is known as the *mammalian brain*.

The structures of the limbic system receive input from all of the sensory systems, but in most animals (and to some degree in humans), the olfactory sense (smell) plays an especially important part in this system. Other parts of the brain that connect closely with the limbic system include the association areas of the CEREBRAL CORTEX involved in higher thought processes and midbrain structures such as the RETICULAR FORMATION (awareness, attention, etc.).

It's possible to recognize this sensory influence on emotions when considering how strong an impact a sentimental song or an odor reminiscent of childhood can have.

The effects of the limbic system are widespread, including tears, sweating, heart rate, hormone release and motor activity (such as facial expressions). Most of the messages sent by the limbic system end up in the hypothalamus located beneath the THALAMUS, at the midline of the CENTRAL NERVOUS SYSTEM. Connected directly to the PITUITARY GLAND below, it controls the body's hormones and regulates instinctive behavior and AUTONOMIC NERVOUS SYSTEM.

The most common symptoms of damage to this area of the brain include abnormalities of the emotions, including inappropriate crying or laughing, easily provoked rage, unwarranted fear, anxiety and depression, and excessive sexual interest.

lithium An ANTIPSYCHOTIC medication used primarily to treat MANIC DEPRESSION, lithium is an element of the periodic table that readily forms salts. Prescribed since 1973 in this country, it was heralded as the first effective treatment for manic depression. While scientists aren't quite sure how this drug works, they believe it may help correct chemical imbalances in neurotransmitters (SEROTONIN and NOREPINEPHRINE) that influence emotion and behavior. While lithium can have a mild antidepressant effect, it is primarily effective for its strong antimanic effects, working best by controlling the "highs" of mania. Lithium can also be effective in the treatment of major DEPRESSION and can boost the effectiveness of other antidepressants when these drugs don't quite get the job done on their own.

Lithium *bromide* was used as a sedative since the early 1900s but fell into disfavor in the 1940s when some heart patients died after using it as a salt substitute. Almost immediately thereafter, Australian psychiatrist John Cade discovered that lithium salts were extremely effective in treating manic depression. Eventually, lithium's popularity grew and by the late 1960s it was widely prescribed in other parts of the world. However, it remained restricted as an experimental drug in the United States until 1971.

Unfortunately, lithium doesn't work well for everyone; it's most effective for those who've had no more than three episodes of mania. About 20 percent of people will have complete remission of mania from taking lithium, and the rest will have varying degrees of relief. For some, they'll experience fewer episodes of mania; those that do occur are shorter and less severe—and they'll feel more stable in between manic episodes. For some people, lithium may just stop working.

Lithium will only work when it is maintained at the correct level in the bloodstream, making regular blood tests necessary.

Side effects More common and less dangerous side effects may include thirst and frequent urination. Some people also gain weight during the first few months they take lithium. Signs of lithium toxicity are: sluggishness, unsteadiness, tremor, muscle twitching, vomiting, or diarrhea. Severe cases of lithium toxicity can cause lasting BRAIN DAMAGE or death. Lithium toxicity can occur not only with a direct overdose but also if a patient's salt and water metabolism becomes imbalanced (such as by an infection that causes anorexia or fluid loss).

lobectomy An operation that involves cutting out a lobe of the brain.

lobotomy A psychosurgical procedure popular during the 1940s and 50s that involved cutting the nerve fibers of the lobe of the brain to permanently tranquilize difficult psychiatric patients.

See also LEUCOTOMY.

locus coeruleus Latin for "blue area," this is an area of the RETICULAR FORMATION that is related to alertness through the synthesis and release of the NEUROTRANSMITTER NOREPINEPHRINE. Stimulants (like amphetamines and cocaine) increase the user's alertness by simulating norepinephine and sometimes raising the concentration of norepinephrine at noradrenergic SYNAPSES.

LSD See HALLUCINOGENS.

L-tryptophan A biosynthetic precursor of SEROTONIN, one of the brain's NEUROTRANSMITTERS.

lucid dreaming The ability to "wake up" inside one's dream without "physically" waking. An EEG of a lucid dreamer shows waking waveforms superimposed on REM (dream-state) waveforms. The body is still asleep, however.

lumbar puncture (LP) The medical term for spinal tap, this is a diagnostic procedure to withdraw and examine the CEREBROSPINAL FLUID (CSF). The procedure was introduced at the end of the nineteenth century as a way to diagnose neurologic disorders.

As other tests have become more sophisticated, the LP is no longer automatically performed in the analysis of all types of CENTRAL NERVOUS SYSTEM disorders. However, it is still used to help diagnose central nervous system infection, tumors in the SUBARACHNOID SPACE, MULTIPLE SCLEROSIS, GUILLAIN-BARRE SYNDROME, and neuroimmunologic disorders.

LPs can also be used to inject drugs into the fluid, including a variety of chemotherapy drugs for the treatment of cancer, and can be used to inject a local anesthetic without causing loss of consciousness. They can also be used to insert a dye that will show up on X-RAY pictures of the SPINAL CORD (called MYELOGRAPHY).

Technique In the 20-minute procedure, the patient lies sideways with knees drawn up, pulling the vertebrae apart. The skin at the base of the spine is anesthetized with a local anesthetic, and a hollow needle is then inserted between two of the vertebrae in the lower part of the spinal canal to remove some cerebrospinal fluid. After the needle is removed, the puncture site is covered. Some patients experience a mild HEADACHE that wears off soon after the procedure.

lysergic acid diethylamide See HALLUCINOGENS.

M

magnetic resonance imaging (MRI) Also called NUCLEAR MAGNETIC RESONANCE (NMR), this diagnostic scanning technique provides high quality cross-sectional images of the brain without using X RAYS or other types of radiation. For many, it has become the preferred technique for brain and SPINAL-CORD imaging. (In fact, only the lower cost and faster imaging time for CAT SCANS keep that technology popular for most brain imaging).

MRI brain scans have several advantages over CAT scans; first, they can easily scan on several planes. In addition, the GRAY and WHITE MATTER differences are more easily defined in an MRI scan. The lack of signal from bone gives MRI an advantage over CAT scans for infarctions in the BRAINSTEM.

MRI is an expensive technique that requires considerable skill to operate; however, the extremely high quality of current images exceeds any other imaging technology. As new computer programs are being developed, imaging time is being shortened and the introduction of paramagnetic "contrast" agents should further enhance imaging and may help shorten scanning time.

The technology is based on an interaction between radio waves and nuclei within the body in the presence of a powerful magnetic field. The machine's powerful electromagnetic first aligns the nuclei of atoms of hydrogen, phosphorus, or other elements and then knocks them out of position by radio waves. When they realign with the magnetic field, they produce a radio signal that can be detected and transformed into a computer-generated image.

There is no known danger with MRI, other than the effect of the electromagnetic field on metal such as implants or metal clips, on magnetic credit-card strips, analog watches, etc. It cannot be used in patients with pacemakers and some aneurysm clips.

magnetite A natural magnetic material, commonly known as lodestone, magnetite is found in the brains of certain animals, from homing pigeons to whales; the animals use the internal magnets to help orient their sense of direction. Recently, scientists at the California Institute of Technology in Pasadena have found magnetite crystals in tissues of the human brain as well.

Brains contain an average of 7 billion crystals of iron magnetite, each either a millionth of an inch or 10 millionth of an inch in width. The total weight of the crystals in the brain are about a millionth of an ounce.

Researchers don't yet know how the magnetite relates to the human nervous system, although some scientists suspect it might provide a clue to the effects of electromagnetic fields (EMFs) and disease. EMFs have been linked to certain disorders such as cancer, but in the past critics have questioned this possibility because they believed the human body contains no magnetic material.

malnutrition Dementing brain disease can be produced by a diet that lacks enough of the B-complex vitamins (especially NIACIN, thiamine, and B_{12}). This is one reason behind the cognitive problems of serious alcohol abusers, who typically lack thiamine because of a poor diet. Recent research suggests that low levels of B_{12} in the blood can lead to SPINAL-CORD degeneration and associated brain diseases.

Malpighi, Marcello (1628–1694) Italian anatomist and pioneer microscopist who was the first to study brain cells by microscope. He concluded that most living materials are glandular and that even the largest organs are composed of tiny glands.

While little is known of his childhood, Malpighi earned doctorates in both philosophy and medicine and taught theoretical medicine at the University of Pisa in 1656. He returned to Bologna in 1659, where he continued to conduct microscopic research and to teach, despite the hostile reception he received from many of his colleagues. As a result of the lack of understanding of his colleagues, he accepted a professorship in medicine at the University of Messina in Sicily in 1662, returning after four years to Bologna, where he continued the microscopic study of the brain in addition to other organs.

In the last 10 years of his life, he was beset by tragedy and failing health. In 1684, scientific opposition reached fever pitch, and his villa was burned, his instruments shattered, and his papers destroyed. In an effort to support the scientist, Pope Innocent XII invited him to Rome in 1691 to be his personal physician, where further honors were showered upon him. He died in Rome three years later.

mammillary bodies   Part of the uppermost portion of the BRAINSTEM; this top surface of the DIENCEPHALON forms the floor on which the mammillary bodies lie. The mammillary bodies may be related to memory function, and they are some of the most commonly reported structures involved in the memory problems common in KORSAKOFF'S SYNDROME. They are generally considered nuclei of the hypothalamus—part of the limbic system. If they are related to memory, it is in some vague, emotional way. Most researchers believe mammillary bodies are related to primitive temperature regulation.

manic-depressive disorder   A form of mental illness, now more correctly referred to as bipolar depression, in which the patient swings between extremes of hyperactivity and deep DEPRESSION. The problem seems to result from imbalance in the activity of certain NEUROTRANSMITTERS (SEROTONIN, DOPAMINE, and NOREPINEPHRINE) that influence emotion and behavior.

While manic depression can be crippling in the acute phase, more than 80 percent of people who are afflicted recover. However, repeated episodes of manic depression can seriously disrupt a person's life and may lead to suicide. Moreover, some experts believe that such recurrent, progressive manic depression is a result of structural changes in the brain as the disease worsens; some physicians recommend keeping some patients on LITHIUM for long periods of time to prevent the almost-impossible-to-reverse deterioration.

Cause   A number of physical illnesses (especially brain disorders), some types of drug abuse, and a family history for the disorder are all established factors. Researchers have located at least one of the defective genes on chromosome 11. One study found that in sets of identical twins, if one twin had manic depression, there was a 50 percent chance that the other twin would develop the disorder. The concordance rate in fraternal twins is only 10 percent, the same as for other siblings. Moreover, adopted children have been found to suffer from manic depression at a rate that matches their birth parents instead of their adoptive parents, although environment and upbringing do play a role in the development of the disease.

Treatment   In severe cases, hospitalization may be required. Lithium is the drug of choice; it works best for people who have had no more than three episodes of mania. About 20 percent of patients will have a complete remission on lithium; the rest will respond in varying degrees. In about 30 percent of manic depressives, lithium smooths out the periods of mania but doesn't control the episodes of depression; in these cases physicians may prescribe Prozac or another selective serotonin reuptake inhibitor (a type of antidepressant). Other patients respond to the anticonvulsants Tegretol or Depakote.

mapping the brain The task of mapping the brain's regions and assigning functions to separate areas is an immense, ongoing task in the field of NEUROLOGY. As early as the 1860s, scientists began to locate specific areas of the brain by noting specific personality or behavior changes in people with EPILEPSY with damage to certain brain areas. Monitoring behavior electrically later enabled scientists to map the motor and sensory areas in both cerebral hemispheres.

During the 1920s, Canadian surgeon Wilder Penfield (see PENFIELD, WILDER) probed the motor, sensory, and "psychic" areas by touching certain areas of the exposed brain with 2- and 3-volt currents fired from an electrode tip. When Penfield touched certain areas, he sparked an activity in remote but functionally related brain regions connected to them.

Scientists have also been able to study the brain by stimulating electrodes implanted deep within the brain and by watching the living brain at work through PET SCANS. PET scans allow scientists to watch the brain's use of sugar and to relate this to specific mental or physical activities.

In addition, it's possible to tag brain cells to find which nerve connects to which, tracing their passage through the brain.

marijuana and the brain Recent research in animals has found dense clusters of receptor sites in the HIPPOCAMPUS for tetrahydrocannibinol, the active ingredient of marijuana (cannabis). This localization of receptors for THC in the hippocampus and nearby LIMBIC-SYSTEM structures helps explain the effects of marijuana, which can range from mild euphoria to weakened short-term memory.

Marijuana contains the active ingredient THC (tetrahydrocannabinol), which is also found in hashish. The leaves are usually smoked, although they can be eaten in food, and they produce feelings of well-being and

calmness that last for about an hour. All forms of cannabis have negative physical effects, including increased heart rate, bloodshot eyes, dry mouth and throat, and increased appetite. Large doses may result in panicky states, phobias, and delusions, although true psychosis rarely occurs. There is evidence that regular users can become physically dependent on the drug.

Use of cannabis may impair or reduce short-term memory and comprehension, alter the sense of time, and reduce ability to perform tasks requiring concentration and coordination. The substance's negative effects on memory have been recorded for some time; in 1845 French psychiatrist Moreau de Tours noted that hashish could gradually weaken the power to direct thoughts at will. More recent studies suggest that the most obvious problem with memory occurs within three hours of smoking, with a direct effect on the hippocampus, the memory center of the brain. Some researchers suggest marijuana may affect the way a person processes and remembers different kinds of information. It appears to interfere with cholinergic transmission, resulting in problems in retrieving words and making it difficult to recall numbers; the ability to store new memories also seems to be affected. Some scientists believe the chronic use of marijuana may cause the same kinds of memory effects as those experienced in patients suffering from brain infections, KORSAKOFF'S SYNDROME and ALZHEIMER'S DISEASE.

Other studies suggest marijuana may interfere with memory because it increases the number of intrusive thoughts (ideas that pass through the mind while the subject is trying to concentrate on a list of words for a research study).

medial temporal lobe An area of the brain important in memory formation. Direct evidence of the importance of this area of the brain comes in the wake of neurosurgery to remove parts of the TEMPORAL LOBE as a treatment for EPILEPSY.

In a series of operations during the mid-1950s, surgeons removed the medial temporal lobe in 10 epileptic patients in order to lessen SEIZURES. While the operations were successful, 8 of the 10 suffered pronounced memory deficits. The most famous of these was known as HM, whose amnesic syndrome is considered to be among the purest ever studied. After the operation, HM was unable to remember anything other than a handful of events since the time of his operation and was described as living in the "eternal present."

The study revealed that AMNESIA was present only in those who had lost both the HIPPOCAMPUS and the AMYGDALA; removal of the amygdala alone did not produce amnesia.

meditation and the brain Meditation is used in an attempt to achieve tranquility, clear headedness, and relaxation by learning to immerse oneself in a single mental task (such as visualizing an object, contemplating a word or sound, or paying attention to one's breath).

Basically, meditation's effects occur as a result of alteration of the brain waves. Different BRAIN-WAVE patterns reflect different states of consciousness. Rapid BETA WAVES are associated with normal arousal; slower ALPHA WAVES indicate a relaxed, meditative state. THETA WAVES, which are still slower, represent drowsiness or deep reverie. DELTA WAVES, the slowest of all, occur during sleep.

Meditation slows and deepens the brain-wave pattern from beta to alpha or (in advanced stages) even to theta, which produces a mildly altered state of consciousness.

medulla One of three parts of the BRAIN-STEM, the medulla looks like a thickened extension of the SPINAL CORD and contains the nuclei of the 9th through the 12th CRANIAL NERVES, receiving and relaying taste sensations from the tongue and relaying signals to speech muscles and in tongue and neck movements. It is situated in the skull, above the PONS and below the spinal cord. The medulla also contains the groups of nerve cells that control the automatic activities of the heartbeat, breathing, blood pressure, and digestion, sending and receiving information about these automatic functions via the VAGUS NERVE. It is also responsible for coughing, sneezing, and gagging.

medulla oblongata Correct name for the MEDULLA.

medulloblastoma A malignant tumor of the CEREBELLUM (a part of the brain located in the lower rear portion of the cranium), one of the most common types of brain tumors found in children. About 50 percent of these tumors are confined to the connecting bridge between the two halves of the cerebellum; the rest actually invade the cerebellum or the BRAINSTEM. The cause of a medulloblastoma is unknown.

Most medulloblastomas occur between the ages of four and eight, with a peak incidence around age 5½. Boys of this age are twice as likely as girls to have this type of tumor, but the sexual difference lessens with age. Several hundred cases of medulloblastoma are diagnosed each year in the United States.

Symptoms Among infants, the only sign is usually increased head size. After age 18 months, the most common symptoms are vomiting and HEADACHE just after awakening (caused by increased pressure within the skull). Other symptoms include irritability, sluggishness, personality change, and impaired attention and memory. Because the cerebellum controls and coordinates activities such as walking and speech, these activities may be affected as the tumor grows; an "ataxic gait" (stumbling, uncoordinated movements) is a common initial symptom.

Depending on the exact location of the tumor, there may be muscle weakness, spasticity, reflex change, limp muscles, stiff neck, imperfect eye coordination, or RAPID EYE MOVEMENTS.

Medulloblastomas are diagnosed with non-invasive tests such as CAT SCANS and MAGNETIC RESONANCE IMAGING (MRI). SPINAL TAPS are never performed if increased intracranial pressure is suspected because of the danger of severe brain damage.

Treatment Medulloblastomas can block the normal flow of SPINAL FLUID, and shunting to remove this fluid may be necessary to decrease the intracranial pressure before the tumor is removed. Surgery can remove most of the tumor, increasing the effectiveness of chemotherapy or radiation. While there is a link between the extent of the excised tumor and subsequent survival, this type of tumor can never be completely removed because stray cells too small for the surgeon to see are almost always present in the surrounding area.

Since the 1920s, radiation therapy has been used to destroy tumor cells that remain after surgery. Irradiation of the entire brain and spine begins about a week after surgery because the tumor may spread throughout the CENTRAL NERVOUS SYSTEM. While this treatment is associated with long-term side effects, some hospitals report up to a 70 percent five-year survival rate for patients whose tumor has apparently been completely removed followed by radiation. High-risk patients also may benefit from chemotherapy.

Poor growth is often the consequence of radiation therapy caused by possible damage to the HYPOTHALAMUS; 80 percent of children treated with radiation have a decreased amount of growth hormone. Radiation damage to the spine may also cause shortness or curvature. The endocrine system may also be damaged. Many children less than four treated with radiation and/or chemotherapy also suffer some degree of decreased intellect, with problems in reading, writing,

and short-term memory. Older children suffer less intellectual damage.

For more information, contact the Association for Brain Tumor Research, 6232 N. Pulaski Rd., Chicago, IL 60646; (312) 286-5571.

melatonin A hormone released by the PINEAL GLAND that induces sleep and influences CIRCADIAN RHYTHMS; experts now believe an abnormal level of melatonin may also suppress mood and mental quickness. The human body is regulated by a biological clock that sets the pace for everyday rhythms of sleep, activity, temperature, and cortisol and melatonin release. Most people maintain a certain flexibility in their biological clock, allowing them to synchronize their system to environmental changes. But experts suspect that some people don't synchronize their clocks so easily. It could be that some people are out of step with the world's 24-hour rhythm, so that melatonin is released too early (causing early-evening sleepiness and early-morning awakening) or too late (causing insomnia and trouble waking up). Normally, melatonin is produced in the dark during sleep, and its production peaks during the winter months.

During the day, melatonin levels are low; at sunset, the cessation of light triggers neural signals that stimulate the pineal gland to begin releasing melatonin. This rise continues for hours, eventually peaking around 2 A.M. in normal, healthy young people and about 3 A.M. in elderly patients. After this, it begins a steady decline to minimal levels again by morning. The delay in timing and decrease in amount of melatonin appears to be a part of the aging process; interestingly, the maximum amount of melatonin released in the bloodstream of the elderly is only about half of that in young adults. This decrease is so predictable that some experts have proposed blood melatonin levels as a measure of biological age. This reduction in melatonin among the elderly may be part of the reason for the sleeping problems and daytime fatigue many senior citizens report.

The melatonin cycle appears to regulate many neuroendocrine functions. When the timing or intensity of the melatonin peak is disrupted by aging, jet lag, etc., many physiological and mental functions are affected. Some of these functions include cognitive ability, memory, and judgment.

There has been some research investigating the possibility of melatonin's ability to slow down the aging process in animal studies. It is being investigated as a treatment to prevent ATHEROSCLEROSIS, reduce triglyceride levels, improve cellular immunity, and increase lifespan. It is also linked with depression; recent research at the University of California at San Diego found that some women who are depressed as a result of PMS (premenstrual syndrome) have lower amounts of melatonin when they sleep. In other studies, manic depressives were found to be extremely sensitive to light; exposure to it caused their melatonin levels to plummet. In addition, the pineal gland appears to be particularly important in the development of SEASONAL AFFECTIVE DISORDER (SAD); treatment of SAD by special lights may ease depression by readjusting the circadian rhythms, thereby normalizing the secretion of melatonin by the brain.

Scientists are studying the possibility of using melatonin as a treatment for jet lag, cancer, sleep disturbances, stress, poor memory, etc. In some studies, melatonin appears to inhibit tumor growth and may be of value in untreatable cancer patients whose disease has spread. There has even been some suggestion that melatonin may help to overcome the negative health consequences of electromagnetic fields.

memory Traditionally understood as the storage and retrieval of information, memory is really not so much a retrieval as an active construction, an abstraction that refers to a *process*—remembering. Memory has not been located in any one place in the brain but is believed to function at the level of levels of neurons scattered in a weblike pattern throughout the brain. In fact, there is no firm distinction between how a person remembers and how a person thinks.

In the brain, NEURONS connect with other cells via junctions called *synapses*; when a neuron sends an electrical signal down its axon, the signal triggers the release of NEUROTRANSMITTERS (special signaling substances) that diffuse across the synapses between cells, attaching themselves to RECEPTORS on the following NERVE CELL. When the neurotransmitter binds to the receptor, this chemical transmission stimulates (or inhibits) the electrical activity of the second neuron; in this way, neurons communicate. The human brain contains about 10 billion of these nerve cells joined together by about 60 trillion synapses.

Bits and pieces of every experience are not stored in one place but are sent out to different regions of the brain: Memories of sound are found in the AUDITORY CORTEX, memories of the appearance settle into the VISUAL CORTEX. Each neuron represents a small bit of the memory, and all the scattered fragments of memory remain physically linked. To be recalled, the memory is called up by the LIMBIC SYSTEM, which pulls different aspects of each memory from the fragments scattered throughout the CORTEX through electrochemical signaling. Consolidation of information into a thought or image seems to require correlated nerve-cell signaling in different parts of the brain.

The backbone of memory could be the parts of the brain cells that receive electric impulses—the DENDRITES, the wisps at the tip of the brain cell that receive signals from the axon terminals of preceding neurons.

Researchers have generally agreed that anything that influences behavior leaves a trace (ENGRAM) somewhere in the nervous system. As long as these memory traces last, they can theoretically be restimulated, and the event or experience that established them will be remembered.

It could be that the HIPPOCAMPUS (part of the limbic system) retrieves a memory using a single moment or sensation to trip off recall of the others: The smell of perfume or the feel of a soft sweater brings with it the memory of *mother*. Each time the memory is called up, the hippocampus strengthens the connections between the various elements of each perception.

False memory This system of recalling memory from consolidating bits of information from all over the brain almost guarantees that people may not always remember accurately. It's quite possible that people may assemble accurate snippets inaccurately. For example, if someone witnessed a car running a red light and someone else later mentions that car running the stop sign, the witness may very possibly reconstruct the memory as a car running a stop sign. Unfortunately, it may be impossible to tease out accurate memories in such a case because there is no structural difference between a memory of a true event and a false one.

Because the origin of a memory (called "source memory") deteriorates more quickly than other aspects of the memory, it is highly prone to suggestion. While not everyone is considered to be suggestible, certain conditions—such as severe emotional stress—can render these people more sensitive to suggestion. This is particularly so during therapy, when comments by a therapist may be internalized and later recalled as actual memory according to psychologist and memory expert Elizabeth Loftus, Ph.D.

HYPNOSIS is especially capable of creating instead of retrieving memories, according to psychiatrist David Spiegel, M.D., of Stanford University. This problem of "false memory" becomes especially important during litigation of repressed memories in abuse cases.

Types of memory Memory is a biological phenomenon with its root firmly in the senses. In fact, there are many different *types* of memories: visual, verbal, olfactory, tactile, kinesthetic, and so on. While people often think of memory as a single phenomenon, in fact there are two distinct mechanisms corresponding to different mental processes—voluntary and involuntary memory. The smell of grandmother's perfume may trigger an involuntary memory if the sensation comes by surprise; it will appear as a voluntary memory if a person chooses to search for it.

If a person's earliest memory is of nestling in the arms of a mother, the person's visual system identified the objects in space—this shape is a sweater, this shape is the mother's face, this is its color, this is its smell, this is how it feels—binding them into the experience of being held by mother. Each of these separate sensations then travels to the hippocampus, which rapidly integrates the perceptions as they occur into a single, memorable experience. The hippocampus then consolidates information for storage as permanent memory in another brain region.

About 60 percent of Americans have primarily a "visual" memory, easily visualizing objects, places, faces, and the pages of a newspaper. The others seem better at remembering sounds or words and the associations they think of are often rhymes or puns.

In addition, some researchers believe there are at least three different types of memory subsystems—sensory, short-term, and long-term memory (although other researchers believe long-term memory is made up of several different types of remembering). While most people think of long-term memory when they say *memory*, in fact these researchers believe information must pass through the first two systems before it can be stored in long-term memory.

Formation of a memory begins with registration of information during perception; the data are then filed in a short-term memory system that seems to be very limited in the amount of material it can store at one time. Unless it is constantly repeated, short-term memory is lost within minutes and is replaced by other material.

The next stage of memory formation is the transference of important material to long-term memory—called *consolidation*—where the process of storage involves associations with words or meanings, with the visual imagery evoked by it, or with other sensory experiences, such as smell or sound.

People tend to store material on subjects they already know something about because the information has more meaning to them. This is why a person with a normal memory may be able to recall in detail many facets about one subject. In addition, people remember words that are related to something they already know because there is already a file in their memory related to that information.

The final stage of memory is retrieving (or recall), in which information stored on the unconscious level is brought up into the conscious mind at will. How reliable this material is, researchers believe, depends on how well it was encoded during stage two.

While most people speak of having a *bad memory* or a *good memory*, in fact most people are good at remembering some things and not so good at remembering others. When a person has trouble remembering something, it's generally not the fault of the entire memory system—just an inefficient component in the memory system.

For example, if a person wanted to remember where he had placed his keys, first he must have become aware of where he put them when he walked in the door. He *regis-* *ters* (takes notice) of what he has done by paying attention to the action of putting his keys down on the hall table. This information is *consolidated*, ready to be retrieved at a later date.

If the system is working properly, he can remember exactly where he left his keys. If he has forgotten where he puts his keys, one of several things could have happened:

- He may not have registered clearly to start with.
- He may not have consolidated what he registered.
- He may not be able to retrieve the memory accurately.

Research indicates that older people have trouble with all three of these stages but are especially troubled with registering and retrieving information.

There are many factors that go into how well a memory is formed, including how familiar the information is and how much attention has been paid. Good health also plays a major part in how well a person performs intentional memory tasks. When mental and physical conditions aren't in peak condition, the entire memory system functions at a slower pace. Attention (a key to memory performance) is diminished and long-term memory weakens. Ideas and images are not likely to be registered as strongly, and memory traces become fainter, making them harder to retrieve or file into long-term memory. In fact, patients who frequently become ill have significantly more memory problems than those who stay in good health, according to a survey of 1,000 subjects by the National Center of Health Statistics.

Techniques available for improving memory generally invoke teaching association techniques that show people how to improve their coding systems. For example, a person might visualize a well-known street and then think of each building as representing a new fact.

People with high IQs usually have good memories, although some people have exceptionally good memories that seem to be unrelated to their intellectual functioning. There are even some people with MENTAL RETARDATION who have profoundly intense memories for specific types of information— the so-called idiot savants.

Research into the biochemical basis of memory itself was first begun during the 1950s, when studies suggested that the complex molecule RNA (ribonucleic acid) served as a chemical mediator for memory. Rat studies showed that when animals were trained to do certain tasks, RNA in certain cells changed. Blocking the rats' RNA did interfere with long-term memory, although no change was apparent in short-term memory. In addition, it appears that active learning that involves the use of memory causes the brain to produce increased amounts of RNA, which in turn increases the amount of protein production. Swedish researchers have discovered that the brains of rats undergoing a learning experience have produced up to 40 percent more RNA than the brains of control rats who had not learned anything.

Today, other memory-enhancing chemicals being studied include CALPAIN, NOREPINEPHRINE, D-AMINO-D-ARGININE VASOPRESSIN (DDAVP) and ADRENALINE.

Calpain seems to be able to digest protein and unblock receptors, facilitating neuronal communication. Calpain is naturally activated by release of calcium from internal stores in the cells, which leads scientists to wonder if calcium deficiency may decrease enzyme activity in older people, leading to memory loss.

Norepinephrine, a neurotransmitter associated with stress, also appears to be linked to memories (especially memories associated with stress).

Adrenaline appears to be a key to locking memories in place in the brain because rats who can't produce adrenaline have poorer recall ability than those who can produce the hormone, and rats who get a booster shot of adrenaline after learning something can remember the information better. This may support the idea that hormone deficiency in older people contributes to memory loss. Adrenaline also boosts attention.

Scientists theorize that hormones like adrenaline act as fixatives, locking up memories of exciting or shocking events. This allows the brain a way to remember important information while discarding trivial bits.

Studying memory   In order to study memory, traditional researchers have used drugs or surgery on animals to affect parts of the brain and then used behavioral tests to measure those effects.

Today, new imaging methods such as X-RAY computerized tomography and MAGNETIC RESONANCE IMAGING (MRI) allow more precise views of these damaged animal brain sections. PET SCANS (POSITRON EMISSION TOMOGRAPHY) have allowed scientists to study the human brain *as it functions* for clues to the relationship between brain structure and function.

memory, disorders of   There is a wide range of specific impairments to memory that can occur from an astonishingly large number of causes, ranging from organic (brain dysfunction) to psychogenic (psychological).

Disorders of memory can be caused by a problem at any of the three stages of memory (registration, long-term memory, and recall). Most problems involve an inability to recall past events because of a failure at the retention or recall state (see AMNESIA). A person who can't store new memories suffers from anterograde amnesia, while a pronounced loss of old memories is retrograde amnesia. These two forms of amnesia may appear together or alone.

Sometimes, however, the problem occurs at the registration stage (for example, depressed people can't remember because their preoccupation with personal thoughts and feelings get in the way of paying attention).

Problems with memory is one of the most common symptoms of impaired brain function; these memory defects may be transitory (such as those after an epileptic SEIZURE) or long term, such as after a severe HEAD INJURY.

In addition, memory problems may be the result of an organic problem in the brain. These could include ALZHEIMER'S DISEASE and the DEMENTIAS, in which cognitive functions are progressively lost. In the early stages of Alzheimer's, there is usually a selective amnesia caused by degenerative processes in the parietemporal-occipital association NEOCORTEX, the CHOLINERGIC BASAL FOREBRAIN, and the LIMBIC SYSTEM structures (such as the HIPPOCAMPUS and AMYGDALA).

Organic amnesia (or global amnesia) is a memory disorder featuring very poor recall and recognition of recent information (anterograde amnesia) and very poor recall and recognition of information acquired before brain damage occurred (RETROGRADE AMNESIA). It is caused by lesions in various brain regions, including the hippocampus and amygdala, by bursting ANEURYSMS, etc.

HUNTINGTON'S DISEASE, an inherited disorder causing involuntary movements, also causes cognitive problems and memory deficits. Huntington's is caused by the increasing atrophy of the CAUDATE NUCLEUS in the BASAL GANGLIA and the frontal association neocortex.

KORSAKOFF'S SYNDROME causes a form of organic amnesia resulting from chronic alcoholism, probably related to thiamine deficiency and poor diet. PARKINSON'S DISEASE is a progressive motor disorder that may also include cognitive problems and poor memory arising from dysfunction of the SUBSTANTIA NIGRA.

Postencephalitic amnesia is caused by a viral infection of the TEMPORAL LOBES of the brain; while the term covers various viruses, the herpes simplex virus is most commonly

the cause. The amnesia in these patients is probably caused by destruction of the hippocampus and amygdala; RETROGRADE AMNESIA is probably caused by the destruction of the temporal association neocortex.

SCHIZOPHRENIA, the most common form of psychosis, affecting 1 percent of the population, has also been linked to memory disorders. However, it is unclear to what extent the memory problems depend on subtype of schizophrenia and to what extent they are the result of the effects of an inability to pay attention to external events.

Brain tumors (see TUMOR, BRAIN) are abnormal growths that destroy brain tissue and put pressure on nearly brain structures. Those causing particular memory problems similar to Korsakoff's syndrome are often found on the floor of the third ventricle near the DIENCEPHALON. But memory deficits are likely to show up in a wide variety of brain tumors.

memory trace   See ENGRAM.

meninges   The three membranes that cover and protect the brain and SPINAL CORD, guarding against shocks, knocks, and vibrations. The tough leathery outer membrane (DURA MATER) lines the inside of the skull, draping loosely around the spinal cord. Next comes the arachnoid mater, an elastic weblike substance separated by the CEREBROSPINAL FLUID-filled ARACHNOID SPACE from the innermost membrane, called the PIA MATER. The pia mater lies directly next to the brain and is much thinner; it closely follows the bumps and wrinkles on the brain's surface.

Infection of the meninges is called MENINGITIS; tumors of the meninges are called MENINGIOMAS.

meningioma   Although these benign tumors are not specifically tumors of the brain, they are classified as such and arise from the middle layer of the MENINGES (protective lining of the brain), usually attaching themselves to the outside layer (DURA MATER).

Constituting 15 to 20 percent of all brain tumors, about one new case per 100,000 is diagnosed each year in the United States among patients of all ages. This type of tumor is slow-growing, sometimes becoming quite large before ever causing symptoms. These tumors are quite rare in children and in African Americans of any age; instead, they occur most often in middle-aged women.

Symptoms   Symptoms vary depending on the size and location of the tumor. HEADACHE is the most common symptom of this type of tumor, although not all tumors will trigger one. A tumor in the FRONTAL LOBE may produce progressive weakness of one area of the body, SEIZURES, or mental changes (such as drowsiness, listlessness, dullness, or personality change). A tumor in the dominant side of the brain (the left side in most right-handed people) can produce speech difficulties such as APHASIA, the loss of the ability to smell, visual problems, or loss of bladder control.

A tumor in the nondominant TEMPORAL LOBE may cause no symptoms at all except for seizures. In the dominant hemisphere, they may cause ANOMIA (problems in recognizing and naming objects).

Tumor in the PARIETAL LOBE may trigger seizures or astereognosis (inability to identify an object by touching it). The tumor may spread to underlying bone, thickening and bulging an area of the skull in childhood, if the bone is still soft.

Diagnosis   Meningiomas can be detected by BRAIN SCANS (CAT or MRI) and by X-RAY, by ELECTROENCEPHALOGRAPH (EEG) and by ARTERIOGRAPHY.

Treatment   Because these tumors are often quite sharply distinct from underlying brain tissue, they can often by completely removed by surgery. If complete removal is not possible, they may be partially removed; because they are so slow-growing, it could be many years before further surgery is necessary. Neither radiation therapy nor chemotherapy is usually used on meningiomas because they do not respond very well to this type of treatment. If a tumor is discovered accidentally during X rays following a HEAD INJURY or because of an odd lump on the head, the surgeon may opt to do nothing but monitor the tumor—especially if the patient is old or in ill health.

The French-made abortion pill RU-486 has shown promise in treating tumors of the brain, among other things; in 1994 a meningioma patient won approval to take the pill, which had been banned in the United States. Approval came after the patient testified before Congress that it was his only available treatment, according to the U.S. Food and Drug Administration.

Prognosis   Complete recovery is possible after surgery, and may take as long as two years or more after surgery. However, like other tumors, meningiomas can recur if not all the cells were removed. While the overall recurrence rate is about 20 percent, a patient's individual risk depends on the location of the original tumor. It is also possible that recurrent symptoms are not caused by a recurrence of the tumor but by damage done to the brain from the original growth.

Because these tumors don't metastasize, they will recur in the same areas as the first tumor. If the original surgery was successful, chances are very good that subsequent ones will also be successful.

For more information, contact the ASSOCIATION FOR BRAIN TUMOR RESEARCH; for address, see Appendix A.

meningitis   An acute infection and inflammation of the MENINGES (the membranes that cover the brain and SPINAL CORD) that can cause symptoms of DEMENTIA. Meningitis usually results from infection by a variety of microorganisms; while viral meningitis is fairly mild, bacterial meningitis is dangerous and can cause dementia and death. In about 8 percent of cases, the disease progresses so rapidly that death occurs during the first 48 hours, despite early treatment with antibiotics. Rarely, some yeasts can also cause meningitis.

Organisms that go on to infect the brain usually travel through the bloodstream from an infection somewhere else in the body, although some may be caused by HEAD INJURY.

The most common forms of bacterial meningitis include neonatal meningitis (see MENINGITIS, NEONATAL), haemophilus meningitis (MENINGITIS, HAEMOPHILUS), meningococcal meningitis (MENINGITIS, MENINGOCOCCAL), and pneumococcal meningitis (MENINGITIS, PNEUMOCOCCAL).

Among the most common problems associated with meningitis include MENTAL RETARDATION, ear and hearing problems, EPILEPSY, HYDROCEPHALUS, LEARNING DISABILITIES, and movement or coordination problems. Because damage is not always noticeable immediately, children who have had meningitis (especially neonatal meningitis) should be checked by a NEUROLOGIST for two years after recovery to identify damage.

Symptoms Fever, severe HEADACHE or vomiting, confusion or drowsiness, and stiff neck—and sometimes SEIZURES. All of these symptoms may not develop early in the condition.

Diagnosis To diagnose the disease, a physician will examine the head, ears, and skin (especially along the spine) for sources of infection, together with samples of pus from the middle ear or sinuses, X-RAYS of chest, skull, and sinuses (or a CT SCAN to detect abscess or deep swelling). The definitive diagnosis is made by analyzing SPINAL FLUID extracted by lumbar puncture for low GLUCOSE level and increased white-blood-cell count in the fluid.

Treatment The most important thing to remember about the treatment of meningitis is speed—suspicious symptoms should be reported as soon as possible. Meningitis is considered to be a medical emergency and is treated with large doses of antibiotics. In some cases, treatment for brain swelling, shock, convulsions, or dehydration may be necessary.

meningitis, haemophilus The most common type of bacterial MENINGITIS in children up to age 10; however, the recent introduction of the Hib vaccine should protect children from haemophilus influenzae type B disease.

Symptoms Onset of symptoms may be gradual instead of sudden, beginning with fever, lack of energy first, followed by lack of energy, HEADACHE, vomiting, stiff neck, drowsiness, and mental confusion.

meningitis, meningococcal A type of bacterial MENINGITIS that is more common in older children and young adults, caused by *Neisseria meningitidis*. While slightly less serious than other types of bacterial meningitis, it is still capable of causing death (about 13 percent), although its damage in survivors is not as long lasting. A vaccine against some forms of the bacteria is sometimes used in areas of epidemic.

Symptoms Symptoms usually begin suddenly, with high fever, lack of energy, HEADACHE, and vomiting, with possible stiff neck, shoulders, and joints. Within 24 to 48 hours, the patient becomes sleepy and confused and may fall into a COMA. There may be convulsions, and about half of patients may have a rash of small red spots or irregular bruising lesions scattered over the whole body. Young children may be irritable and restless during the early stages.

meningitis, neonatal A particularly dangerous type of bacterial MENINGITIS that may affect as many as 40 or 50 out of every 100,000 newborns. If the disease is contracted during the first week of an infant's life, it is fatal 50 percent of the time; half of the survivors will have BRAIN DAMAGE.

Infants often pick up the disease during delivery from their mothers, from the birthing staff, or from equipment in the delivery room. Premature or low-birth weight babies are particularly at risk because of an immature immune system.

Neonatal meningitis is usually caused by either *Streptococcus group B* or *Escherichia coli* bacteria.

Symptoms Infants may show no signs of disease or infection, other than irritability, poor appetite, and fluctuating temperature. Any unexplained fever or sign of infection in newborns—especially those at risk for meningitis—should be treated with suspicion.

meningitis, pneumococcal The less-common but most-dangerous of all types of bacterial MENINGITIS, this type causes a death rate of more than 30 percent and leaves survivors with extensive, lasting BRAIN DAMAGE. Caused by the *Streptococcus pneumoniae*, it strikes anyone from infancy to adults, usually after a respiratory infection or HEAD INJURY.

Symptoms Symptoms usually begin suddenly with high fever, lack of energy, HEADACHE, and vomiting, with possible stiff neck, shoulders, and joints. Within 24 to 48 hours, the patients become sleepy and confused and may fall into a COMA. There may be convulsions.

meningocele A form of SPINA BIFIDA, this is a protrusion of the MENINGES (protective covering) of the SPINAL CORD caused by a congenital problem with the spine. Meningocele is less serious than myelocele (protrusion of the spinal cord and the meninges).

mental illness A general term describing problems with one or more functions of the mind, such as perception, memory, or emotion, that causes suffering to the patient or others. Mental illness is different from sub-

normality, in which a person fails to develop normal intellectual capabilities.

Mental illness is broadly divided into neurosis, in which the patient can appreciate reality, and psychosis, in which the ability to appreciate reality is missing. Neuroses appear to be related to environment, upbringing, and personality, whereas psychoses appear to be problems caused by complex biochemical brain disease.

See also MENTAL ILLNESS FOUNDATION; NATIONAL ALLIANCE FOR THE MENTALLY ILL; NATIONAL ALLIANCE FOR RESEARCH ON SCHIZOPHRENIA AND DEPRESSION.

Mental Illness Foundation A national support group that works to inform people about MENTAL ILLNESS. Founded in 1983, the group publishes a quarterly newsletter and a directory that lists mental illnesses and provides information on how to contact related associations. For address, see Appendix A.

mental retardation Subnormal intellectual capacity with associated problems in at least two of 10 areas of adaptive behavior, including communications, self-care, home-living skills, social skills, leisure, health/safety, self-direction, functional academics, community use, and work. The term implies a harmful process that occurred before birth or early in life.

Classification Individuals with mental retardation may be classified according to their intellectual capacity as mildly, moderately, or profoundly retarded.

Mildly retarded, or "educable," have IQ scores between 55 and 70 (approximately 75 percent of the retarded population). They may never reach more than third or fourth grade level in educational skills, but after reaching adulthood they should be able to function in society with some degree of supervision.

The moderately retarded, or "trainable," have IQs between 45 and 55; most are capable of learning self-care skills but will never achieve significant academic standards. They may live at home and attend sheltered workshops; those who live in a group setting may require considerable supervision. About 20 percent of the retarded population are moderately retarded.

The severely (IQ 25–45) and profoundly (IQ less than 25) retarded are completely dependent on others for their care. Some may be bedridden and never become socialized. These two groups make up only 5 percent of the total mentally retarded population.

While the above classifications have been used for many years, they have been challenged more recently by some experts in the field, who have proposed that the mentally retarded individuals be classified in one of only two groups—mild (IQ between 50 and 70) and severe (IQ below 50).

Causes The more severe forms of mental retardation usually have a specific physical cause, and their incidence is about the same in all socioeconomic levels. About one-fourth are caused by DOWN SYNDROME, another quarter by other inherited or congenital conditions (such as BRAIN DAMAGE, PHENYLKETONURIA, amino-acid disorders, lysosomal storage diseases, mitochondrial diseases, inherited metabolic disease, CENTRAL NERVOUS SYSTEM infection, tumors, CEREBRAL PALSY), and one-third are caused by trauma or infection at birth or early childhood. About 15 percent of cases are unknown, although FRAGILE X SYNDROME may account for some of these cases.

On the other hand, mild mental retardation appears to have no physical cause but seems to be hereditary. Poverty and malnutrition may contribute to the problem.

Symptoms There may be no outward psychological symptoms in the mildly retarded other than slowness in mental tasks; emotions may be expressed in a childlike way. In addition, HYPERACTIVITY, AUTISM, and repetitive involuntary movements are about four times more common in this group.

In those who are severely retarded with no speech, EPILEPSY and neurological problems are common, together with incontinence and self-injury.

Treatment Early therapy to boost motor and verbal skills may allow more and more children to avoid institutionalization and become moderately self-sufficient, but there is no specific way to eliminate intellectual deficits. Family counseling may be imperative to preserve a stable home life.

See also ASSOCIATION FOR CHILDREN WITH DOWN SYNDROME; ASSOCIATION FOR CHILDREN WITH RETARDED MENTAL DEVELOPMENT; ASSOCIATION FOR RETARDED CITIZENS; CENTER FOR FAMILY SUPPORT; FEDERATION FOR CHILDREN WITH SPECIAL NEEDS; JARC; MENTAL RETARDATION ASSOCIATION OF AMERICA; NATIONAL ASSOCIATION OF DEVELOPMENTAL DISABILITIES COUNCILS; NATIONAL DOWN SYNDROME CONGRESS; NATIONAL DOWN SYNDROME SOCIETY; PARENTS OF CHILDREN WITH DOWN SYNDROME; PILOT PARENTS; YOUNG ADULT INSTITUTE AND WORKSHOP.

Mental Retardation Association of America A national support group working for the improvement of the quality of life for the mentally retarded and promoting research aimed at preventing MENTAL RETARDATION. The group also works for adequate national appropriations, for supportive legislation and implementation of statutes and regulations to benefit the mentally retarded, to assist federal government agencies that serve the retarded to assure quality programming and new services, for informing the public, and for providing referral services. The association advocates alternative quality programs through support of both community-based and institutional services and informs parents of the right to a choice of quality services. The association also encourages the development of small familylike homes, constructed and furnished according to accepted community standards, on the campuses of our state institutions as well as in communities throughout the country. The group also supports mentally retarded persons in their legal, moral, and human rights and seeks recognition of the rights and responsibilities of parents. For address, see Appendix A.

See also THE ARC; ASSOCIATION FOR CHILDREN WITH DOWN SYNDROME; ASSOCIATION FOR CHILDREN WITH RETARDED MENTAL DEVELOPMENT; CENTER FOR FAMILY SUPPORT; FEDERATION FOR CHILDREN WITH SPECIAL NEEDS; JARC; NATIONAL ASSOCIATION OF DEVELOPMENTAL DISABILITIES COUNCILS; NATIONAL DOWN SYNDROME CONGRESS; NATIONAL DOWN SYNDROME SOCIETY; PARENTS OF CHILDREN WITH DOWN SYNDROME; PILOT PARENTS; VOICE OF THE RETARDED; YOUNG ADULT INSTITUTE AND WORKSHOP.

mental status examination A diagnostic assessment of a person's orientation to time and place and general level of functioning (intellectually, emotionally, and socially) following trauma. The examiner observes general appearance, attitudes, and behavior and tries to assess orientation by asking "What is your name?" or "What day is it?" The examiner tests mental grasp by asking a person to complete a basic mental task, such as counting backward.

mesencephalon See MIDBRAIN.

Mesmer, Franz Anton (1734–1815) An Austrian physician whose system of treatment (known as MESMERISM) was the forerunner of modern-day hypnosis. While still a student at the University of Vienna in 1766, Mesmer discovered the work of the Renaissance mystic physician Paracelsus. He tried to uncover a link between astrology and human health as a result of planetary forces transmitted through a subtle invisible fluid. By 1775, Mesmer began to teach that a person may transmit universal forces to others in the form of "animal magnetism" and based his

therapeutic sessions on those beliefs. During these sessions, several people sat around a vat of dilute sulfuric acid while holding hands or iron bars sticking out of the solution.

Three years later, his beliefs became increasingly unpopular with other physicians and he was forced to leave Austria for Paris, where he continued to maintain a lucrative practice in mesmerism. However, here too physicians did not accept his beliefs. In 1784 King Louis XVI appointed a special scientific commission, which included U.S. statesman and inventor Benjamin Franklin, guillotine inventor J.I. Guillotin, and chemist A.L. Lavoisier, to investigate Mesmer's methods.

Their report found no scientific basis in his methods, noting that his cures were probably the result of a person's own beliefs and imagination, but it was the French Revolution that ended his Parisian practice and sent him into exile in London. Still, those he had taught continued to practice. Among his former students was the Marquis de Puysegur of Buzancy, who treated a young peasant who went into a state that would be today described as a hypnotic trance. Because it was like sleep but more like sleepwalking, Puysegur called the state *artificial somnambulism*; the term later became associated with a highly hypnotizable person. But despite the peasant's alertness during the trance, when he awoke he had no recollection of what had happened. Puysegur had discovered posthypnotic amnesia, which had never before been described, and took the peasant to Paris to meet Mesmer just before Mesmer left for London.

After Mesmer died in 1815, his followers were known as *mesmerists* and their technique was known as *mesmerism*.

mesmerism Also known as *animal magnetism*, this eighteenth-century system of treatment was the forerunner of modern-day hypnosis. Mesmerism was named for Austrian physician Franz Anton Mesmer (see MESMER, FRANZ ANTON) who developed the practice while trying to uncover a link between astrology and health as a result of planetary forces transmitted through a subtle invisible fluid. By 1775, Mesmer began to teach that a person may transmit universal forces to others in the form of "animal magnetism" and based his therapeutic sessions on those beliefs. During these sessions, several people sat around a vat of dilute sulfuric acid while holding hands or iron bars sticking out of the solution. After he died in 1815, his followers were known as *mesmerists* and their technique was known as *mermerism*. One of his followers, Abbe Faria, renamed somnambulism *lucid sleep* and criticized Mesmer's theory that some sort of fluid transferred from the operator to the patient. He was one of the first to understand that the ability of a person to enter lucid sleep depended more on the patient than on the mesmerist. During the nineteenth century, mesmerism was renamed *hypnotism* after the Greek god of sleep (Hypnos), and the practice began to receive attention from the medical community of the time.

microcephaly An abnormally small head, usually associated with MENTAL RETARDATION, that is linked with fetal BRAIN DAMAGE during rubella (German measles) or if the mother is exposed to X RAYS early in pregnancy. Microcephaly may also be caused by brain damage during birth or after injury or disease in early infancy. There is no treatment for this condition.

midbrain Also known as the MESENCEPHALON, this is one of the three divisions of the BRAINSTEM. Found in the upper part of the brainstem situated above the PONS, the midbrain serves as a connecting link between the HINDBRAIN and the FOREBRAIN. The midbrain is the origin of the cranial nerves that control five of the six muscles that move the eye and the muscle that controls the size and reactions of the pupils; it helps maintain balance and receives information about positioning of muscles around eyes and jaw.

The mesencephalon is made up of three main parts: the tectum (containing auditory and visual relay stations, called the inferior and superior colliculi), the tegmentum (containing the midbrain RETICULAR FORMATION that controls attention, the SUBSTANTIA NIGRA and the red nucleus, both of which are involved in motor control.

migraine The severe HEADACHE known as migraine, with accompanying symptoms of nausea, diarrhea, visual disturbances, and *depression*, attack about 8 million Americans— 75 percent of them women. They are believed to be linked to changes in the levels of ESTROGEN and SEROTONIN. Depression and STRESS also contribute to migraines.

Because of the suspected role of serotonin in migraine attacks, some doctors have been successful in treating them with small doses of one of the new antidepressants, Prozac, Zoloft, or Paxil, which act exclusively on the serotonin system.

What's clear is that the old belief of a "migraine personality" is untrue—migraines are *not* associated with those who are ambitious, orderly, obsessive, and rigid. These character traits were first proposed in 1937 and have been perpetuated ever since as a stereotypical explanation for a migraine attack. While it may be true that some migraine sufferers may develop a tense personality in reaction to their illness, this tension may really be a way to control their lives, which are often disrupted by these headaches.

milacemide (2-n-pentylaminoacetamide) Some studies have shown that this nootropic drug appears to improve human selective attention, word retrieval, numeric memory, and vigilance. Milacemide crosses the blood-brain barrier, where it is converted in the brain to glycinamide and then glycine and interacts with brain receptors associated with long-term potentiation of memory.

In one study, milacemide enhanced the speed and accuracy of word retrieval in healthy humans, although the effect was selective. Source memory (memory of the context in which a fact was learned) improved significantly, but item memory (memory of the fact itself) did not.

However, the drug appears to enhance memory only in normal subjects; according to studies, it was not effective in the treatment of ALZHEIMER'S DISEASE patients. It is not currently approved by the Food and Drug Administration for use in the treatment of age-associated memory impairment.

mild head injury Even the mildest bump on the head is still capable of doing damage to the brain; in fact, research suggests that 60 percent of patients who sustain a mild brain injury are still having symptoms after three months.

Mild head-injury symptoms can result in a puzzling interplay of behavioral, cognitive, and emotional complaints that make it difficult to diagnose. Although research is still limited, studies have found that symptoms following even the mildest head injury can linger, causing ongoing discomfort and interfering with personal lives.

But until recently, diagnostic tools were not sensitive enough to detect the subtle structural changes that can occur and sometimes persist after mild head injury. A small minority are plagued by symptoms, including HEADACHE, dizziness, confusion, and memory loss, that may continue for months. Typically, CAT SCANS have yielded negative results for this group of patients. But studies involving MAGNETIC RESONANCE IMAGING (MRI) and brain electrophysiology indicate that contusions and diffuse axonal injuries associated with mild head injury are likely to affect those parts of the brain that relate to functions such as memory, concentration, information processing, and problem solving.

A 1981 study of 424 patients diagnosed with mild head injury showed that many had recurrent problems with deviant behavior, headaches, dizziness, and cognitive problems; only 17 percent of these patients were symptom-free three months after the accident. A separate 1987 study found that 47 percent of these subjects still had symptoms three months after the accident. A third study in 1989 reached similar conclusions.

Only 12 percent of patients with mild head injury are hospitalized overnight, and instructions they receive upon leaving the emergency room do not address behavioral, cognitive, and emotional symptoms that can occur after such an injury.

Diagnostic tests

CAT scans While CAT scans are widely available in emergency rooms to assist in the diagnosis of neural HEMATOMAS, many experts believe these scans may not pick up the subtle damage following a mild head injury.

MRI Many researchers believe MRI is more sensitive in diagnosing many brain lesions beyond a basic hematoma. For example, MRI is more sensitive in detecting the diffuse axonal or shearing injury, and contusions often seen in mild head injury.

Quantitative EEG (qEEG) In many patients, neither CAT nor MRI can detect the microscopic damage to white matter that occurs when fibers are stretched in a mild, diffuse axonal injury. In this type of mild injury, the AXONS lose some of their covering and become less efficient, but MRI only detects more severe injury and actual axonal degeneration. Mild injury to the WHITE MATTER reduces the quality of communication between neurons in any part of the brain. A quantitative EEG is an enhanced form of an EEG in that the signals from the brain are played into a computer, digitized, and stored. This type of

EEG can measure the time delay between two regions of the CORTEX, and the amount of time it takes for information to be transmitted from one region to another.

Evoked potentials This electrophysical technique is not generally useful in patients with less-serious mild head injury. EPs are not sensitive enough to document any physiologic abnormalities, although the patient may be having symptoms. If testing is done within a day or two of injury, the EP may pick up some abnormalities in BRAINSTEM auditory-evoked potentials.

Neuropsychological testing These tests may show positive results when imaging tests and neurologic exams are negative. In some patients with persistent symptoms following mild head injury, neuropsychological tests are part of a comprehensive assessment. The tests can also provide information when litigation is an issue.

Future tests PET (POSITRON EMISSION TOMOGRA-PHY), which evaluates cerebral blood flow and brain metabolism, may provide useful information on functional pathology. SINGLE PHOTO EMISSION COMPUTED TOMOGRAPHY (SPECT) is less expensive than PET and might provide data on cerebral blood flow after mild head injury.

Patients who do experience symptoms are advised to seek out the care of a specialist; unless a family physician is thoroughly familiar with medical literature in this newly emerging area, there is a great chance patient complaints will be ignored, according to MHI experts. Instead, patients with continuing symptoms following a mild head injury are advised to call a local head-injury foundation, which can then refer patients to the best nearby practitioner.

minimal brain dysfunction An outdated term for minor delay or dysfunction in the development of motor skills and the ability to use the senses properly. This general term has been used in the past to describe disor-ders now called LEARNING DISABILITIES or ATTEN-TION DEFICIT HYPERACTIVITY DISORDER (ADHD).

molecular neurobiology The study of genes, proteins, and other microscopic elements of NEURONS and other cells making up the brain and NERVOUS SYSTEM.

Mongolism See GENETIC DISORDERS OF THE BRAIN.

monoamine oxidase (MAO) An enzyme found in most tissues of the body that triggers the oxidation and breakdown of a large number of monoamines (such as EPINEPHRINE, NOREPINEPHRINE, and SEROTONIN).

monoamine oxidase (MAO) inhibitors and the brain Antidepressants known as MONOAMINE OXIDASE *inhibitors* work by blocking the breakdown of monoamines (SEROTONIN, NOREPINEPHRINE, and DOPAMINE) by an enzyme in the brain called *monoamine oxidase.* When the NEUROTRANSMITTERS are not broken down, they start piling up in the brain—and because DEPRESSION is associated with low levels of these monoamines, it's not surprising that *increasing* the monoamines eases depressive symptoms.

Unfortunately, monoamine oxidase doesn't just break down those neurotransmitters; it's also responsible for mopping up another amine called tyramine, a molecule that affects blood pressure. When monoamine oxidase becomes blocked and the monoamine levels rise, levels of tyramine begins to rise, too. While a hike in neurotransmitters may be beneficial, an increase in tyramine can be disastrous. Excess tyramine can cause a sudden, sometimes fatal, increase in blood pressure which is so severe that it can burst blood vessels in the brain.

Every time a person eats chicken liver, aged cheese, broad-bean pods or pickled herring, tyramine levels increase in the brain. Normally, MAO enzymes take care of this potentially harmful tyramine excess. But if a person is taking a MAO *inhibitor*, the MAO enzyme can't stop tyramine from building up. This is exactly what happened when the drugs were first introduced in the 1960s. Because no one knew about the tyramine connection, a wave of deaths from brain hemorrhages swept the country. Other patients taking MAO inhibitors experienced severe HEADACHES caused by the rise in blood pressure. These early side effects were particularly disturbing because nobody knew why they were happening.

The mystery was solved when a British pharmacist noticed that his wife, who was taking MAO inhibitors, had headaches when she ate cheese. But the early MAOIs were considered so dangerous (they also can damage liver, brain, and cardiovascular systems) that even when the MAO-tyramine connection was finally understood, these drugs were taken off the American market for a time. (A related European antidepressant drug, Deprenyl, is marketed in this country as an anti-Parkinson medication; it requires less stringent dietary precautions.)

Eventually the MAOIs were reintroduced in this country despite the tyramine risk because some depressed people don't respond to any other medication. Nevertheless, MAO inhibitors are usually the antidepressant of last resort.

See SELECTIVE SEROTONIN REUPTAKE INHIBITORS.

mood See EMOTIONS AND THE BRAIN; LIMBIC SYSTEM.

morphine and the brain Morphine is the main component of opium and was first isolated in 1805 by a German chemist who named the opiate after Morpheus, the Greek god of dreams. Since then, chemists have been able to make other types of OPIATES by slightly altering the morphine molecule. For example, heroin is made by adding two acetyl groups to the morphine molecule, which enable the heroin to enter quickly into the brain, causing the much-desired "rush."

Scientists discovered that the brain contains special opiate RECEPTORS that allow opiate molecules to act on human BRAIN CELLS. Morphine and other opiates resemble molecules produced by the brain itself, called ENDORPHINS or ENKEPHALINS (Greek for "in the head"). Scientists found a high concentration of opiate receptors in the SUBSTANTIA GELATINOSA, which is where pain nerves first connect with the SPINAL CORD. There were also clusters of opiate receptors in the THALAMUS, which is partly involved with deep, lasting pain—the kind that the opiates work best in controlling. There were more opiate receptors in the MIDBRAIN, where pain signals are processed.

Opiates relieve pain not by eliminating it, but by making the patient indifferent to it. The reason is that the morphine acts not on the nerves that transmit pain sensations to the brain, but on the brain and spinal-cord centers that integrate incoming pain information.

The location of the opiate receptors also explains some of the other effects of morphine and its derivatives. For example, heroin addicts typically exhibit tiny pinpoint pupils in the eyes; this is because there are many opiate receptors in the pretectal nuclei, located in the brain area that controls pupil size.

In addition, opiates can kill by interfering with breathing because there are many opiate receptors in the medulla, pons and the nucleus of the solitary tract, areas of the brain controlling breathing.

Addiction/tolerance While a drug addiction does have psychological factors, there are also physiological reasons behind these side effects. When an addict constantly supplies morphine to the NERVE CELLS, they bind to opiate receptors in the brain, triggering a cutback in the body's own production of endorphins. Tolerance occurs because the normal production of endorphins stops and the body then needs more and more outside opiates to meet its needs.

When the drug is stopped, withdrawal symptoms occur because the body needs some time to start to produces its own opiates to replace those supplied from the drug. The brain can't function normally because some of its neuromodulators are missing, and the addict will experience the side effects of withdrawal (agitation, sleeplessness, DEPRESSION, unusual pain sensitivity, stomach cramps, and diarrhea) until the body's endorphin production returns to normal.

motor aphasia See BROCA'S APHASIA.

motor area See MOTOR CORTEX.

motor association The oldest form of memory in the biological world, this type of memory is responsible for the fact that once a human learns to ride a bicycle, the motor memory of the experience is never forgotten.

Birds and mammals can remember both sensory and motor associations, but animals farther down the evolutionary ladder (such as fruit flies, cockroaches, and flatworms) can form only motor associations.

Research with cabbage butterflies in 1986 revealed that motor associations enhance survival; while individual butterflies visit flowers of one species, the motor memories of experienced butterflies enable them to work more quickly and obtain more nectar from flowers. Because each flower requires a different method to obtain nectar from it, cabbage butterflies who can select one single species are more productive. Scientists know that recognition depends on memory and not on instinct because different cabbage butterflies favor different species; experiments have shown that if necessary, cabbage butter-

flies will change to a new species and become faithful to those flowers.

motor cortex Part of the CEREBRAL CORTEX (pre-central gyrus) that extends from ear to ear across the roof of the brain, concerned with movement and coordination. It lies just in front of the SENSORY CORTEX (post-central gyrus). Each hemisphere's motor cortex controls the muscles on the opposite side of the body so that if the function of the right motor cortex is impaired, muscles on the left side of the body will be paralyzed.

A variety of regions in the CENTRAL NERVOUS SYSTEM send input to the motor cortex: the sensory cortex, the premotor and supplementary motor areas, the BASAL GANGLIA, and the CEREBELLUM.

The corticospinal tract connects the motor cortex to the motor neurons in the SPINAL CORD and BRAINSTEM; this descending tract also branches out to other structures important in motor activity. Damage to this tract can cause a loss of voluntary movement below the damaged area, although reflex activity will persist because reflex resides segmentally in the spinal cord.

motor homunculus The term (Latin for "little men") for the map representing the body parts and their relative size according to how much of the MOTOR CORTEX is devoted to each. If you electrically stimulate area to area in the motor cortex, different parts of the body respond. If you draw a map of these activated body areas as they are represented in each region of the motor cortex, you will see a distorted image of a man—a homunculus.

motor nerve A nerve devoted to carrying impulses outward from the CENTRAL NERVOUS SYSTEM to activate a muscle or gland, also called efferent fibers.

motor-neuron disease A progressive degenerative disease of the nerves that control muscles usually beginning in middle age, causing muscle weakness and wasting. Speech or swallowing may deteriorate, with wasting and weakness in muscles of the tongue, hands, and other parts of the body. It primarily affects the motor cells of the SPINAL CORD, the motor nuclei in the BRAINSTEM, and the corticospinal fibers. The three distinct forms of motor-neuron disease include AMYOTROPHIC LATERAL SCLEROSIS (ALS), progressive muscular atrophy, and progressive bulbar palsy. Though the latter two conditions start with patterns of muscle weakness different from ALS, they usually develop into that disease.

Two types of motor-neuron disease (usually inherited) affect much younger patients: infantile progressive spinal muscular atrophy (Werdnig-Hoffmann paralysis) affects infants at birth or shortly after with weakness progressing to death in several months to several years, with rare exceptions. A milder form, chronic spinal muscular dystrophy, begins from childhood through adolescence and causes progressive weakness that may never cause serious problems. The cause is unknown.

See also DEGENERATIVE DISEASES.

Treatment Weakness usually spreads to the muscles needed for breathing within four years, but exceptions do occur. Some people have lived more than 20 years after the initial diagnosis. While scientists have no way to slow the degeneration of the nerves, they may be able to lessen disability. Care is usually aimed at lessening discomfort.

motor neurons The final neuron in the brain-to-muscle pathway that carry nerve impulses to muscles, controlling muscular activity.

See also DEGENERATIVE DISEASES; MOTOR-NEURON DISEASE.

motor system disease See MOTOR NEURON DISEASE.

MRI The abbreviation for MAGNETIC RESONANCE IMAGING.

multi-infarct dementia One of the two most common incurable forms of mental impairment in old age, caused by a series of small STROKES that result in widespread death of brain tissue. Multi-infarct dementia causes a step-by-step degeneration in mental ability, with each step occurring after a stroke; memory (especially of recent events) is affected first.

Multi-infarct dementia accounts for about 20 percent of the irreversible cases of mental impairment. In the early stages before severe damage has been done, the person usually is aware of impaired ability, which can lead to frustration and DEPRESSION.

Cause Multi-infarct dementia (and the strokes that cause it) are usually the result of an underlying medical condition, such as high blood pressure and artery damage.

Diagnosis Those who are suspected to have multi-infarct dementia should have thorough physical, neurological, and psychiatric evaluations, including a complete medical exam and tests of mental state together with a BRAIN SCAN. The brain scan can rule out curable diseases and may also show signs of normal age-related changes in the brain, such as shrinkage.

Treatment Prevention is really the only effective treatment for multi-infarct dementia; patients with high blood pressure, TRANSIENT ISCHEMIC ATTACKS, or earlier strokes should continue treatment for these diseases to minimize the chance of developing DEMENTIA.

While there is no cure for multi-infarct dementia, careful use of drugs can lessen agitation, anxiety, and depression and improve sleep. Proper nutrition is especially important, and the patient should be encouraged to maintain normal daily routines, physical activities, and contact with friends. Stimulate the patient by providing information about time of day, place of residence, and what is going on in the home and the world; this can help prevent brain activity from failing at a faster rate. Memory aids, such as a visible calendar, lists of daily activities, safety guidelines, and directions to commonly used items, may also help people in their day-to-day living.

multiple sclerosis A degenerative disease of the CENTRAL NERVOUS SYSTEM believed to involve the immune system, which attacks the MYELIN (protective covering of nerve fibers), disrupting function and causing paralysis and, in some patients, memory loss as a result of dysfunctioning FRONTAL and TEMPORAL LOBES. The severity of the disease varies considerably among patients.

The disease usually appears in early adult life in women more than in men and among whites more often than among blacks or Asians. The disease occurs in one in every 1,000 people in temperate zones. Some people have a single attack with no recurrence; others have periods when the disease is active (called exacerbations) and times when they are symptom-free (remissions). Finally, some have a chronic, progressive form of the disease that becomes increasingly severe.

Cause The cause of MS is unknown, but it is thought to be an autoimmune disease in which the body's own defense system treats myelin as an invader, gradually destroying it. While MS is not considered to be a genetic disorder, there seems to be a genetic factor because relatives of affected people are eight times more likely than others to contract the disease. It is believed that the environment may also play a part; the area in which a child spends the first 15 years of life affects future risk of contracting the disease. (MS is five times more common in temperate-zone continents such as the United States and Europe.) It is believed by some that this environmental relationship may involve a slow virus, picked up during a susceptible time of early life, that triggers an autoimmune disorder in which the body attacks its own tissue.

Recent research suggests that some kinds of antibodies in the immune system may help repair myelin, which may explain the disease's remissions. These antibodies may promise a treatment or even a cure in the future if the antibody level can be increased.

Symptoms Symptoms vary widely depending on the part of the brain that is affected. They can include tingling, numbness, muscle weakness, muscle cramps, lack of coordination, paralysis, blurry or double vision, abnormal fatigue, confusion, forgetfulness, incontinence, and impaired sexual function; memory loss does not often appear immediately but may occur years later.

Diagnosis Confirmation of the disease usually comes only after other diseases have been ruled out; a NEUROLOGIST may perform tests to help confirm the diagnosis, including LUMBAR PUNCTURE (removal of a fluid from the spinal canal for lab analysis) or testing electrical activity in the brain via BRAIN SCANS.

Treatment At present, there is no cure. However, the drug interferon beta-1b (brand name: Betaseron) reduces the number of flare-ups in people with relapsing-remitting MS. Research suggests that the drug can help those who are mildly disabled, are still able to walk, and have frequent worsening of symptoms. Flare-ups include blurred vision, slurred speech, and problems with strength or coordination. The drug does not reverse existing neurologic problems or prevent permanent disability.

This is the first drug to offer more than symptomatic relief, and it has been put on the "accelerated approval" path by the U.S. Food and Drug Administration. This means that while it is being distributed, it is in short supply and patients must apply to receive the drug from physicians. In 1995, Betaseron is expected to be available to anyone with relapsing-remitting MS.

Side effects of Betaseron include inflammation at the injection site, flulike symptoms, and severe DEPRESSION.

Corticosteroid drugs may alleviate some acute symptoms, and other drugs may help incontinence and depression.

Prognosis MS does not shorten life span, and most people with the disease can lead fairly normal lives. Recent studies have found that, contrary to earlier beliefs, pregnancy does not worsen symptoms and does not affect the long-term course of the disease. However, some experts caution that a parent with MS may not have the physical stamina to care for a baby or an active child and may need some child care help. For more information, contact the NATIONAL MULTIPLE SCLEROSIS SOCIETY; for address, see Appendix A.

Multiple Sclerosis Foundation A national support group that provides funding for research into the cause, prevention, treatment, and cure of MULTIPLE SCLEROSIS. The foundation provides information, referral and support services, and health-care options. Founded in 1986, the foundation publishes a quarterly newsletter and brochures. For address, see Appendix A.

See also MULTIPLE SCLEROSIS SOCIETY.

muscular dystrophy A term covering a group of common neuromuscular diseases characterized by progressive weakening and wasting of skeletal muscles. They are caused by the death of muscle fibers, cellular reaction and replacement of muscle tissue by connective tissue. There is no cure; treatment is supportive.

Muscular Dystrophy (MD) Association National volunteer health agency fostering research into the cause and cure of neuromuscular diseases, including muscular dystrophies, MOTOR-NEURON DISEASES (including AMYO-

TROPHIC LATERAL SCLEROSIS), inflammatory myopathies, diseases of neuromuscular junction (including MYASTHENIA GRAVIS), diseases of the peripheral nerve (including FRIEDREICH'S ATAXIA and charcot-marie-tooth), metabolic diseases of muscle, and myopathies due to endocrine abnormalities.

The association supports international programs of more than 400 research awards, major university-based neuromuscular disease research and clinical centers, and 240 outpatient clinics in hospitals in the United States and Puerto Rico.

Services for patients in local chapters include diagnostic exams, follow-up medical evaluations, wheelchairs, physical therapy, and summer camps.

Founded in 1950, the association publishes a newsletter, research updates, and literature. For address, see Appendix A.

myasthenia gravis A chronic neurologic disease affecting the neuromuscular transmission of the voluntary muscles characterized by marked fatigue and weakness of certain muscles. The fatigue is so profound that muscles are temporarily paralyzed. It primarily affect teenagers and young adults (women are more often affected, in a 3 to 2 ratio) and adults over age 40. The disease is rare, affecting only two to five people per 100,000 people each year.

Cause The body's immune system attacks and destroys the cholinergic RECEPTORS in muscles. These receptors bind acetylcholine, the neurotransmitter released from motor neurons. As a result, nerve impulses are normal but the muscle can't respond.

Symptoms This disease is extremely variable in the ways in which it affects different people and in the same person at different times. The affected muscles become worse with use, but they may recover completely with rest. Patients typically experience remissions interspersed with relapses of the condition. In addition to fatigue and weakness, symptoms include drooping of the upper eyelid, double vision, and speech problems. Patients with this disease tire even when so slight an exertion as combing the hair, chewing, or talking. Between 15 and 20 percent of patients complain of arm and hand muscle weakness; leg muscle weakness is less common. Progressive weakness of the diaphragm and nearby muscles may produce breathing problems or myasthenic crisis, which is an acute emergency.

Myasthenic crisis is the sudden onset of muscular weakness in myasthenia gravis patients and is usually the result of undermedication, or lack of medication. It may also result from progression of the disease, emotional upset, systemic infection, some drugs, surgery, or trauma. Symptoms of this crisis include sudden breathing problems and an inability to swallow or speak. Weakness of respiratory and laryngeal muscles can depress breathing and obstruct the patient's airway if not treated promptly.

In mild cases, the patient can lead a comparatively normal life. In a few patients, however, the disease's progression can't be stopped; paralysis of the throat and respiratory muscles may be fatal.

Treatment In some patients with mild conditions, regular medication helps transmit nerve impulses to muscles and is often enough to restore the patient's condition to near normal. Anticholinesterase drugs increase the concentration of available acetylcholine, helping to activate what receptors are left; this yields an increase in the response of the muscles to nerve impulses, thereby improving strength. These drugs do not cure the disease but do improve symptoms. Drugs in current use include pyridostigmine bromide (Mestinon), ambenonium chloride (Mytelase), and neostigmine bromide (Prostigmin). Most patients prefer Mestinon because it provides fewer side effects.

Side effects include abdominal cramps, nausea and vomiting, and diarrhea.

Other treatment includes immunosuppressive therapy to remove circulating antibodies, including the administration of corticosteroids, plasmapheresis (blood plasma exchange), and surgical removal of the thymus. Plasmaphersis temporarily reduces circulating harmful antibodies and can markedly improve some patients' condition; it does not treat the underlying disorder.

Because the thymus appears to be involved in the production of harmful antibodies, in severe cases its removal causes substantial remission of the disease and sometimes appears to cure the problem.

myelin The white cells (fatty material composed of lipids and proteins) that form a protective sheath around some types of nerve fibers and help facilitate electrical impulse transmission. Myelin also acts as an electrical insulator, increasing the efficiency of nerve conduction. It is myelin that gives the white color to the WHITE MATTER of the brain, composed primarily of myelinated nerve fibers.

The abnormal breakdown of myelin, such as in MULTIPLE SCLEROSIS, is called demyelination, and seriously disrupts normal impulse conduction.

myelin sheath The protein covering that surrounds axonal fibers.

See also MULTIPLE SCLEROSIS; MYELIN.

myelogram An X-RAY examination of the brain and SPINAL CORD to look for tumors or spinal-cord injury. The technique begins with a LUMBAR PUNCTURE (spinal tap), in which a small amount of CEREBROSPINAL FLUID is removed and replaced with a contrasting fluid that will show up on X-ray film. The patient is tiled while a series of X rays are taken at different angles; most of the contrast fluid is then removed. The study is performed to see if excess myelin is in the CSF; this can indicate demyelination.

Side effects The procedure is uncomfortable, and common side effects include nausea, vomiting, flushing, pressure, HEADACHE, and some pain (especially when the fluid is removed). While serious side effects are rare, they may include possible infection and allergy to the contrast dye.

myelography A specialized method of X-RAY examination of the spinal canal that involves injection of a radiopaque contrast medium into the SUBARACHNOID SPACE. The X rays that results are called myelograms. This technique is used to recognize tumors of the SPINAL CORD and other conditions that compress the nerve roots. See MYELOGRAM.

The procedure may cause feelings of pressure or nausea, although these effects should be minimized. Afterward, patients may experience a HEADACHE because of changes in the pressure of the CEREBROSPINAL FLUID (CSF); lying down will help alleviate this headache, which is usually brief.

Before the test, most patients are hospitalized, and no food or drink are given for several hours beforehand. A sedative may be given; the procedure usually takes between 45 and 90 minutes.

While noninvasive tests such as CAT SCANS or MAGNETIC RESONANCE IMAGING provide good resolution for diagnosis of spinal problems, myelography may be preferred because of its sharp resolution; fluid obtained during the procedure may provide additional information about cancer, inflammation, and evidence of infection.

Technique In the procedure, a needle is inserted between two of the lower vertebrae and a small amount of cerebrospinal fluid is withdrawn. Contrast media is injected slowly through the LUMBAR-PUNCTURE needle, and a series of X rays are taken to show the configuration of the space around the spinal cord and whether it is distorted by a protruding disc or bony spur. The table is tilted to move the medium to the location of the suspected disorder in the spine. Most contrast dyes are absorbed by the blood and excreted in the urine and do not usually have to be removed when the procedure is over.

Risks Some conditions (tumors or herniated discs) may be made worse by the change in CSF pressure, requiring an emergency operation. Significant complications are
rare.

myelomeningocele A severe and common form of SPINA BIFIDA.

N

naloxone A chemical which can bind to the opiate receptor sites in the brain instead of ENDORPHIN but which has no pain-controlling ability. An opiate antagonist, it binds to an opiate receptor without activating it. By binding, it blocks true endogenous opiates from binding and activating.

narcolepsy An often-inherited physical disorder of the brain characterized by irresistible daytime sleep attacks and drowsiness, automatic behavior, cataplexy, sleep paralysis, hypnagogic hallucinations, and disrupted nighttime sleep. In narcolepsy, the RAPID EYE MOVEMENT (REM) STATE OF SLEEP appears during waking cycles; attacks of sleepiness may last up to an hour long and can be severely disabling. About three-quarters of patients also have cataplexy (the sudden loss of muscle tone while awake). Other symptoms include vivid HALLUCINATIONS when falling asleep or awakening.

Recent research suggests that abnormal levels of DOPAMINE may be an underlying cause of the condition. Preliminary studies with a drug that increases the activity of dopamine, a chemical associated with alertness, has suggested promising results. Other treatment includes regular naps together with stimulant drugs to control drowsiness accompanied by antidepressants to suppress cataplexy.

See also AMERICAN NARCOLEPSY ASSOCIATION; NARCOLEPSY AND CATAPLEXY FOUNDATION OF AMERICA.

Narcolepsy and Cataplexy Foundation of America A national support group for those with NARCOLEPSY that disseminates information to public and professionals, encourages formation of support services, maintains a library, and publishes brochures. For address, see Appendix A.

See also ASSOCIATION OF SLEEP DISORDERS CENTER; NARCOLEPSY AND CATAPLEXY FOUNDATION OF AMERICA.

narcotics and the brain Narcotics (drugs that induce stupor and relieve pain) primarily include MORPHINE and other derivatives of opium, although the term also applies to other drugs that depress brain function, such as general anesthetics and hypnotics. In legal terms, a narcotic is any addictive drug that can be illegally abused.

Morphine and morphinelike narcotics have been largely replaced as sleeping drugs because of their ability to cause dependence and tolerance, but they are still used for relief of severe pain.

National Alliance for the Mentally Ill (NAMI) A national alliance of self-help and advocacy groups concerned with severe and chronic mentally ill individuals. The group's objectives are to provide emotional support and practical guidance to families and to educate and inform the public about mental illness. The alliance conducts consumer advocacy activities at the local, state, and national levels to enact legislation and to promote funding for institutional and community-based settings for the seriously mentally ill. It also refers callers to its more than 600 state and local affiliates.

In addition, the alliance monitors and assures quality treatment, rehabilitation, and support services; promotes research; disseminates information and resources; and operates a speakers' bureau. Founded in 1979, the group has 130,000 members and publishes brochures, handbooks, and newsletters. For address, see Appendix A.

See also MENTAL ILLNESS; NATIONAL ALLIANCE FOR RESEARCH ON SCHIZOPHRENIA AND DEPRESSION; SCHIZOPHRENIA.

National Alliance for Research on Schizophrenia and Depression A professional organization that raises funds for research on SCHIZOPHRENIA, DEPRESSION, and other mental illnesses. Affiliated with the NATIONAL ALLIANCE FOR THE MENTALLY ILL, the NATIONAL DEPRESSIVE AND MANIC DEPRESSIVE ASSOCIATION, and the NATIONAL MENTAL HEALTH ASSOCIATION, the group was founded in 1986 and publishes a quarterly newsletter. For address, see Appendix A.

National Association of Developmental Disabilities Councils A group of state and territorial councils that work to improve the lives of people with developmental disabilities and that promotes cooperation and communication among federal agencies, state governments, volunteer groups and other organizations, and individual state and territorial councils. The association also educates and informs the public about the needs of those with developmental disabilities and works within the Washington, D.C., community to represent the views of developmental disabilities councils. Serving as an information clearinghouse, the group develops small groups of experts to consider issues of special concern. Founded in 1975, the group publishes a monthly newsletter, monographs, and reports.

See also ASSOCIATION FOR CHILDREN WITH DOWN SYNDROME; ASSOCIATION FOR CHILDREN WITH RETARDED MENTAL DEVELOPMENT; ASSOCIATION FOR RETARDED CITIZENS; CENTER FOR FAMILY SUPPORT; FEDERATION FOR CHILDREN WITH SPECIAL NEEDS; JEWISH ASSOCIATION FOR RETARDED CHILDREN; MENTAL RETARDATION ASSOCIATION OF AMERICA; NATIONAL DOWN SYNDROME CONGRESS; NATIONAL DOWN SYNDROME SOCIETY; PARENTS OF CHILDREN WITH DOWN SYNDROME; PILOT PARENTS; VOICE OF THE RETARDED; YOUNG ADULT INSTITUTE AND WORKSHOP.

National Ataxia Foundation A professional organization open to any individual who wishes to contribute to the eradication of ATAXIA, a genetic disease characterized by the degeneration of the nerves in the SPINAL CORD and the CEREBELLUM, causing a loss of coordination and disturbance in gait. The foundation provides information and referrals and publishes various materials, including a quarterly newsletter, videos, and brochures.

The group hopes to make an early diagnosis of ataxia by locating all potential victims and encouraging them to have an examination, to educate the public and the helping professions about ataxia, to initiate basic research, and to coordinate the efforts of worldwide research centers. The foundation members hope to locate a possible biochemical or structural abnormality underlying this condition; to this end, the foundation holds clinics for the identification of new cases of ataxia among those recognized as potential patients and provides service and information to ataxia patients and their families. Founded in 1957, the group has 1,000 members. For address, see Appendix B.

National Attention-Deficit Disorder Association A national support group for those who have attention deficit disorders (ADD), their families, and local support groups which want national affiliation. The association seeks to promote a greater public awareness of the needs of those with ADD and tries to address educational, psychological, and social needs. Founded in 1989, the group publishes a bimonthly newsletter. For address, see Appendix A.

National Brain Injury Research Foundation A research group that sponsors research on brain injuries, sponsors charitable and educational programs, maintains library and speakers' bureaus, and bestows awards. Founded in 1987, the group has 2,500 members and holds a semiannual conference. It publishes the semiannual newsletter *JMA Bulletin*; the quarterly *Journal of Head*

Injury, and brochures. For address, see Appendix A.

National Center for Learning Disabilities
A national voluntary organization promoting increased public awareness of LEARNING DISABILITIES that provides referrals to volunteers, parents, and professionals working with the learning disabled. The center publishes a state-by-state guide to programs, schools, services, and organizations, including information such as warning signals, rights, work, glossary, etc. Founded in 1977, the group has 4,000 members and publishes a triennial newsletter and an annual magazine. For address, see Appendix A.

See also ASSOCIATION FOR CHILDREN AND ADULTS WITH LEARNING DISABILITIES; COUNCIL FOR LEARNING DISABILITIES; LEARNING DISABILITIES ASSOCIATION OF AMERICA; NATIONAL NETWORKER; ORTON DYSLEXIA SOCIETY; TIME OUT TO ENJOY (TOTE);

National Coalition for Research in Neurological Disorders A professional association that represents health agencies and professional societies concerned with obtaining funds for neurological research. The group provides information about the fields of NEUROLOGY and NEUROSURGERY, and lobbies for increased funding for training and research in neurological disorders. Founded in 1952, the group has 57 members and publishes a quarterly *NCR News.* For address, see Appendix B.

National Down Syndrome Congress A national support group for families of those with DOWN SYNDROME (DS), educators, health professionals, and other interested individuals. The organization answers questions from parents for assistance with health concerns and refers them to local groups. The congress works to promote the welfare of persons with Down syndrome. The congress promotes the belief that persons with DS have the right to a normal and dignified life, particularly in the

areas of education, medical care, employment, and human services. The group examines issues of social policy and conditions that limit the full growth and potential of children and adults with Down syndrome. The group assists parents on possible solutions to the needs of the child with DS, coordinates efforts and activities of local parents' organizations, and acts as a clearinghouse of information.

Founded in 1973, the group has 5,000 members and publishes a newsletter 10 times a year. For address, see Appendix A.

See also ASSOCIATION FOR CHILDREN WITH DOWN SYNDROME; ASSOCIATION FOR CHILDREN WITH RETARDED MENTAL DEVELOPMENT; CENTER FOR FAMILY SUPPORT; FEDERATION FOR CHILDREN WITH SPECIAL NEEDS; JARC; MENTAL RETARDATION ASSOCIATION OF AMERICA; NATIONAL ASSOCIATION OF DEVELOPMENTAL DISABILITIES COUNCILS; NATIONAL DOWN SYNDROME SOCIETY; PARENTS OF CHILDREN WITH DOWN SYNDROME; PILOT PARENTS; VOICE OF THE RETARDED; YOUNG ADULT INSTITUTE AND WORKSHOP.

National Down Syndrome Society A national support group devoted to research into the causes and treatment of DOWN SYNDROME that works to increase public awareness of the condition, raises funds to support all areas of Down syndrome research, and sponsors educational programs. The group provides information and referral for families and professionals and develops programs and services for families and for individuals with Down syndrome. Founded in 1979, the group publishes a directory of parent support groups and early intervention programs, brochures, and booklets. For address, see Appendix A.

See also ASSOCIATION FOR CHILDREN WITH DOWN SYNDROME; ASSOCIATION FOR CHILDREN WITH RETARDED MENTAL DEVELOPMENT; CENTER FOR FAMILY-SUPPORT; FEDERATION FOR CHILDREN WITH SPECIAL NEEDS; JARC; MENTAL RETARDATION ASSOCIATION OF AMERICA; NATIONAL ASSOCIATION OF DEVELOPMENTAL DISABILITIES COUNCILS; NATIONAL DOWN

SYNDROME CONGRESS; PARENTS OF CHILDREN WITH DOWN SYNDROME; PILOT PARENTS; VOICE OF THE RETARDED; YOUNG ADULT INSTITUTE AND WORKSHOP.

National Foundation for Brain Research
A foundation dedicated to preventing and curing disorders of the brain, this group collects, organizes, and disseminates information relating to the 1990s as the Decade of the Brain. The group maintains the Decade of the Brain Coalition, which strives to achieve by the end of the decade a large increase in federal funding for research on the brain. It also hopes to increase public awareness of the importance of brain research by producing educational TV programs, distributing reports and pamphlets, and operating traveling museum exhibits.

The foundation publishes the quarterly newsletter *Decade of the Brain News* and sponsors an annual Decade of the Brain symposium in Washington, D.C. For address, see Appendix A.

National Headache Foundation
A national support group that offers membership information, sends literature on headaches and their treatment, provides a list of headache specialists, and provides relaxation tapes. For address, see Appendix A.

National Head Injury Foundation
A national support group for people concerned with HEAD INJURY that encourages formation of support groups, acts as an information clearinghouse, and makes referrals. For address, see Appendix A.

National Hydrocephalus Foundation
A national support group for patients with HYDROCEPHALUS, their families, and interested others. The foundation hopes to eliminate the stigma associated with the disease, provide information, define and resolve specific problems of families, collect information about hydrocephalus, and inform parents of

their children's educational rights. The group refers adult hydrocephalics or parents of hydrocephalics to appropriate services, makes referrals, maintains a library, and conduct symposia with physicians in the field. Founded in 1979, the group has 500 members and publishes a quarterly newsletter and a video. For address, see Appendix A.

National Institute of Neurological Disorders and Stroke (NINDS)
One of the federal National Institutes of Health that is responsible for conducting and disseminating research into the brain and related disorders. The institute publishes various materials for both public and health professionals. For address, see Appendix B.

National Multiple Sclerosis Society
This national support group for patients with MULTIPLE SCLEROSIS (MS) and their families stimulates, supports, and coordinates research into the cause, treatment, and cure of MS. The group provides services for patients, helps establish MS clinics and therapy centers, and sponsors public education. The society sponsors the Project Rembrandt, a biennial competition for artists with MS, and maintain numerous committees including international research and medical programs. The society provides information and referrals and offers community services, counseling, training programs for caregivers, swimming programs, vocational rehabilitation, and loans medical equipment. The group maintain a 1,000-volume information resource center and library containing 17,000 reprints, maintains a speakers' bureau, and compiles statistics.

Founded in 1946, the group has 470,000 members and publishes a quarterly magazine. For address, see Appendix A.

National Networker
A national support group for learning disabled adults, for professionals, and for others interested in prob-

lems of LEARNING DISABILITIES. The group seeks to educate, to compile statistics and provide information about LD, and to provide a peer counseling network to help members develop themselves as leaders in this field. Founded in 1982, the group has 2,500 members and publishes a quarterly newsletter. For address, see Appendix A.

See also COUNCIL FOR LEARNING DISABILITIES; LEARNING DISABILITIES ASSOCIATION OF AMERICA; NATIONAL CENTER FOR LEARNING DISABILITIES; ORTON DYSLEXIA SOCIETY; TIME OUT TO ENJOY (TOTE).

National Neurofibromatosis Foundation A national support group for patients with NEUROFIBROMATOSIS (also called Von Recklinghausen's disease) and their families, health-care workers, teachers, and others. The foundation hopes to provide patients and families with information; helps find medical, social, and genetic counseling; provides information to health professionals; and supports scientific research on the cause, prevention, and treatment.

The foundation holds symposia and workshops and compiles statistics. Founded in 1978, the group has 5,500 members and publishes a quarterly newsletter and a quarterly research newsletter. For address, see Appendix A.

National Parkinson Foundation A national support group that provides information, makes physician referrals and provides written materials. For address, see Appendix A.

National Reye's Syndrome Foundation A support group for researchers, health professionals, and families of children who have had REYE'S SYNDROME. The group provides information and raises funds for research into the cause, treatment, cure, and prevention of the disease. The foundation provides support and guidance to families experiencing the syndrome, helps federal and state agencies

obtain data on cases, and encourages government funding. The foundation offers a resource clearinghouse, financial aid programs, support groups, and referral services.

Founded in 1974, the group has 10,000 members and publishes a semiannual newsletter. For address, see Appendix A.

National Spinal Cord Injury Association National support organization for patients with spinal-cord injury and for health-care professionals by supporting research for a cure for paralysis from spinal-cord injury, providing prevention and education programs and services, and helping individuals reach their personal goals. The association sponsors In Touch With Kids, a network of parents of children with spinal-cord injury or disease. The group also conducts recreation, advocacy, support groups, and peer counseling programs and maintains a placement service. Founded in 1948, the group has 9,000 members and publishes an annual directory, a quarterly journal, and a variety of fact sheets. For address, see Appendix A.

See also AMERICAN PARALYSIS ASSOCIATION; AMERICAN SPINAL INJURY ASSOCIATION; SPINAL CORD SOCIETY.

National Stroke Association A national support group for STROKE survivors and their families, health-care professionals, and institutions and the lay community that seeks to reduce the incidence and impact of stroke by promoting research, educating the public, and providing a network for stroke survivors. The group serves as an information referral clearinghouse on stroke and provides information on prevention, treatment, rehabilitation, resocialization, and research. The association also offers guidance in developing stroke support groups and clubs, maintains a speakers' bureau, and compiles statistics. The association also operates the Dwight D. Eisenhower Institute for Stroke Research and maintains a stroke Information and Referral Center.

Founded in 1984, the association has 72,000 members and publishes a quarterly newsletter, a quarterly journal, and various other materials. For address, see Appendix A.

National Tay-Sachs and Allied Diseases Association, Inc. A support group that offers information on education, family service, prevention, and research programs concerning TAY-SACHS and other degenerative lysosomal and brain diseases in infants and children. The association serves as a referral service on all aspects of Tay-Sachs, promotes mass screening programs and appropriate legislation, and sponsors International Quality Control and Reference Sample Center for TSD labs. The group offers support groups and services for parents, compiles statistics, and operates a speakers' bureau.

Founded in 1956, the group has 5,000 members and publishes books, a semiannual newsletter and makes available sound and slide or video materials. For address, see Appendix A.

National Tuberous Sclerosis Association A national support group for families affected by TUBEROUS SCLEROSIS, a genetically inherited disease characterized by EPILEPSY, MENTAL RETARDATION, behavioral problems, tumors, or skin lesions. The group offers a nationwide network of volunteer state representatives and encourages and provides grants for research into the diagnosis, cause, management, and cure of this disease. The association provides information and conducts educational programs for medical and allied professionals. The group answers questions about the disease and makes parent-to-parent contact referrals. Founded in 1975, the group has 750 members and publishes a quarterly newsletter and semiannual re-

source newsletter. For address, see Appendix A.

natural opiates See ENDORPHINS; LIMBIC SYSTEM.

neocortex The part of the brain that processes reason, logic, language, mathematics, and speculation about the future and influences those behavior patterns set in motion by the more primitive parts of the brain. Many mammals also have a large neocortex.

neostriatum See STRIATUM.

nerve cells See NEURONS.

nerve conduction velocity study A diagnostic technique in which the motor or sensory nerves are stimulated at different points and the velocity of the conduction of propagated impulse is measured. This test measures the velocity of the fastest conducting fibers (the large myelinated AXONS). There is normal velocity if the MYELIN is intact; slowed conduction can be caused by demyelination or destruction of large myelinated fibers.

This test is particularly useful in diagnosing GUILLAIN-BARRE SYNDROME or conditions such as carpal tunnel syndrome.

nerve-growth factor (NGF) Among the many *neurotrophic factors*, this is a naturally occurring hormone that stimulates the growth of NEURITES (tiny projections of a growing NEURON carrying information between cells). Nerve-growth factor is one of the human-growth factors currently being studied for its medical potential to restore function in the aging. Human-growth hormone, another growth factor, is also being investigated for its potential to strengthen the elderly.

Growth factors (there are at least eight different varieties currently being studied) each have a different target cell in the body,

TYPES OF USAGE FOR GROWTH-FACTOR HORMONE

Nerve-Growth Factor: Alzheimer's disease
Basic fibroblast-growth factor: Wound healing and Parkinson's disease, stroke
Brain-derived neurotrophic factor: Parkinson's disease
Neurotrophin-3: Nerve damage following trauma, chemotherapy, or diabetes, and in the treatment of Alzheimer's disease.
Neurotrophin-4/5: Alzheimer's and Parkinson's diseases
Ciliary-neurotrophic factor: Lou Gehrig's disease
Glial-growth factor: Peripheral neuropathy
Glial-maturation factor: Nerve injuries

and each has a possible role in protecting the body's nerve cells against damage from diseases such as ALZHEIMER'S, PARKINSONS, and LOU GEHRIG'S.

In addition, scientists at the University of California at San Diego found that in a variety of learning and memory tests, it was shown that infusions of nerve-growth factor into the brain could improve learning capacity and increased the size of brain cells that had previously shrunk. In Sweden, a human Alzheimer's patient is reportedly being treated with a similar approach.

Some scientists are now developing a new class of drugs called K252 compounds, which are designed to boost the body's production of nerve-growth factor. Other studies are investigating a possible treatment for Parkinson's disease, amyotrophic lateral sclerosis (Lou Gehrig's disease), and STROKE patients.

The problem with using the different growth factors are that most of these protein molecules are large and difficult to handle and must be pumped directly into the brain because they will not cross the blood/brain barrier. Researchers hope that new kinds of drug delivery systems, such as patches and nasal sprays, may simplify transport problems with these growth factors.

nerve impulse Also known as nerve signal, this is the electrical message carried by the neurons.

nerve signal See NERVE IMPULSE.

nervous system A vast network of cells that carry information (coded as NERVE IMPULSES) to and from all parts of the body. The system is divided into the CENTRAL NERVOUS SYSTEM (the brain and SPINAL CORD) and the PERIPHERAL NERVOUS SYSTEM (PNS) (the nervous tissue outside the cranium and vertebral column). The PNS includes the AUTONOMIC NERVOUS SYSTEM, which is further divided into the sympathetic and PARASYMPATHETIC NERVOUS SYSTEMS. The basic functional unit of the nervous system is the nerve cell, or NEURON.

neural graft A transplant of neural tissue from a healthy brain to a damaged are of the brain or spinal cord.

neural plate Ectoderm found lying along the central axis of the early embryo that forms the NEURAL TUBE and, eventually, the CENTRAL NERVOUS SYSTEM.

neural tube defects A group of defects occurring at birth caused by a failure of the NEURAL TUBE to close properly. During fetal development, a ridge of neurallike tissue develops along the embryo's back. As the fetus develops, this material differentiates into the SPINAL CORD and peripheral nerves at the lower end and the brain at the upper end. A developmental problem during this time can cause abnormalities ranging from a total lack of brain (ANENCEPHALY) to SPINA BIFIDA. In spina bifida, the bony arches of the spine don't close, leading to CSF leaks. More severe defects of these bones lead to more serious neurological conditions.

A MENINGOCELE refers to the protrusion of the MENINGES through the opening in the spine, with a constant risk of damage and infection to the meninges. In a MENINGOMYELO-CELE, the nerve roots and the spinal cord are exposed, and there is a constant risk of infection; this condition is accompanied by paralysis and numbness in the legs and urinary incontinence. There is also usually HYDROCE-PHALUS (fluid in the brain) and ARNOLD-CHIARI MALFORMATION as well. If the neural tube fails to fuse at the cranial end (called *cranium bifidum*), the child will be born with severe mental and physical disorders.

This type of birth defect can be caused by women who use HOT TUBS or saunas during early pregnancy; this practice nearly triples the chances of giving birth to babies with spina bifida or brain defects, according to research.

neurapraxia   A temporary loss of nerve function characterized by tingling, numbness, and weakness. It is caused by compression of a nerve, but since there is no structural damage, the nerve and the patient should recover completely.

neurasthenia   An outdated term meaning "nervous exhaustion." It was used to describe a group of physical and psychological symptoms including irritability, fatigue, HEADACHE, dizziness, ANXIETY, insomnia, DEPRESSION, and sensitivity to noise that can be caused by organic damage (such as HEAD INJURY) or by neurosis.

neurinoma   Alternate name for ACOUSTIC NEUROMA.

neurite   Tiny projections that sprout from a growing neuron; these neurites may become DENDRITES or axons. If the developing neurite is to become an axon, it may release transmitters from its terminals *before* making synaptic contact. Researchers have shown how this helps shape dendrite arrangement of neurons the cell in question will eventually contact.

neuroanatomy   One of the oldest of the neurosciences, this is the study of the physical structure of the nervous system from gross anatomy of the brain to the microscopic study of NEURONS.

neurobiology   The study of the biology of the brain.

neuroblastoma   A type of tumor that usually develops in the adrenal glands, although few do develop within the brain itself. The outlook for this type of tumor is hard to predict because they range from being relatively benign to highly malignant. About one-third of affected patients survive at least five years after treatment.

Symptoms   Weight loss, aches and pains, paleness, irritability, diarrhea, or high blood pressure.

Treatment   Removal of the tumor followed by radiation therapy and anticancer drugs.

neurochemistry   The study of the biochemical processes in the brain.

neurocranium   Rare term for the part of the skull that houses the brain.

neurodevelopmental treatment   A form of therapy for those who suffer from CENTRAL NERVOUS SYSTEM disorders that cause abnormal movement. The technique attempts to initiate or refine normal stages and processes in the development of movement.

See also NEURODEVELOPMENTAL TREATMENT ASSOCIATION.

Neurodevelopmental Treatment Association   A group of physical and occupational therapists, speech pathologists, special educators, physicians, parents, and others interested in NEURODEVELOPMENTAL TREATMENT (NDT), a form of therapy for those who suffer from CENTRAL NERVOUS SYSTEM disorders that cause abnormal movement.

The group informs members of new developments in the field, disseminates ideas to eventually improve fundamental independence, and locates articles related to NDT.

Founded in 1967, the group has 4,000 members and holds an annual convention in the first weekend in May. It publishes the bimonthly *NDTA Newsletter* and a bibliography. For address, see Appendix A.

neuroectodermal tumor One of the two most common types of brain tumor in children, found in an area of the brain that controls coordination, arising in the cells that originally line the neural tube. Recent research has suggested that some of these tumors in children may be related to their mothers' lack of multivitamins during pregnancy. Scientists also believe there may be some similarity between the development of neural tube defects and the development of neuroectodermal tumors.

In interviews at the Children's Hospital of Philadelphia, a comparison of the diets of 332 mothers' diets showed that the cancer patients' mothers were less likely to have taken multivitamins during the first six weeks of pregnancy. The diets also contained less vitamin C and beta-carotene, and fewer fruits and vegetables.

Children of the women who ate the most fruits and vegetables had a 72-percent lower neuroectodermal-tumor risk than children of mothers who ate the least; mothers who ate the most vegetables cut the risk by 63 percent. Specifically, children whose mothers ate high amounts of vitamin A had a 41-percent risk, a 58-percent risk for mothers who took high levels of vitamin C, and a 62-percent risk for those whose mothers took a high levels of folate. Taking multivitamins during the first six weeks of pregnancy was associated with a 44-percent drop in risk for these tumors.

The study's scientists suggested that the protective benefit of fruits and vegetables may be primarily obtained from folate more than other nutrients. Folate had previously been found to prevent serious NEURAL TUBE DEFECTS.

neuroepithelioma A malignant form of GLIOMA, this is a tumor of the retina that commonly spreads into the brain.

neurofibrillary tangles Accumulations of fibrous filamentary material within the brain's NEURONS which show up heavily with the use of a silver stain. Neurofibrillary tangles are one of the hallmarks of ALZHEIMER'S DISEASE. The tangles were first described by German neuropathologist Alois Alzheimer in 1906; his finding was the one that differentiated Alzheimer's disease from other neurological problems. Because his first diagnosis was of a fairly young patient, the disease was regarded for a long time as a form of *presenile dementia.* It is now recognized as the same pathological brain atrophy present in many patients as they age.

neurofibromatosis This uncommon genetic disorder (also known as *von Recklinghausen's disease* or *elephant man's disease*) is characterized by soft, fibrous swellings growing from nerves in the skin and elsewhere. If the swellings (neurofibromas) occur in the CENTRAL NERVOUS SYSTEM, they can cause EPILEPSY and other complications, including visual or hearing problems. In addition, there may be coffee-colored spots (*café au lait*) on the skin of the trunk and pelvis.

Treatment There is no cure for this disease. Surgical removal of the neurofibromas is necessary only if they are causing complications.

neuroglial cells Special cells that are packed around and between the NEURONS,helping to support the delicate nervous tissue. The neuroglial ("nerve glue") cells make up about half the volume of the brain;

in addition to support for neurons, they regulate the ionic environment outside neurons. Ionic balance is critical to electrical function.

neurohormone A hormone that acts as a NEUROTRANSMITTER, such as adrenalin (epinephrine).

neuroleptic malignant syndrome (NMS)
An uncommon, extremely dangerous reaction to antipsychotic (neuroleptic) drugs characterized by sudden high fever with sweating, high blood pressure, delirium, muscle rigidity, racing heart, and breathing problems. Afterwards, patients often report feelings of impending doom. Untreated, the condition has a mortality rate of nearly 30 percent.

Early diagnosis and intervention has reduced the death rate from this syndrome. Its exact cause is still unknown, but scientists do know that the main problem comes from high doses of antipsychotic drugs–especially when the drugs are given quickly or injected. Any patient who is dehydrated or agitated or who suffers from mood disorders appears to be an increased risk.

Antipsychotic medication can be given again to most patients despite an episode of NMS; usually, the drugs are given at least two weeks after recovery, beginning with a low dose that is gradually increased. Vital signs should be monitored daily and levels of creatine phosphokinase measured once or twice in the first two weeks.

Prevention Health-care workers should monitor the patient's fluid intake, blood levels of iron, lithium, blood urea nitrogen (BUN), and creatinine. The room should be kept cool and high doses of antipsychotics should be avoided.

Treatment Once neuroleptic symptoms appear, antipsychotic drug administration should be stopped, and symptoms treated.

neurolinguistics The study of how information is received through the senses, processed in the NEURONS and neural pathways of the brain (especially the language areas) and expressed in language and behaviors.

neurological exam A simple systematic assessment of the function of various parts of the NERVOUS SYSTEM that can be performed in a *neurologist's* office and cause no pain. The most important part of a neurological exam is the description of symptoms and how they developed. Some of the routine tests for nervous system function include *tendon reflexes* (see REFLEXES), *Babinski reflexes*, *muscle strength*, *muscle tone*, *sensory function*, and *mental status*.

Tendon reflexes can be tested by tapping the knee with a rubber-tipped hammer. This test evaluates motor-nerve function, spinal-cord connections, and peripheral-nerve conditions. Light stroking of the underside of the foot may produce an involuntary movement of the big toe, called the Babinski reflex; this can suggest an abnormality in the nerve tracts that originate in the brain. Because muscle weakness can be a manifestation of neurological disorder, tests of muscle strength may be part of a neurological exam. To test muscle *tone*, the physician moves the arm or leg and assesses ease and range of movement. Both legs may be tested, for example, to check for differences between the two sides of the body. Spasticity, rigidity, or flaccidity may suggest problems in the nerves controlling different muscle groups.

Because sensations of pain, heat and touch travel through the sensory nerves to the central nervous system, sensory tests are an important part of a neurological exam. The sensory functions can be tested by asking patients what they feel when the skin is touched by a pinprick, a hot or cold object, or a tuning fork. Because nervous system disorders can affect the eyes and the senses of taste, hearing, and smell, tests of these senses can be important. Eye testing is especially useful; pupil size and difference in size, range of eye movement, gaze, and field of vision can help diagnose disturbances in nerves affecting vision.

Physicians will also evaluate gait, posture, coordination, and sense of balance by assessing a patient's ability to stand, walk, or move the body in a particular way.

Finally, a patient's mental status may be evaluated by asking questions to determine orientation in place and time and to determine whether judgment or memory are disturbed.

neurologist A specialist in the diagnosis and treatment of diseases and disorders of the nervous system. Neurologists conduct examinations (such as ELECTROENCEPHALO-GRAPHY or LUMBAR PUNCTURE) of patients' nerves, reflexes, motor and sensory functions, and muscles to determine the cause and extent of a problem.

neurology A medical specialty concerned with the diagnosis and treatment of functional or organic disorders of the brain, SPINAL CORD, and nerves. The science of neurology has developed over the past 200 years, beginning with the study of nerve function in animals during the eighteenth century by Stephen Hales and Robert Whytt. However, it was not until the mid- nineteenth century that clinical neurology was first studied. During this period, new information was learned about the causes of APHASIA, EPILEPSY, and motor problems caused by BRAIN DAMAGE.

When the ELECTROENCEPHALOGRAPH was invented in the 1920s by Hans Berger, the ability to record electrical brain activity facilitated the diagnosis of neurological disease. Together with the analysis of CEREBROSPINAL FLUID and the development of cerebral angiography, neurologists were able to more precisely diagnose and treat brain problems.

In the early 1970s, the development of CAT SCANS and of MAGNETIC RESONANCE IMAGING (MRI) in the 1980s yielded detailed views of the inside of the brain, which further improved the diagnosis of brain disease.

neuroma A benign tumor of nerve tissue that may affect any nerve in the body, usually from an unknown cause. Occasionally, a neuroma develops after a nerve injury.

See also ACOUSTIC NEUROMA.

neurometrics A method for diagnosing brain disorders by comparing auditory evoked potentials (AEP) from several different regions of the brain with tracings taken from normal, healthy human brains.

neuron Another name for *nerve cell*, a neuron is the basic functional unit of the NERVOUS SYSTEM. In the brain, neurons are responsible for information processing, converting chemical signals to electrical signals and then back to chemical signals again.

There are about 50 million neurons in the CEREBRAL CORTEX, 40 billion more in the CEREBEL-LUM, and another 10 billion in the rest of the brain and SPINAL CORD—about the same as there are stars in the galaxy. Each neuron has up to 60,000 SYNAPSES. The average number of neurons varies dramatically and seems to have nothing to do with general intelligence (some animals have more neurons than humans do). Apparently, quantity is less important than the quality of the connections between them.

A neuron consists of a compact cell body made up of the nucleus, several long branched extensions (DENDRITES) and a long fiber (the AXON) with twiglike extensions at its end. Neurons are the major type of cell that makes up the brain and nervous system, carrying signals to and from the brain and performing all of the brain's work. Each neuron receives electrical impulses through dendrites, which lie adjacent to one another in a gigantic web whose tiny branches direct signals toward the body of the nerve cell.

If enough arriving signals stimulate the neuron, the neuron fires, sending this electrical pulse down its axon, which connects through synapses into the dendrites of other cells.

Information is carried inside a neuron by electrical pulses, but once the signal reaches the end of the axon it must be carried across the synaptic gap by chemicals called NEURO-TRANSMITTERS. On the other side of the synapse is another dendrite, containing RECEP-TORS that recognize these transmitting molecules. In a series of complicated steps, the receptor biochemically opens an ionic channel. Charged ions pass through this open channel; the movement of ions generates an electrical current which changes the voltage of the post-synaptic neuron. If the shift is positive enough, this neuron will fire an action potential of its own.

At the same time, the first neuron emits enzymes into the cleft that terminate the transmission and reabsorb any excess transmitter chemicals left in the synapse.

A single neuron can receive signals from thousands of other neurons, and its axon can branch repeatedly, sending signals to thousands more. While researchers have long understood the mechanism of neurons, it's only recently that they have begun to understand how these cells might be able to store memories.

Most researchers agree that when a person experiences a new event, a unique pattern of neurons is activated in some way and within the entire configuration of brain cells, certain cells "light up." Unlike the wiring in the home, however, the brain's circuits are not permanent; as knowledge is acquired, circuits break apart and reform, constantly rewriting themselves and influencing our representations in the world.

The amazing ability of brain cells to make just the right connections may have been gained at the expense of their ability to reproduce; almost all other cells in the body can regenerate, and when these cells die they are replaced by others. Only in the brain are cells irreplaceable. We are born with almost all of the brain cells we will ever have, and those that die (about 18 million a year between ages 20 and 70) are lost forever.

neuropathology A neurology specialty concerned with the causes and effects of neurological conditions instead of their diagnosis and treatment, which is usually handled by a NEUROLOGIST or a NEUROSURGEON.

neuropathy A general term meaning pathological status of neurons. It is also called *neuritis*, and refers to a disease or damage to the peripheral nerves which connect to the brain and SPINAL CORD, to the sense organs, muscles, glands, and internal organs. Neuropathy is characterized by numbness and weakness, pain or tingling, depending on which nerves are affected.

Most neuropathies occur from damage or irritation to the AXONS (the conducting fibers that make up nerves) or to the fatty substance called MYELIN that insulates the axons. An axon's myelin sheath may suffer damage ranging from thinning to total loss, which may either slow or completely block the passage of electric signals.

Some cases of neuropathy may have no obvious cause; other instances may be triggered by dietary deficiencies, diabetes, alcoholism, etc. Nerves may also become acutely inflamed after a viral infection, such as in GUILLAIN-BARRE SYNDROME, or they may result from autoimmune disorders like systemic lupus erythematosus. They may also be found secondary to cancerous tumors such as lung cancer or lymphomas. A group of neuropathies may also be inherited.

Symptoms Precise symptoms depend on whether the affected nerve fibers are SENSORY or MOTOR NERVES. Sensory nerve damage may cause sensations of cold, numbness, and tingling, whereas motor damage may lead to muscle wasting and weakness. AUTONOMIC NERVOUS SYSTEM damage may cause blurred vision, sweating problems, faintness, and problems with stomach, bladder, intestinal, and sexual functions.

Treatment Treating the underlying disorder will help. If treatment is successful and the damaged nerve cells contain intact cell bodies, a full recovery from neuropathy is possible.

neuropeptides Connected sequences of proteins. Normally, they are produced by the PITUITARY GLAND and function as NEUROTRANSMITTERS. They include ADRENOCORTICOTROPHIC HORMONE (ACTH), melanocyte-stimulating hormone (MSH) and VASOPRESSIN. Some researchers believe ACTH seems to improve sustained attention and diminish DEPRESSION in DEMENTIA patients, and vasopressin is also being studied as a possible memory enhancement drug. There are at least 100 known neuropeptides.

neuropharmacology See PSYCHOPHARMACOLOGY.

neuropsychiatry The branch of medicine that deals with the relationship between psychiatric symptoms and neurological disorders that are usually types of brain disease, infections, or tumors. In addition, neuropsychiatry is concerned with subtle forms of BRAIN DAMAGE that may underlie psychotic illness.

neuropsychological   assessment Tests that can evaluate the extent of BRAIN DAMAGE and memory deficits, including assessment of language, memory, perception, reasoning, emotion, self-control, and planning. This kind of testing was first used as a way to distinguish between those whose abnormal behavior was caused by brain dysfunction and those whose problems were caused by psychological factors. Disorders caused by

brain dysfunction are called organic; psychological disorders are referred to as functional or psychogenic.

Early tests were based on the assumption that there were common characteristics in all organic impairments and gave a general assessment of "organicity" instead of details about the status of different mental functions.

Although the idea of *brain damage* as a single concept persists, in fact there is not one simple test that can uncover the often-diffuse problems experienced by those who have brain problems. Because brain damage may cover lesions of different sizes and shapes, different causes in different areas of the brain, uncovering the evidence requires a more sophisticated, comprehensive assessment. In order to properly rehabilitate a patient with brain deficits, it is imperative to have a clear picture of the patient's cognitive strengths and weaknesses to help choose the treatment technique and to measure response to treatment.

neuropsychologist A clinical psychologist with special training in NEUROLOGY as well as intensive training in psychological assessment. The relationship of NEUROPSYCHOLOGY to other neurosciences is an evolving one and may include not only discriminating patients who are brain injured, but may also define the nature and extent of brain damage, may assess treatment programs and patients' progress, and may plan rehabilitation programs.

neuropsychology The clinical and experimental field devoted to the study, understanding, assessment, and treatment of behavior directly related to the function of the brain. While NEUROPSYCHOLOGISTS work most often with those whose brains are abnormal, neuropsychologists also investigate individual differences within normal people due to different brain functions or organization.

Neuropsychology is a field somewhere between psychology and NEUROLOGY, closely related to behavioral neurology. Many experts in the field are trained by neurologists in medical settings instead of receiving primary training in psychology.

Experimental neuropsychology deals with both human and animal models and tries to delineate the relationship between the brain and behavior. While the fields of clinical and experimental neuropsychology may seem to be similar, the goals of the two are significantly different; while clinical neuropsychology tries to find rules and procedures effective with large numbers of patients with poorly defined disorders, experimental neuropsychology works with patients who have precisely determined disorders as a way of exploring brain-behavior relationships.

neurosurgeon   A physician who specializes in operations involving the brain and nerves, using laser-powered scalpels, operating microscopes and a range of other technological aids.

neurosurgery   The surgical treatment of disorders of the nervous system. While neurosurgery is ineffective against many generalized NERVOUS SYSTEM disorders (such as MULTIPLE SCLEROSIS), it can be effective against nerve failure due to specific structural changes.

Conditions that may respond to neurosurgery include HEAD INJURY, brain ABSCESSES, tumors, abnormalities of the blood vessels supplying the brain, bleeding inside the skull, some birth defects (such as HYROCEPHALUS), intracranial pressure, SPINAL-CORD compression, intracranial hemorrhage, and nerve damage caused by illness or accidents. NEUROSURGEONS also are involved in the surgical treatment of intractable pain.

The development of neurosurgery has been aided by improvements in anesthesia, scanning techniques, radiology, and antiseptics.

Neurosurgical Society of America   A professional group of specialists in neurological surgery. Founded in 1948, the group has 162 members who sponsor an annual scientific meeting. For address, see Appendix B.

neurosyphilis   Infection of the brain or SPINAL CORD that is found in untreated SYPHILIS many years after the patient first becomes infected. Spinal-cord damage from this disorder may cause poor coordination, urinary incontinence, and abdominal and limb pain. Infection in the brain may lead to DEMENTIA, muscle weakness and, sometimes, extensive neurological damage (called "general paralysis of the insane").

neurotensin   A   painkilling   NEUROTRANSMITTER.

neurotoxic drugs   Any drug that causes damage to the nervous system. These include anticonvulsants (hydantoin), carbamazepine, chloramphenicol, cisplatin, cycloserine, disulfiram, isoniazid, lincomycins, LITHIUM, metronidazole, mexiletine, nitrofurantoin, pemoline, pyridoxine, quinacrine, and quinine.
See also NEUROTOXIN.

neurotoxin   A   poisonous   or   destructive compound that damages nervous tissue. While hundreds of substances have neurotoxic properties, the most common are heavy metals, solvents, pesticides, and drugs (such as alcohol, street drugs, and prescription drugs). Neurotoxins also can be found in the venom of some snakes, and they are released by some types of bacteria, such as those that cause tetanus.

Metals recognized as neurotoxins include lead, mercury, and manganese; industrial settings are common sites for metal neurotoxic poisoning. Fungicides containing mercury have caused mass poisonings; mercuric chloride wastes, which appear as methyl mercury in fish and shellfish, led to serious outbreaks in Japan. Manganese intoxication in the United States has been recognized among those who work in mining, ore crushing, and ferromanganese alloy industries, primarily from inhaling dust particles or fumes. Toxicity may appear between 4 months to 15 years after exposure.

Solvents found in some industries may cause characteristic nerve damage; some harmful solvents include n-hexane, methyl-n-butyl ketone, and toluene.

Chemicals The actual numbers of neurotoxins in the environment vary widely. Of the 65,000 industrial chemicals registered with the Environmental Protection Agency, for example, estimates range from a low of 2,000 (between 3 and 5 percent) to 18,000 (28 percent). The March of Dimes estimates that between 5 and 10 percent of birth defects are caused by environmental effects, but they have no estimates on the number of neurological birth defects are caused by neurotoxins.

Gases including carbon monoxide and methyl chloride have neurotoxic effects, and as many as 39 separate *insecticide* compounds account for a large number of poisonings among farm workers.

Most commercial products have not been tested for neurotoxicity, which means that permissible exposure limits (PEL) have not even been set.

See also ALZHEIMER'S DISEASE; DEMENTIA; HEADACHES; LEARNING DISABILITIES; NEUROTOXIC DRUGS; PARKINSON'S DISEASE; PERIPHERAL NEUROPATHY; TOXIC ENCEPHALOPATHY; TOXIC MOOD DISORDER.

Symptoms The hallmarks of neurotoxicity are mood and personality changes, but other symptoms may vary depending on what control centers in the brain are damaged. Symptoms may include memory problems, emotional changes, or physical damage (such as brain swelling). Other symptoms of neurotoxic nerve damage are weakness, numbness, or paralysis of a part of the body served by the affected nerve.

Lead, the most significant environmental hazard, according to the Environmental Protection Agency (EPA) causes a range of symptoms including learning disabilities. Solvents may cause symptoms within two months of exposure and include muscle weakness, sensitivity to touch, slowed MOTOR and SENSORY NERVE function, impaired mental functions, toxic mood disorders, and severe manic depression. Exposure to mercury (a metal that damages a variety of brain areas) may cause cerebellar disorders, irritability, visual problems, deafness, mental disturbances, ANXIETY, and HALLUCINATIONS or delirium. Manganese toxicity causes apathy, memory problems, progressive problems with walking and motor control, and speech disturbances. Chronic disorders may remain indefinitely.

How they work Neurotoxins interfere with the performance of the NERVOUS SYSTEM—that delicate network of cells that process information transmitted from sensory organs. The nervous system also controls all the body's major functions, including personality, mood, and thought; even a minor interference with the system can have significant effects on everyday performance. Neurotoxins can be inhaled, ingested, or absorbed through the skin, mucous membranes, and the conjunctivas of the eyes. Once ingested, its effects depends on the type of neurotoxin involved, the amount ingested, frequency of exposure, and whether exposure is chronic or acute.

Neurotoxins damage the nervous system by disrupting the NEURONS, their MYELIN nerve sheath that covers the neuron, or the NEUROTRANSMITTERS (chemical messengers in the brain). The nervous system is especially vulnerable to damage because neurons can't regenerate once they are lost. In addition, certain brain regions and nerves in the brain are directly exposed to chemicals in the blood, and many neurotoxic substances readily cross the BLOOD-BRAIN BARRIER. Finally, because the nervous system depends on a delicate electrochemical balance, it's not hard for neurotoxic substances to interfere with function.

Diagnosis Neurotoxicity is extremely hard to diagnose because the brain feels no pain and because the brain is responsible for such a wide variety of functions, low-level toxicity may go unnoticed. Mental, behavioral, or nervous systems may be attributed not to neurotoxicity but to aging or psychological causes, and the public is often not aware that commercial products can in fact affect brain function.

There are specific blood and urine tests for neurotoxins. Testing for most substances with hair samples is considered inconclusive and experimental. While it has been proven unreliable, some physicians and commercial labs still use this test.

High-risk groups The developing fetus is particularly sensitive to neurotoxins because its nervous system is in the process of growing, dividing, and making important connections and because the blood-brain barrier is not yet fully formed. In later stages of fetal development and after birth, exposure to alcohol or lead, for example, can lead to lowered intelligence levels, motor or sensory problems, learning disabilities, and behavior problems. During childhood, the nervous system is still in a state of rapid development, and young children are still vulnerable to neurotoxin damage.

The elderly are also at risk for damage from neurotoxins because of structural and chemical changes in the body beginning at about age 60. Aging leads to a natural decrease in nerve cells, and exposure to neurotoxins can speed up this process of attrition. Aging also alters the way the body metabolizes drugs and chemicals, and a neurotoxin that may have only a slight impact on a younger adult can have a far more serious effect on an elderly person.

In addition, employees of neurotoxic chemical companies are particularly vulnerable to neurological diseases if they don't take proper precautions. Because of this, federal regulations require that protective measures (such as ventilation systems or protective clothing) be used. Unfortunately, some companies ignore the law, some employees may ignore the rules, and some protective systems fail. In addition, the neurotoxic properties of many substances have not yet been adequately studied. For these reasons, neurological disturbances are one of the 10 major forms of occupational hazards, according to the National Institute of Occupational Safety and Health.

In the workplace While the National Institute of Occupational Safety and Health (NIOSH) recognizes that neurotoxicity is a major cause of occupational disease, they have established safety standards for only 72 substances specifically related to neurotoxicity. Moreover, the EPA tends to concentrate on cancer-causing substances and has issued only a few regulations specifically limiting the use of chemicals for their neurotoxic potential. This lack of regulatory control may be due in part to the fact that the field of neurotoxicity is fairly new; it did not exist as a formal area of study until the early 1970s.

Workers who experience risk of neurotoxic chemical exposure include agricultural employees, degreasers, dentists, dry cleaners, electronics workers, hospital workers, lab workers, painters, plastics workers, printers, rayon workers, steelworkers, transportation workers, and hobbyists.

neurotransmitter A chemical released at the SYNAPSE (space between neurons) of a neuron which relays a nerve signal from one NERVE CELL to another. When a neurotransmitter is released into the synapse, it moves across the space and attaches to a RECEPTOR in the membrane of a neighboring NEURON. Some neurotransmitters stimulate the release of neurotransmitters from other neurons, while others inhibit the release of neurotransmitters.

Neurons responsible for the same functions contain the same kinds of neurotransmitters; for example, neurons responsible for moving muscles all contain ACETYLCHOLINE, whereas all those in charge of hunger contain NOREPINEPHRINE. In addition, there are both *excitatory* and *inhibitory* neurotransmitters in the brain. Excitatory neurotransmitters include acetylcholine, EPINEPHRINE, norepinephrine, and SEROTONIN; inhibitory neurotransmitters include ENDORPHINS and ENKEPHALINS, gamma-aminobutyric acid (GABA), SUBSTANCE P, and GYLCINE.

Neurotransmitters are made from the protein in food; this protein is first broken down in the stomach and intestines into smaller substances called AMINO ACIDS. These amino acids enter the blood, where they are absorbed by the brain, which uses the amino acids to make neurotransmitters. It is the correct balance of the neurotransmitters in the brain that is responsible for proper function. Any deficiencies in nutrients will upset the level of certain neurotransmitters and interfere with the behaviors or actions for which they are responsible. On the other hand, a problem (such as DEPRESSION) can be corrected by altering the balance of the neurotransmitters; this is precisely what antidepressant medication is designed to do. Different neurotransmitters are manufactured by different nutrients in the diet; therefore, too much or too little of any one nutrient may lead to an abnormal level of neurotransmitters in the brain.

The most common neurotransmitters include acetylcholine, norepinephrine, dopamine, GABA, and serotonin.

New Adult Reading Test (NART) A list of 50 words of increasing difficulty that can establish premorbid intelligence in those of high-average or superior intelligence. Psychologists trying to assess brain damage must somehow quantify loss without knowing how well the person performed before problems began. For example, a person with an IQ of 140 before BRAIN DAMAGE occurred could lose 20 or 30 points and still test as "average." If the person's previous intellectual ability was known, subsequent IQ testing would reveal a significant loss of intellectual ability.

NART was developed to take advantage of the fact that language tends to persist despite brain damage. The test was devised on the basis of research show that patients with DEMENTIA were able to pronounce unusually spelled words (such as *ache*) despite gradual deterioration in other intellectual spheres.

Scores on this test are considered to be a good predictor of intelligence before deterioration took place in those with high-average or superior intelligence.

nicotine A stimulant drug in tobacco that causes dependence; while this drug has no medical use, some of its derivatives are used as potent insecticides.

After inhaling, the nicotine in smoke passes quickly into the blood (nicotine in chewing tobacco is absorbed more slowly through the mouth); once in the blood, nicotine acts on cholinergic receptors of the NERVOUS SYSTEM until it is broken down by the liver and excreted in urine.

Neurotransmitter	Action
acetylcholine	Affects: short-term memory, thirst, body temperature, motor function
epinephrine (adrenaline)	Affects: fight-or-flight response
norepineprhine	Affects: long-term memory, hunger, sleep/wake cycle
serotonin	Affects: emotions, sleep, satiety
endorphins/ enkephalins	Affects: emotions, pain, pleasure, appetite
GABA	Affects: everything
substance P	Affects: pain

The nicotine contained in cigarettes somehow alters brain chemistry, producing a feeling of well being, which reinforces the smoking habit. It acts primarily on the AUTONOMIC NERVOUS SYSTEM, which controls involuntary body activity (such as breathing and heart rate). Its effects depend on dosage and past usage and vary from one person to the next. A person who is not used to smoking will be more quickly affected, responding with nausea, vomiting, and slowed heart rate; in habitual smokers, however, the drug boosts heart rate, narrows blood vessels, and stimulates the nervous system, resulting in more energy, alertness, and concentration. Excess amounts of nicotine can cause vomiting, seizures, and sometimes death.

In 1988, U.S. Surgeon General C. Everett Koop stated that he believed that tobacco is "addicting in the same sense as drugs such as heroin and cocaine." Experts believe a person continues to smoke despite evidence of significant health damage in order to achieve the same brain chemical activity that is associated with pleasure.

nimodipine (Nimotop) A possible "memory drug" which has been used successfully to treat STROKE victims and is being studied for the treatment of ALZHEIMER'S DISEASE and age-associated memory impairment. The drug is a calcium-channel blocker, which means that it alters the flow of calcium ions through cell membranes, increasing brain blood flow and blocking excess calcium in the part of the brain associated with memory and learning. Nimodipine also seems to increase ACETYLCHOLINE levels.

It was approved by the Food and Drug Administration in 1989 to treat hemorrhagic stroke, as it improves blood flow in the brain and lessens oxygen deprivation.

In recent studies, Italian researchers noted a 69.5 percent increase in mental performance among 40 patients aged 65 and 80 years old who were suffering minor to medium signs of mental aging. Twenty percent showed no change, and 9.5 percent worsened slightly.

Vanderbilt University researchers found that nimodipine was effective in improving memory, DEPRESSION, and general state of mind in 178 elderly patients in cognitive decline.

See also MEMORY ENHANCEMENT.

NMDA receptor A receptor for the AMINO ACID called GLUTAMATE, which is found in every cell in the body and that plays a central role in brain function. Recent research suggests that glutamate may also be responsible for brain damage as a result of oxygen deprivation following a STROKE. NMDA is named after a synthetic form of glutamate (N-methyl-D-aspartate) used in research. NMDA receptors play heavily in learning and memory systems of the brain.

NMR The abbreviation for nuclear magnetic resonance.

See MAGNETIC RESONANCE IMAGING.

nondominant hemisphere The brain hemisphere that is not dominant for speech.

nootropics A class of drugs designed to improve learning and memory without other CENTRAL NERVOUS SYSTEM effects. The name *nootropic* was taken from the Greek *noos* (mind) and *tropein* (toward).

There is some disagreement about which drugs are to be considered nootropics, but experts usually agree that they include the PYRROLIDONE DERIVATIVES (piracetam and oxiracetam, pramiracetam, and aniracetam).

The mechanism by which these drugs seem to work is not known, although some studies suggest they affect the part of the nervous system that uses ACETYLCHOLINE as a NEUROTRANSMITTER. There also appears to be some involvement with adrenal steroid production in the adrenal CORTEX.

No nootropic drug has been approved by the U.S. Food and Drug Administration; they are available to patients outside of the United States.

noradrenaline Another name for NOREPINEPHRINE.

norepinephrine A NEUROTRANSMITTER secreted by the adrenal gland and found in the AUTONOMIC NERVOUS SYSTEM (part of the nervous system concerned with control of involuntary bodily functions). Chemically, norepinephrine is a CATECHOLAMINE (a class of compounds that affect the nervous and cardiovascular systems, metabolic rate, and body temperature) and is closely related to EPINEPHRINE. It is also released as a neurotransmitter by sympathetic nerve endings located in the area of the MIDBRAIN called the LOCUS CERULEUS. Isolated in the 1930s, norepinephrine was the second neurotransmitter to be discovered.

Norepinephrine's primary function is to help maintain a constant blood pressure by constricting certain blood vessels when blood pressure drops. This action explains its use as an emergency injection in the treatment of shock or severe bleeding. Among its many other actions, it is responsible for the FIGHT-OR-FLIGHT RESPONSE to danger or stress and is responsible for constricting small blood vessels and increasing blood pressure, increasing blood flow through the arteries of the heart, increasing the rate and depth of breathing, and relaxing the smooth muscle in intestinal walls. It also helps to control emotion and mood.

normal pressure hydrocephalus (NPH) Also known as "water on the brain," this uncommon disorder involves an obstruction in the normal flow of CEREBROSPINAL FLUID, which causes a buildup of cerebrospinal fluid on the brain. It is called "normal pressure" hydrocephalus because the pressure in the spinal fluid is normal, unlike most cases of water on the brain.

NPH can present with all of the symptoms of classic ALZHEIMER'S DISEASE, especially the DEMENTIA. A CAT SCAN will show the ventricles of the brain are enlarged from an excessive amount of fluid on the brain. Other symptoms include urinary incontinence and difficulty in walking. Presently, the most useful diagnostic tools include the imaging techniques, such as MRI (MAGNETIC RESONANCE IMAGING).

NPH is caused by any of several factors including MENINGITIS, ENCEPHALITIS, and HEAD INJURIES. In addition to treatment of the underlying cause, the condition may be corrected by a neurosurgical procedure (inserting a shunt) to divert the fluid from the brain.

NPH is treated with a surgical procedure called a ventricular-atrial shunt to eliminate the fluid. About 50 percent of cases are cured with this treatment. While its cause is unknown, it is believed to result from an interference of the circulation of fluid in the brain. The condition may also be caused by a brain hemorrhage or inflammation that blocks the fluid; in these cases, shunting doesn't provide relief.

nuclear magnetic resonance (NMR) See MAGNETIC RESONANCE IMAGING (MRI).

nucleus accumbens A region in the LIMBIC SYSTEM where there are a large number of DOPAMINE NEUROTRANSMITTERS, which are involved in various brain functions, including movement and emotion. Much of the effects of cocaine and amphetamines occur in this part of the brain, which may be permanently damaged by abuse of these drugs. Chronic administration of these drugs in animals has produced such permanent damage; at its worst, the result may be a psychotic condition much like SCHIZOPHRENIA, which is also believed to be related to dopamine.

nucleus basalis of Meynert An area near the optic chiasm (where the optic nerves cross) that enters into the CEREBRAL CORTEX. When this area is destroyed, it causes a drop in ACETYLCHOLINE activity in the cortex similar to ALZHEIMER'S DISEASE. Scientists suspect that the beginning of Alzheimer's disease may be related to a slow death of cells in the nucleus basalis, which may lead to the formation of the plaques also seen in the disease.

O

occipital cortex See VISUAL CORTEX.

occipital lobes The rear region of the CERE-BRUM that receives sensory information from the eyes. Damage to this part of the brain causes visual problems or blindness.

ocular dominance columns Cells in each of these columns, found in the PRIMARY VISUAL CORTEX, process information from either the right or the left eye; there is no mixing of right-left eye information within columns.

oculomotor nerve Also known as the third cranial nerve, this nerve (together with the fourth and sixth cranial nerves) is responsible for eye movements.

See also CRANIAL NERVES.

olfactory bulbs Interior lobes of the brain concerned with the sense of smell. The two olfactory bulbs lie on top of a thin body plate in the roof of the nose and connect to the brain via the OLFACTORY NERVE. Scent particles enter the nose, stimulating smell receptors at the top of the nasal cavity, sending electro-chemical signals through holes in the eth-moid bone to an olfactory bulb; from there, it travels to several brain regions in the lower, more primitive part of the FOREBRAIN. Connec-tions with the LIMBIC SYSTEM explains the emo-tional aspects of smell and may explain why some smells can quickly trigger powerful memories. On the other hand, links with the HYPOTHALAMUS can trigger strong physical re-actions (such as nausea and vomiting) in response to unpleasant smells. Olfactory con-nections with the RETICULAR FORMATION explain the stimulating action of smelling salts.

See also SMELL, SENSE OF.

olfactory fatigue The loss of the ability to detect a certain smell. The amount of time

that olfactory fatigue remains varies; it is a more extreme version of "smell adaptation," which is the temporary loss of the ability to smell an odor that returns in a few minutes after the cause is removed. Some scientists believe olfactory fatigue occurs when the brain modifies the sense of smell by transmit-ting signal to the nerves, which pick up the "smell" message; the more a person is ex-posed to these odors, the less he or she notices them.

See also SMELL, SENSE OF.

olfactory nerve Also known as the first cranial nerve, the olfactory nerve carries the sensation of smell via nerve impulses from the nose to the brain. Smells are detected by hairlike nerve endings (called RECEPTORS) in the mucous membrane lining the top of the nasal cavity. Nerve fibers travel from the receptors through holes in the nasal cavity roof, ultimately forming two structures called the OLFACTORY BULBS. From here, the nerve fibers make their way to the olfactory centers in the brain.

If the olfactory nerves are injured (usually by a HEAD INJURY), the sense of smell may be impaired or completely lost.

See also CRANIAL NERVES; SMELL, SENSE OF.

oligodendroglioma A rare type of slow-growing primary BRAIN TUMOR that affects sev-eral hundred American patients a year—usu-ally young or middle-aged adults.

See also ASSOCIATION FOR BRAIN TUMOR RE-SEARCH, FRIENDS OF BRAIN TUMOR RESEARCH, NA-TIONAL INSTITUTE OF NEUROLOGICAL DISORDERS AND STROKE.

Symptoms Symptoms are the same as for other brain tumors, including HEADACHE, lack of coordination, vomiting, weak facial mus-cles, swallowing or speaking problems, eye/vision problems, ear or hearing problems, paralysis, or personality changes.

Diagnosis A wide variety of tests can be used to diagnose brain tumors, including MYELOGRAM, ANGIOGRAM, BRAIN SCANS (such as CAT SCAN, PET SCAN, MRI, etc.). Other tests include LUMBAR PUNCTURE (spinal tap), ELECTROENCEPHALOGRAPH (EEG), and biopsy.

Treatment Surgical removal of the tumor may lead to a complete cure; about one-third of patients live for five years or more.

opiates The active element in heroin, morphine, and opium, which are similar in structure to the ENDORPHINS found naturally in the brain.

optical aphasia The inability to name the object that one sees. Recognition survives, because a victim of optical aphasia seeing a bowl of soup can lick his or her lips or smile but would not be able to name what is seen. Other recognition survives, too, so that if he or she can taste or smell the soup, the victim can name it; it is only the *visual* recognition that is lacking.

See also APHASIA.

optic chiasm The point at which the right and left optic nerves cross.

optic nerve Also known as the second cranial nerve, this nerve carries impulses from the eyes to the brain.

See also CRANIAL NERVES.

optic neuritis A condition characterized by an abrupt loss of vision (usually over two or three days) caused by the demyelination of the OPTIC NERVE. Pain in the eye is common, and there is often loss of color vision.

In one study, the risk of MULTIPLE SCLEROSIS (MS) in patients with one attack of optic neuritis was 34 percent in men and 74 percent in women. Early age at onset of the optic neuritis increased the risk of MS, but multiple attacks of optic neuritis did not increase MS risk.

The chance of recovering vision is very good; about half of all patients recover their vision within a month, and 75 percent of all patients recover their sight within six months. Neither pain nor papillitis (nerve inflammation or swelling) alters the prognosis for recovery.

Treatment Intravenous steroids methylprednisolone followed by prednisone speeded up return of vision, but only marginally.

optic tectum The roof of the rear part of the CEREBRUM, which is concerned with visual processes.

organic brain syndrome A disturbance of consciousness, intellect, or mental functioning of physical (organic) as opposed to psychiatric origin without a precise known physical cause, but which is believed to be a chemical abnormality in the brain. Possible causes include degenerative diseases such as ALZHEIMER'S DISEASE, metabolic imbalances, infections, drugs, toxins, vitamin deficiencies, or the effects of brain trauma, STROKE, or tumor.

Symptoms In the acute phase of the condition, symptoms can range from a slight confusion to stupor or COMA and may include disorientation, memory impairment, HALLUCINATIONS, and delusions. The chronic form of the syndrome causes a progressive decline in intellect, memory, and behavior.

Treatment Treatment is more likely to be successful with the acute form of organic brain syndrome if the underlying cause can be identified; in chronic cases, irreversible BRAIN DAMAGE may already have occurred.

organic mental disorders A group of mental disorders with a known or presumed physical cause, such as BRAIN TUMOR, drug abuse, HEAD INJURY, metabolic disorders, etc. Physicians generally make a distinction between organic mental disorders (when the cause is known) and ORGANIC MENTAL SYN-DROMES, when the cause is not known.

A wide variety of disorders can be caused by this problem, such as HALLUCINATIONS, DE-LUSIONS, DELIRIUM, DEMENTIA, and mood disorders.

organic mental syndrome Psychological or behavioral symptoms with unknown cause that are linked to brain dysfunction. A person would be diagnosed with an organic mental syndrome, for example, if he or she has DELIRIUM or DEMENTIA from an unknown cause. Symptoms could be due to a wide variety of problems, such as a STROKE, substance abuse, poisoning, BRAIN TUMOR, or neurological disease. Once the source of brain dysfunction is discovered, the person's mental problems is rediagnosed as an OR-GANIC MENTAL DISORDER.

Orton Dyslexia Society, The A professional group for professionals in the fields of NEUROLOGY, pediatrics, psychiatry, education, social work, and psychology; parents; or other persons interested in the study, treatment, and prevention of the problems of DYSLEXIA. The group answers questions about dyslexia and makes referrals to other members and support groups. Written materials are also available. The society also provides a focal point for activities and ideas generated in various fields as they relate to problems of language development and learning. The society is named for Dr. Samuel T. Orton, a pioneer in the field. Founded in 1949, the group publishes an annual journal and a quarterly newsletter. For address, see Appendix B.

osmoreceptors A group of cells in the HY-POTHALAMUS and lower BRAINSTEM that monitor the concentration of salts and proteins in the blood. If the blood concentration increases, the osmoreceptors trigger nerve impulses to the hypothalamus, which increases the release of VASOPRESSIN from the PITUITARY GLAND, instructing the kidneys to restrict the release of urine until the blood concentration returns to normal.

oxiracetam One of a class of NOOTROPIC drugs and an analog of PIRACETAM. A few findings suggest oxiracetam enhances vigilance and attention, with some effects on spontaneous memory and improvements in concentration.

In one Italian study, researchers assessing the drug's danger of birth defects gave pregnant mice oxiracetam from the beginning of their pregnancies until birth. Instead of having a toxic effect, the drug appeared to benefit the offspring of the treated mothers. These offspring—who had never received the oxiracetam directly—showed signs of being more curious at one month of age than the offspring of controls who had received a placebo. At three months, the treated offspring were performing significantly better in memory tests than the offspring of controls.

In a test of 272 humans, demented patients who received oxiracetam showed significant improvements in memory and concentration after three months of therapy.

Oxiracetam is currently being investigated for the treatment of ALZHEIMER'S DISEASE at a number of centers around the country, but it is not currently available in the United States for other than experimental use.

See also MEMORY ENHANCEMENT.

oxytocin One of two hormones secreted by the pituitary gland that initiates labor, stimulates uterine contraction, and plays a part in lactation. This neuropeptide also is involved in grooming and social behavior and may play a role in one type of obsessive-compulsive disorder (OCD). According to research, high levels of oxytocin in the brain are found among patients diagnosed with

OCD who do not have a family history of TOURETTE'S SYNDROME, one form of OCD.

In recent studies, scientists collected CEREBROSPINAL FLUID from 29 people with OCD, 23 people with Tourette's syndrome, and 31 healthy controls. Levels of oxytocin rose dramatically in the group of OCD sufferers but not in those who had no personal or family history of tic disorders or the control group. Moreover, those with the most severe OCD symptoms had the highest levels of oxytocin.

P

Paget's disease A common disorder of middle age in which bone formation is disrupted, weakening and thickening bones of the skull, among others. Because the disease is prevalent in some parts of the country more than others, it is suspected to be caused by a viral infection. Paget's disease affects about 3 percent of the population over age 40; the disorder tends to run in families and affects more men than women.

Paget's disease is usually diagnosed from an X RAY that has been taken for some other reason. Changes in the skull may lead to a distortion of the facial bones, producing a leonine appearance, and to inner-ear damage that may cause deafness, ringing in the ear, vertigo, or HEADACHE. Enlarged vertebrae may press on the SPINAL CORD, causing pain and sometimes paralysis.

Treatment Most people don't require treatment other than painkillers. Surgery may be needed to correct deformities.

pain The experience of pain involves almost every part of the brain, the SPINAL CORD, and the PERIPHERAL NERVOUS SYSTEM, the immune system, endocrine glands, and the metabolic system.

Basically, pain is caused when peripheral nerves are activated by a stimulus to the skin or internal organs. When a pain nerve is stimulated, an electrical signal runs down its AXON. The outer wall of a NERVE CELL is a membrane full of fluid that contains salts (including sodium, potassium, and chloride ions). All are electrically charged particles, and the membrane is surrounded by body fluid that also contains charged particles.

When the neuron is stimulated by pain, its membrane allows a large amount of positively charged sodium ions to enter the cell at the point of stimulation, which changes the properties of the neighboring part of the membrane, allowing sodium ions to enter there as well. The result is a wave of electrochemical activity that moves rapidly down the neuron. The pain information is transmitted electrochemically to the spinal cord, where it is processed and sent to numerous brain regions. In the brain, specific relay nuclei transmit the information to the sensory part of the CEREBRAL CORTEX and to nonspecific nuclei that send out the information to other brain regions.

Information about pain reaches brain regions involved in emotion, sensory perception, body movement, and hormonal release. The pain system also involves a wide range of different NEUROTRANSMITTERS and a group of PEPTIDES (including ENDORPHINS) that are similar to morphine.

The intricacy of the pain system can explain how wounded people may not be consciously aware of their pain and how amputees can still feel pain in the amputated part—despite its absence.

Recent research has suggested that the brain mechanisms behind pain in musculoskeletal areas, skin, and internal organs are different.

painkillers Medications that reduce a person's sensitivity to pain, including general and local anesthetics, aspirin, and opiate derivatives.

General anesthetics act on the BRAINSTEM to induce loss of consciousness, whereas local anesthetics deaden pain by affecting nerve membranes, blocking the transmission of impulses to a body area served by a sensory nerve. Other types of mild, general painkillers—such as aspirin—apparently act on pain centers in the THALAMUS deep inside the brain, traveling through the blood to all parts of the NERVOUS SYSTEM.

Analgesics are drugs that block pain

without interfering with consciousness; for intractable pain, physicians may prescribe morphine or another derivative from opium.

Painkillers, anesthetics, and analgesics can be given by injection into the blood, which very quickly distributes the drug throughout the body; by inhalation, through the rectum, via the SPINAL CORD (an epidural), which enters the CEREBROSPINAL FLUID bathing the brain, or by mouth.

paleocortex An evolutionary early region of the CORTEX; it is the olefactory cortex of the cerebrum. It is composed primarily of the piriform cortex and the parahippocampal gyrus.

paleomammalian The second layer of Paul MacLean's triple brain, equivalent to the LIMBIC SYSTEM, and the seat of emotions.

paradoxical sleep Another word for RAPID-EYE-MOVEMENT SLEEP (REM), a deep state wherein dreaming takes place.

parasympathetic nervous system (PNS) One of two parts of the AUTONOMIC NERVOUS SYSTEM, the PNS is responsible for slowing and steadying the body's internal activity, such as heart and breathing rates, by releasing ACETYLCHOLINE. These effects are almost the opposite of the efforts of the SYMPATHETIC NERVOUS SYSTEM. Parasympathetic nerves also increase blood flow to the stomach, liver, intestines, and other organs involved in digestion. In addition, these nerves activate other mechanisms of eating and digestion, including increased salivation, the release into the stomach and intestine of digestive juices, and stimulation of muscles in the intestinal wall to promote the movement of food through the digestive system.

Moreover, parasympathetic nerve fibers contract the pupil and allow the eye to focus on close objects.

The parasympathetic nervous system is made up of one chain of nerves passing from the brain and another leaving the lower SPINAL CORD. The parasympathetic nervous system also helps to maintain erection of the penis in sexually aroused men.

Parents of Children with Down Syndrome A national support group that offers parent-to-parent counseling, support, and information for new parents of Down Syndrome children, information on doctors, hospitals, and professionals. The group also promotes membership in the ASSOCIATION FOR RETARDED CITIZENS and maintains a speakers' bureau. Founded in 1966, the group has 150 members and publishes two monthly newsletters. For address, see Appendix A.

See also ASSOCIATION FOR CHILDREN WITH DOWN SYNDROME; ASSOCIATION FOR CHILDREN WITH RETARDED MENTAL DEVELOPMENT; ASSOCIATION FOR RETARDED CITIZENS; CENTER FOR FAMILY SUPPORT; FEDERATION FOR CHILDREN WITH SPECIAL NEEDS; JARC; MENTAL RETARDATION ASSOCIATION OF AMERICA; NATIONAL ASSOCIATION OF DEVELOPMENTAL DISABILITIES COUNCILS; NATIONAL DOWN SYNDROME CONGRESS; NATIONAL DOWN SYNDROME SOCIETY; PILOT PARENTS; VOICE OF THE RETARDED; YOUNG ADULT INSTITUTE AND WORKSHOP.

parietal cortex Part of the CEREBRAL CORTEX that regulates special perception; it also contains short-term memory for the perception of motion.

parietal lobes The upper portion of the CEREBRUM to the rear of the CEREBRAL HEMISPHERES and above the TEMPORAL and OCCIPITAL LOBES. The parietal lobes (together with the upper temporal and occipital lobes) serve for processing higher sensory and language function.

Parkinson Disease Foundation A professional organization to raise funds for scientific research into the cause, prevention, and cure of PARKINSON'S DISEASE and supports its own labs. The group provides information on patient care and rehabilitation, including a list of clinics where treatment is available, and a list of patient self-help groups. It also supports a brain bank to permit anatomical and chemical studies. In addition, the group sponsors scientific meetings and conducts training programs. Founded in 1957, the group has 85,000 members and publishes booklets, brochures, and a quarterly newsletter. For address, see Appendix B.

parkinsonism A neurologic disorder characterized by a masklike face, rigidity, and slowed movements. The term is used for Parkinson's disease–type symptoms, but is of other etiology. While Parkinson's disease has no known cause, other types of parkinsonism may be caused by ANTIPSYCHOTIC DRUGS, ENCEPHALITIS LETHARGICA, CARBON-MONOXIDE poisoning, CEREBROVASCULAR DISEASE, and the use of certain illegal drugs.

See also BASAL GANGLIA.

Parkinson's (or Parkinson) disease A brain disorder that causes muscle tremor, stiffness, and weakness; there is evidence that motor deficits may be accompanied by cognitive problems including poor memory. The disease was first described by James Parkinson (1755–1824) of London. (Parkinson was a pupil of John Hunter, the physician who inoculated himself with SYPHILIS and later died as a result of his experiment.)

Parkinson's disease is caused by atrophy of NERVE CELLS in the substantia nigra of the BASAL GANGLIA of the brain and a resulting decrease in activity of the NEUROTRANSMITTER called DOPAMINE. About one in 200 people are affected by the disease, with 50,000 new cases each year. Incidence of Parkinson's is lower among women and smokers.

Symptoms Parkinson's disease usually begins with a slight tremor, followed by a stiff, shuffling walk, trembling, a rigid stoop, and a fixed expression. The intellect is unaffected until late in the disease, although speech may become slow; DEPRESSION is common.

Diagnosis Symptoms mimic a wide range of other disorders, including adverse drug reactions, carbon-monoxide poisoning, STROKE, HEAD INJURY, and BRAIN TUMORS. While initial symptoms are so mild they may be easily overlooked, as the disease progresses it becomes so clearcut a physician may be able to diagnose the condition by a simple examination. However, other possible disorders should be excluded via tests (CT or MRI SCANS or blood work).

Treatment Although there is no cure for Parkinson's disease, physicians usually prescribe exercise, special aids, and encouragement. Drugs may minimize symptoms but cannot halt the degeneration of the brain. LEVODOPA, which the body converts into DOPAMINE, is usually the most effective drug and is often the first one tried. But the beneficial effects of L-dopa often suddenly wear off, when another drug may be given. L-dopa may then be reintroduced several weeks later. Other drugs include bromocriptine and amantadine. They may also receive ANTICHOLINERGICS; however, patients who exhibit DEMENTIA in Parkinson's disease have also been shown to have a deficiency in their cholinergic system and the use of these drugs can therefore worsen the symptoms of the dementia.

Sometimes, a surgical operation on the brain may reduce the tremor and rigidity, but it is reserved for the young, active sufferers who are otherwise in good health.

Without treatment, the disease progresses during 10 to 15 years to severe weakness and incapacity; about one-third of patients eventually go on to develop dementia. Experiments with transplants of dopamine-replacing adrenal tissue are now being conducted.

See also UNITED PARKINSON FOUNDATION; APPENDIX A.

Parkinson's Educational Program A national support group that serves as a clearinghouse for information on PARKINSON'S DISEASE, syndrome, and PARKINSONISM. The group also helps establish local support groups through the country, maintains an information exchange program with 32 other countries, and provides information to the public and professionals. Founded in 1982, the group supports 500 local groups and publishes materials, a glossary of definitions, publications catalog, a monthly newsletter, and a monthly physician referral list and also offers patient-support group information. For address, see Appendix A.

Parkinson Support Groups of America A national group for self-help groups whose members are PARKINSON DISEASE patients and their relatives and friends. The group provides encouragement, companionship, physical therapy, and counseling and offers programs and activities to help people with Parkinson's in improving the quality of their lives. Members try to define the needs of support groups and their members, makes recommendations, and supplies resources necessary for and encourages research into the cause and treatment of Parkinson's disease.

The group provides information and promotes legislative and administrative efforts, plans symposia with health-care professionals, and sponsors speakers' bureau. Founded in 1981, the group has 150 members and publishes a bimonthly newsletter. For address, see Appendix A.

Penfield, Wilder (1891–1976) Canadian neurosurgeon who discovered during the 1950s that stimulating various areas of the CORTEX produced a range of responses from patients; however, only stimulation of the TEMPORAL LOBES elicited meaningful, integrated experiences, including sound, movement, and color. Interestingly, some of these memories that popped up during stimulation were unremembered in the normal state. Furthermore, the memories Penfield stimulated appeared to be far more detailed, accurate, and specific than normal recall.

Penfield did not set out to study memory; he wanted to reduce SEIZURES in epileptic patients by removing the damaged tissue in the brain that triggered the seizures. Penfield knew that the seizures always were preceded by a "mental aura" (a warning sensation the patient experiences before a seizure). He hoped to open a skull of fully conscious patients and move a stimulating electrode across the brain to deliver a weak electrical shock to various areas to find the site on the brain that produced the mental aura. If he found such a site, he reasoned, he could destroy it and end the seizures.

While his technique was often successful, his discovery of the ability to stimulate memories radically altered ideas that were popular at the time about how the brain worked. Stimulating one side of the brain brought back a certain song to one patient, the memory of a moment in a garden listening to a mother calling her child in another. Interestingly, stimulating the same point elicited the same memory every time. It seemed that Penfield had found an ENGRAM—the site in the brain where memory was stored.

As a result of his findings, Penfield believed that the brain makes a permanent record of every item to which a person pays conscious attention, although this record may be forgotten during day-to-day life.

People First International A national support group that seeks to provide developmentally disabled persons with training in leadership skills and advocacy. The group also offers consultation and helps new groups get started. Founded in 1974, the group publishes films, videos, and books. For address, see Appendix A.

See also ASSOCIATION FOR CHILDREN WITH DOWN SYNDROME; ASSOCIATION FOR CHILDREN WITH RE-

TARDED MENTAL DEVELOPMENT; CENTER FOR FAMILY SUPPORT; FEDERATION FOR CHILDREN WITH SPECIAL NEEDS; JARC; MENTAL RETARDATION ASSOCIATION OF AMERICA; NATIONAL ASSOCIATION OF DEVELOPMENTAL DISABILITIES COUNCILS; NATIONAL DOWN SYNDROME SOCIETY; PARENTS OF CHILDREN WITH DOWN SYNDROME; PILOT PARENTS; VOICE OF THE RETARDED; YOUNG ADULT INSTITUTE AND WORKSHOP.

peptides   A class of substances made up of chains of AMINO ACIDS joined end to end. Some NEUROTRANSMITTERS are peptides.

peripheral nervous system (PNS)   All parts of the NERVOUS SYSTEM lying outside of the CENTRAL NERVOUS SYSTEM (the brain and SPINAL CORD). The PNS comprises the nerves extending to every part of the body and includes the cranial nerves and the spinal nerves. The part of the PERIPHERAL NERVOUS SYSTEM that controls involuntary movements and vegetative functions is called the AUTONOMIC NERVOUS SYSTEM, which is divided into the SYMPATHETIC and the PARASYMPATHETIC NERVOUS SYSTEMS. Because the PNS is not protected by the BLOOD-BRAIN BARRIER, as is the central nervous system, the PNS is far more vulnerable to neurotoxic damage.

peripheral neuropathy   Damage to the nerves of 'the PERIPHERAL NERVOUS SYSTEM, caused by a number of diseases and one of the most common results of poisoning with NEUROTOXINS. Damage can occur either to MOTOR NERVES (causing muscle weakness) or to sensory nerves (interfering with sensations of touch to cold, heat, pain, and pressure, or causing pain). Often neurotoxic exposure causes damage to both types of nerves. This condition can develop either quickly, with intense symptoms, or accumulate slowly over a long period of time.

During the 1930s, widespread outbreak of peripheral neuropathy was caused by solvent contamination of Ginger Jake, a popular tonic used as a digestive aid and to treat flu and menstrual problems. Normally, ingredients included ginger, castor oil, and a large amount of alcohol. However, varnish was substituted for the more expensive castor oil by one unscrupulous distributor, and as many as 100,000 people were diagnosed with "Ginger Jake syndrome"—symptoms ranging from numbness to permanent paralysis.

Symptoms   The first signs of peripheral neuropathy are often cramps in the legs, problems in climbing stairs, or problems in grasping heavy objects. Other symptoms include continual numbness and tingling in the feet similar to the "pins-and-needles" feeling when a leg or foot is compressed and "falls asleep." In severe cases, there may be paralysis.

personality   The concept of *personality* is complex, taking into account a whole range of a person's traits and behaviors. Psychologists define *personality* as an enduring tendency to act and feel in particular ways.

There is evidence that part of the CEREBRAL CORTEX known as the PREFRONTAL CORTEX in the FRONTAL LOBE plays a role in personality traits such as planning and organizational ability, ethical and moral sense, and overall emotional control.

One of the best examples of the relationship between the PREFRONTAL CORTEX and personality is in the unfortunate example of Phineas A. Gage, who was injured when a 3-foot iron rod pierced his skull during an explosion in 1848. Incredibly, he did not die, but his left frontal lobe was destroyed when the bar entered the skull. Before the accident, he had been a well-liked, calm, and steady worker, but afterward his friends noticed extreme personality changes. He became deeply disagreeable, tactless, profane, and restless. It appeared that a sort of civilizing influence over his personality had been lost when his frontal lobe was obliterated. Interestingly, alcohol appears to mimic this type of prefrontal control over behavior because intoxication can lead to similar personality changes such as increased profanity, vulgarity, aggression, and loss of sexual restraint.

Some researchers have begun to study the effect of certain NEUROTRANSMITTER levels on personality. Initial results suggest that the levels of DOPAMINE seem to correlate with the degree of extroversion.

Of course, personality is more than the sum total of a person's NEUROTRANSMITTERS; it is shaped by a variety of factors, including genetic and environmental influences. Family size, income, position within the family (eldest or youngest, for example), nutrition, and body size or shape can all affect personality.

pesticides and the brain One of many NEUROTOXINS that can adversely affect the NERVOUS SYSTEM, damaging and inhibiting the enzyme acetylcholinesterase, which is essential for proper neuromuscular function.

Of the many different types of pesticides commercially available, the organophosphates (originally developed as nerve gas during World War II) are the most commonly used; they include malathion, disulfotan, and dementon. Even a tiny amount of exposure to organophosphate may cause toxic mood disorders and NEUROPATHY; concentrated exposure can kill. Most neurological damage is reversible, once exposure has ended.

The most common way for a person to become poisoned with pesticides is by skin absorption—especially farm workers and those who work in pesticide manufacturing plants. Many people may be exposed at home by spraying in gardens or to prevent bug infestations. Pesticides can also contaminate groundwater or food.

PET scan Positron emission tomography is an imaging technique used to record and create images of the chemical activity in regions of the brain that are used primarily as a research tool. This type of scan creates computerized images of the distribution of radioactively labeled GLUCOSE in the brain in order to show brain activity. The more active a part of the brain is, the more glucose it uses. PET sensors are arrayed around the head of a patient, who sits with the head behind black felt to keep out distractions. The scan can pinpoint the source of the radioactivity (and heightened activity). These data are sent to computers that produce two-dimensional drawings showing the neural "hot spots." While PET accurately tracks brain function, it can resolve brain structures less than a half-inch apart.

PET scans are especially helpful for investigating the brain, where they can be used to detect tumors, to pinpoint the location of epileptic activity, and to investigate brain function in mental illness.

PET scans of labeled drugs that attach to specific RECEPTORS can show the distribution and number of those receptors.

See also BRAIN SCANS; CAT SCAN; NUCLEAR MAGNETIC IMAGING; SQUID; SPECT.

petit mal seizure A type of epileptic seizure that occurs during childhood and adolescence but rarely in adulthood. These seizures are characterized by a momentary loss of awareness resembling a daydream.

This type of seizure may last up to 30 seconds at a time and may occur hundreds of times daily.

See also EPILEPSY; GRAND MAL SEIZURE.

phenylalanine An AMINO ACID from which the brain manufactures norepinephrine, which plays a major role in learning and memory. It is converted into TYROSINE in the body; in the inherited disease PHENYLKETONURIA, the enzyme that converts phenylalanine into tyrosine is defective. Unless phenylalanine (a natural constituent of most protein foods) is eliminated from the diet, it builds up in the brain and causes severe MENTAL RETARDATION.

phenylketonuria (PKU) A genetic inborn error of metabolism in which a child has a defect in the liver enzyme that normally converts the amino acid PHENYLALANINE into a useful form; as a result, it builds up in the blood, which can block normal brain development and cause severe mental retardation. At birth, every American baby is tested for PKU with the Guthrie (PKU) test; a few drops of blood from the heel will reveal excess phenylalanine in the blood.

The disease affects at least one in every 16,000 babies, most often those of northern European background (Jews, Asians, and Africans are less commonly affected).

Untreated, the condition can cause MENTAL RETARDATION by age 1, if not properly treated or resistant, PKU can lead to behavior problems and LEARNING DISABILITIES.

See PKU PARENTS. For address, see Appendix A.

Treatment Diet low in foods with phenylalanine, such as cow's milk, meat, regular formula, and other protein-rich food; regular monitoring of blood phenylalanine levels; no aspartame sweeteners. Special formulas are available that contain no phenylalanine; as the child ages, he or she should follow a low-protein, vegetarian diet. Most cases of PKU respond to this diet, but experts don't agree on how long a person needs to follow this diet. Many children go off the diet when they enter adolescence; women with PKU must be sure to follow a low-protein diet during pregnancy to avoid causing irreparable BRAIN DAMAGE to the fetus.

phenytoin (Trade name: Dilantin) This well-known treatment for EPILEPSY may also improve intelligence, concentration, and learning, according to some studies. In the United States, the only approved use for this drug is to control various types of SEIZURES, which it does by stabilizing electrical activity in cell membranes. It is a cerebral vasodilator.

Excess amounts of the drug has the opposite effect on memory, intelligence, and reaction time. Many patients are allergic to the drug.

phosphatidylserine A component of BRAIN-CELL membranes that keeps fatty substances soluble.

In studies of phosphatidylserine and ALZHEIMER'S DISEASE, University of Munich researchers noted some improvement in EEG readings but little improvement in measures of DEMENTIA.

phrenology The belief that there is a relationship between the structure of the skull and structural characteristics of the brain. Phrenology first become popular when the French surgeon La Peyronine first noted odd behavior following specific brain injuries. By 1819, Dr. Franz Joseph Gall (see GALL, FRANZ JOSEPH) invented the science of phrenology by dividing the brain into 27 separate "faculty areas," enabling a person's personality to be deduced by the corresponding bumps on the skull. For the next 50 years, everyone began to judge their fellows by the shape of their forehead. Dr. Gall also introduced the then radical idea that the mind was primarily based in the brain.

physostigmine A drug, used as eyedrops in the treatment of glaucoma, that also may produce mild memory improvement among ALZHEIMER'S DISEASE patients. Physostigmine also reverses memory loss following the administration of SCOPOLAMINE in normal subjects. Physostigmine is believed to improve memory by inhibiting acetylcholinesterase, a substance that breaks down ACETYLCHOLINE, which is important in a range of memory processes.

In one study, scientists tested physostigmine with 20 Alzheimer's patients as they performed a "famous faces" test, a digit span, and recognition of verbal and pictorial information. Physostigmine enhanced performance on the recognition task but not on the famous-faces or digit-span tests. These findings are similar to others which found only a modest improvement in memory with physostigmine.

The drawback to the drug is that it has a narrow dose range over which it has beneficial effects.

pia mater The innermost layer of the membranes surrounding and protecting the brain that dips into all the furrows and SULCI of the brain. Made up of fine tissue and mesothelial cells, it also contains many blood vessels that supply the brain. Sometimes, the pia mater and the ARACHNOID are regarded as one membrane, which is then called the pia-arachnoid or leptomeninges.

Pick's disease A type of DEMENTIA almost impossible to distinguish from ALZHEIMER'S DISEASE except on autopsy, although it occurs far less frequently. In Pick's disease, BRAIN CELLS have "Pick's bodies," which consist of a miscellaneous collection of parts of the normal cell. Although the parts are recognizable, their normal relationships have been disrupted.

On average, patients contract this disease at about 55 years, with death following within seven years. After the midfifties, new cases of Pick's disease become infrequent; there have only been three cases of Pick's disease reported in patients over 70.

Pick's disease usually begins in the FRONTAL LOBES, featuring early change of personality and social behavior instead of the memory changes usually noticed in Alzheimer's disease patients, although these will eventually follow. Some patients become mute. The spatial problems often seen in Alzheimer's disease are not usually present in early stages of Pick's disease, although they will develop eventually.

Pilot Parents A national support group for parents, professionals, and others concerned with providing emotional support to new parents of children with special needs. The group sponsors a parent-matching program that allows parents who have had sufficient experience and training in the care of their own children to share their knowledge and expertise with parents of children recently diagnosed. The group also provides information concerning developmental disabilities, medical services, and supportive agencies within communities. The group maintains speakers' bureaus and a library and conducts educational programs. Although activities are conducted on a local level, the program serves as a model for similar groups that are being organized throughout the United States. Founded in 1971, the group has 340 members and publishes a monthly newsletter. For address, see Appendix A.

See also ASSOCIATION FOR CHILDREN WITH DOWN SYNDROME; ASSOCIATION FOR CHILDREN WITH RETARDED MENTAL DEVELOPMENT; ASSOCIATION FOR RETARDED CITIZENS; CENTER FOR FAMILY SUPPORT; FEDERATION FOR CHILDREN WITH SPECIAL NEEDS; JARC; MENTAL RETARDATION ASSOCIATION OF AMERICA; NATIONAL ASSOCIATION OF DEVELOPMENTAL DISABILITIES COUNCILS; NATIONAL DOWN SYNDROME CONGRESS; NATIONAL DOWN SYNDROME SOCIETY; PARENTS OF CHILDREN WITH DOWN SYNDROME; VOICE OF THE RETARDED; YOUNG ADULT INSTITUTE AND WORKSHOP.

pineal gland A tiny structure within the brain responsible for secreting the hormone MELATONIN, responsible for inducing sleep and regulating CIRCADIAN RHYTHM, affecting mood, and mental quickness. The amount of this hormone that is secreted varies over a 24-hour period and is greatest at night. It is believed that the secretion of this hormone is controlled by nerve pathways from the retina; light affects the secretion.

Because the pineal gland is not duplicated

in each hemisphere, philosopher Rene Descartes chose this site as the place where the body and soul are integrated.

The gland is located deep within the brain, just below the back part of the CORPUS CALLOSUM, the band of fibers that connects the two halves of the CEREBELLUM. Tumors occur rarely in the pineal gland.

pinealoma A tumor of the pineal body often found in children. It is treated most often by radiation therapy because surgery can be difficult and cases must be selected carefully. Pinealomas are very responsive to radiation; a SHUNT to relieve the intercranial pressure may also be necessary. This treatment is often very effective and cures the problem.

piracetam A drug belonging to a group of drugs called NOOTROPICS; piracetam appears to improve the learning ability of animals and protect against memory loss in the absence of oxygen (ANOXIA) by improving the transmission of impulses between NEURONS. In addition, some studies indicate that mixing piracetam with CHOLINE may boost the brain's metabolism and improve memory function.

In a recent study of 84 geriatric patients with nonvascular senile cognitive deterioration, piracetam was found to be better than a placebo at enhancing several cognitive abilities, including attention, memory, and behavior, especially at 6 gram/day doses.

Scientists are studying a range of possibilities behind piracetam's action, including stimulation of GLUCOSE metabolism, enhanced phospholipid levels or protein biosynthesis, and increased cholinergic and dopaminergic stimulation.

When older mice were given piracetam for two weeks, scientists discovered they had a 30 to 45 percent higher density of muscarinic cholinergic receptors in the FRONTAL CORTEX than before. Researchers concluded that piracetam, unlike other drugs, appears to have a regenerative effect on the NERVOUS SYSTEM. This could also explain, according to the study authors, why mixing choline with piracetam enhances its memory attributes. While piracetam is derived from the NEUROTRANSMITTER GABA (gamma amino butyric acid), there is no evidence that piracetam works through the GABAergic system; in fact, some research suggests that the GABA system may inhibit memory.

Piracetam also seems to produce resistance to several neurotoxic substances and stimulate learning through influences on the HIPPOCAMPUS and CORTEX while enhancing oxygen utilization.

pituitary adenomas A tumor of the PITUITARY GLAND that may occur commonly in young- or middle-aged adults. Surgical excision is usually quite effective; it may not be possible to remove all of a larger tumors; therefore, radiation may be necessary in addition.

pituitary gland Located just below the HYPOTHALAMUS, this gland produces many hormones as well as ENDORPHINS. In conjunction with the hypothalamus, they essentially run the endocrine system. This "master gland" secretes hormones that control the hormone secretion by other endocrine glands. It is controlled by the hypothalamus, which is adjacent to the pituitary. It affects the growth of bones, muscles, the thyroid, adrenal cortex, secretion of testosterone and estrogen, development of follicles, ovulation, water balance, blood pressure, and uterine contraction.

pituitary tumors About 10 percent of BRAIN TUMORS are pituitary tumors, most of which are benign. However, because of the location of the PITUITARY GLAND in a bony enclosure at the base of the skull, a tumor must grow upward, where it often presses on the optic nerve and causes visual problems.

The most common type of pituitary tumor is the endocrine inactive tumor, which destroys some of the hormone-secreting cells in the pituitary gland as it grows, causing hypopituitarism. This often results in problems with sexual function, reduced sperm production, and interrupted menstrual periods.

Other types of tumors in this gland may result in the excess production of a particular hormone, depending on the location of the tumor. These excess hormones can include too much growth hormone (causing gigantism or acromegaly), excess thyroid-stimulating hormone (causing hyperthyroidism), or excess ACTH (causing Cushing's syndrome), too much prolactin (causing abnormal milk production), or too much antidiuretic hormone (causing diabetes insipidus).

Treatment Surgical removal of the tumor, radiation therapy, replacement of missing hormones, or a combination of these approaches. The drug bromocriptine may be used to treat hormone-secreting tumor because it suppresses the production of some of these hormones.

PKU See PHENYLKETONURIA.

PKU Parents An organization of parents and professionals involved with children who have PHENYLKETONURIA (PKU). The group provides support for parents, offers information and information exchange, and publishes a quarterly newsletter. For address, see Appendix A.

planum temporale Part of the brain that is involved in understanding speech; in most healthy people, it is much larger in the left hemisphere. In fact, many parallel areas in the CORTEX are larger in one HEMISPHERE than the other.

plasticity A NEURON'S ability to change structurally or functionally, often in a permanent way, which enables the brain to recover functions lost through damage. Plasticity is responsible for a wide variety of events, including drug tolerance, but scientists aren't sure how the brain actually accomplishes these facts. Understanding how the NERVOUS SYSTEM performs these examples of plasticity would provide valuable clues to the way that the nervous system learns and remembers. Because one of the most distinctive features of learning is persistence, an analysis of a neuron's plasticity is important to the study of learning.

Electrical stimulation, neuronal disease, and enriched learning environments have all shown the ability to produce changes in the brain's SYNAPSES.

pleasure centers Deep within the HYPOTHALAMUS is a structure which appears to be associated with pleasure. The existence of this structure has been proven primarily through animal research; rats with electrodes connected to this region would incessantly press a lever to stimulate the region and experience pleasure. A similar area in the hypothalamus in humans has been found during NEUROSURGERY.

These pleasure centers involve certain NEUROTRANSMITTERS of the LIMBIC SYSTEM, and it is the action of these chemicals that is mimicked by psychoactive drugs. DOPAMINE and NOREPINEPHRINE (two neurotransmitters found in NEURONS of the limbic system) are released by the use of cocaine and AMPHETAMINES. Opiate receptors are also found throughout the limbic system, and these are also stimulated by morphine, heroin, and other narcotics. Scientists believe that these drugs cause a sense of euphoria by stimulating one or more of these pleasure centers in the brain.

pneumoencephalography A technique used in the X-RAY diagnosis of diseases inside the skull, in which air is introduced into the VENTRICLES of the brain to displace the

CEREBROSPINAL FLUID. X-ray photos can show the size and condition of the ventricles and the SUBARACHNOID SPACES.

polioencephalitis A type of viral brain IN-FECTION that attacks the GRAY MATTER of the CEREBRAL HEMISPHERES and the BRAINSTEM. The term is now usually restricted to infections of the brain by the POLIOMYELITIS virus.

polioencephalomeyitis Any viral infection of the CENTRAL NERVOUS SYSTEM, such as RABIES, that affects the GRAY MATTER of the brain and the SPINAL CORD.

poliomyelitis An infectious viral brain IN-FECTION once known as infantile paralysis, but today more widely known as polio, that kills motor NEURONS in the SPINAL CORD and BRAIN-STEM. The virus is excreted in the feces of an infected person, from where it may be spread directly or indirectly via fingers to food. Air-borne transmission also occurs.

While the disease is most common where sanitation is poor, epidemics may occur even in hygienic conditions where individuals have not acquired immunity to the disease during infancy or through vaccination.

Since the development of effective vac-cines in the 1950s in the United States, polio has virtually been eliminated from the United States and Europe. Cases do occur in people who have not been fully vaccinated, and polio remains a serious risk for unvaccinated travelers visiting southern Europe, Africa, or Asia.

Of those who have been paralyzed, more than half eventually make a full recovery. More than a quarter suffer minor permanent muscle weakness, and less than a quarter are left with a severe disability. Fewer than 1 in 10 patients dies; those who do are primarily adults and those with a severely infected brainstem.

In some cases, years after extensive paral-ysis with some recovery, there is a "post-polio" degeneration with new weakness and pain in some of the recovered muscles.

Symptoms This viral infection causes problems ranging from slight disability to total paralysis. About 85 percent of children infected with the virus have no symptoms at all; the rest have a short illness with a slight fever, sore throat, HEADACHE, and vomiting that lasts for a few days, after which most children recover completely.

In *abortive poliomyelitis*, only the throat and intestines are infected, and the symptoms resemble stomach ache or flu. In *nonparalytic poliomyelitis*, the symptoms are accompanied by muscle stiffness (especially in neck and back). *Paralytic poliomyelitis* is much less common and includes weakness and even-tual paralysis of the muscles. After a short period of apparent health, there is a major illness with symptoms of MENINGITIS, with fever, severe headache, stiff neck and back, and aching muscles. This progresses (often in just a few hours) to extensive paralysis of muscles. If infection spreads to the brain-stem, there are problems in swallowing and breathing. In *bulbar polio*, the muscles of the respiratory system are involved, and breathing is affected.

Treatment There is no specific drug treat-ment for polio other than to treat symptoms. Bulbar polio may require the use of a respi-rator. In cases of paralysis, physical therapy is required to prevent muscle damage while the virus is active; later, it may retain muscle function.

Prevention Either the Sabin vaccine (oral) or the Salk vaccine (injected) is considered to be highly effective in preventing the develop-ment of polio. In the United States, infant-sare now routinely vaccinated against this disease, during infancy at 2, 4, and 18 months, with an optional extra dose at 6 months and a booster at 5 years. The vaccine contains all three types of poliovirus, and immunity develops against each in turn. There are two alternative types of vaccine:

IPV (inactivated polio vaccine), which contains dead viruses and is given by injection, and OPV (oral poliovirus vaccine), which contains live but harmless strains of virus and is given by mouth. OPV is the vaccine of choice in the United States, except for children who have an immunodeficiency disorder, which lowers resistance to infection. There is an extremely small risk (about one in 5 million) of the live vaccine causing polio in the vaccinated person or in a close contact.

pons One of the three divisions of the BRAIN-STEM, the pons receives sensations from facial skin and from the eyes, nose, mouth, and teeth. The pons tells the jaw muscles to chew, controls the outer eye muscle that moves the eye to the side, receives taste sensations from the front of the tongue, works the muscles that control facial expressions, receives nerve impulses from sounds that enter the ear, receives signals from the cochlea, and causes secretion of saliva and tears.

positron emission transaxial tomography (PETT) scan See PET SCAN.

postcentral gyrus A part of the brain where touch and pressure sensation is perceived; also known as somatosensory cortex.

postconcussion syndrome A syndrome of symptoms following even a mild bump on the head that can include dizziness and memory loss for as much as six months or longer after a HEAD INJURY. Research has shown that suggests that 60 percent of patients who sustain a mild BRAIN INJURY are still having symptoms after three months.

The fact that a head injury can produce symptoms throughout the body has been known for at least the past 3,000 years; the Edwin Smith Surgical Papyrus, written between 2,500 and 3,000 years ago, contains information about 48 cases; eight describe

head injuries that affect other parts of the body.

Mild head injury symptoms can result in a puzzling interplay of behavioral, cognitive, and emotional complaints that make it difficult to diagnose. Although research is still limited, studies that do exist have found that symptoms following even the mildest head injury can linger, causing ongoing discomfort and disrupting personal lives.

Symptoms following a head injury may be due both from the direct physical damage to the brain and also to secondary factors affecting the brain such as lack of oxygen, swelling, and vascular disturbances. An injury that pierces the skull may also cause a brain INFECTION.

The kind of injury the brain receives during a closed head injury depends on the type of accident; whether or not the head was unrestrained on impact and the direction, force, and velocity of the blow. If the head is resting on impact, the maximum damage will be found at the impact site; a moving head will cause a "contrecoup" injury, where the damage will occur on the side opposite the point of impact.

Both kinds of injuries, however, cause swirling movements throughout the brain, tearing nerve fibers and causing widespread vascular damage. There may be bleeding in the CEREBRUM or SUBARACHNOID SPACE leading to HEMATOMAS, or else brain swelling may raise pressure inside the cranium, cutting off oxygen to the brain.

After a head injury, there may be a period of impaired consciousness followed by a period of confusion known as posttraumatic amnesia. For some reason, the physical and emotional shock of an accident can interrupt the transfer of all information that happened to be in the short-term memory just before the accident; this is why some people can remember information several days before and after an accident but not information right before the accident occurred. Both the length of time of unconsciousness and post-traumatic amnesia have been linked to how well a person recovers after a head injury.

Until recently, diagnostic tools weren't sensitive enough to detect the subtle structural changes that can occur and sometimes persist after mild head injury. Typically, CAT SCANS have not been helpful with this group of patients who struggle with symptoms after their injury. But studies involving MAGNETIC RESONANCE IMAGING (MRI) and brain electrophysiology indicate that contusions and diffuse axonal injuries associated with mild head injury are likely to affect those parts of the brain that relate to functions such as memory, concentration, information processing, and problem solving.

In fact, a study of 424 patients diagnosed with mild head injury showed that many had recurrent problems with deviant behavior, HEADACHES, dizziness, and cognitive problems; only 17 percent were symptom-free three months after the accident.

Only about 12 percent of patients with mild head injury are hospitalized overnight, and instructions given upon release from the emergency room usually don't address behavioral, cognitive, and emotional symptoms that may occur after such an injury.

Diagnostic tests While CAT scans are widely available in emergency rooms to help in the diagnosis of neural hematomas, many experts believe these scans may not pick up the subtle damage following a mild head injury.

Many researchers believe that MRI is more sensitive in diagnosing many brain lesions beyond a basic hematoma. For example, an MRI is more sensitive in detecting the diffuse axonal or shearing injury and contusions often seen in this type of brain accident.

In many patients, neither CT nor MRI can detect the microscopic damage to WHITE MATTER that occurs when fibers are stretched in a mild, diffuse axonal injury. In this type of mild injury, the AXONS lose some of their covering and become less efficient, but MRI only detects more severe injury and actual axonal degeneration. Mild injury to the white matter reduces the quality of community between different parts of the CEREBRAL CORTEX. In these cases, a quantitative EEG may be used. This type of assessment is different from an EEG in that the signals from the brain are played into a computer, digitized, and stored. This type of EEG can measure the time delay between two regions of the CORTEX and the amount of time it takes for information to be transmitted from one region to another.

The study of evoked potentials is an electrophysical technique not generally useful in patients with less serious head injury. Evoked potentials are not sensitive enough to document most physiologic abnormalities, although the patient may be having symptoms. If testing is done within a day or two of the injury, the EP may pick up some abnormalities in brainstem auditory-evoked potentials.

Neuropsychological tests may show positive results when imaging tests and neurologic exams are negative. In some patients with persistent symptoms following mild head injury, neuropsychological tests are part of a comprehensive assessment. The tests can also provide information when litigation is an issue.

POSITRON EMISSION TOMOGRAPHY (PET SCAN), which evaluates cerebral blood flow and brain metabolism, may provide useful information on functional pathology following mild head injury. SINGLE PHOTO EMISSION COMPUTED TOMOGRAPHY (SPECT) is less expensive than PET and might provide data on cerebral blood flow.

Patients who do experience symptoms should seek out the care of a specialist; unless a family physician is thoroughly familiar with medical literature in this newly emerging area, experts caution that there is a great chance that patient complaints will be ignored. Patients with continuing symptoms after a mild head injury are advised to call a local head-injury foundation, which can refer patients to the best local practitioner.

posterior cerebral arteries, infarction of

Patients who have had infarctions of the posterior cerebral arteries may experience problems in short-term memory, inability to learn new facts and skills, and RETROGRADE AMNESIA. Often, memory problems are associated with visual-field defects.

See also CEREBROVASCULAR ACCIDENTS; SUBARACHNOID HEMORRHAGE.

posture
When the upper body sags, rounding the shoulders, hanging the head and jutting out the chin, it creates kinks in the spine that squeeze the two arteries passing through the spinal column to the brain. This kink can reduce blood supply to the brain, causing "fuzzy thinking" and forgetfulness, especially in older people.

potassium
The most important ion in the brain. Potassium ions allow brain cells to discharge, sending messages to other neurons.

pramiracetam
This NOOTROPIC drug enhances the functioning of the cholinergic system in much the same way as its relative, PIRACETAM, but it is effective at much lower doses. In one study, subjects with ALZHEIMER'S DISEASE showed enhanced intelligence and memory following administration of pramiracetam. However, it is not yet approved by the FDA.

prefrontal cortex
Located in the telencephalon, this brain structure is important in judgment, planning, tact, impulse control, and abstract thinking. In addition, the prefrontal cortex is intimately connected with the LIMBIC SYSTEM. Moreover, input to the prefrontal cortex from the THALAMUS, HYPOTHALAMUS, and MIDBRAIN seem to provide information about the internal emotional and motivational states; these influences, together with other information synthesized by the prefrontal cortex from incoming sensory information, help to give meaning and significance to external events.

Researchers suspect that the prefrontal cortex plays a role in structuring behavior by helping prepare sensory and motor systems for action, by holding some information in a flexible memory. Relatively more developed in humans than any other species, there is an enormously complex interaction between this area and other parts of the brain. When this area is damaged, doctors can't point to any one particular skill or function that is lost; rather, it appears as if an essential quality of "being human" is lost.

In recent research, scientists tested chess players who answered increasingly complex questions designed to identify parts of the brain used for a particular type of thinking. Results of the study suggested that the prefrontal cortex is where the brain plans and processes events or thoughts that are considered as a unit.

pregnenolone
A simple steroid that, in recent research trials, seems to enhance memory in rats and restore normal levels of neurotransmitters (such as ACETYLCHOLINE) which decline during aging. The drug has been tested in humans as a treatment for arthritis and was found to produce no side effects. The hormone was used during the 1940s to treat rheumatoid arthritis but had been abandoned when physicians discovered that cortisone was far more effective.

Pregnenolone is one of several steroid drugs researchers are investigating for possible memory enhancement properties. While several rat and mice studies have seemed to suggest a link between memory improvement and the steroid, the mechanism by which steroids influence memory and learning remains little understood. Scientists suggest pregnenolone might enhance memory because it serves as a raw material for the production of all steroid hormones used in storing information in memory. Concentrations of many of these steroids decline with age; by restoring these levels, pregnenolone may bring back memory abilities that had begun to erode.

Neurologists in California are currently studying pregnenolone's effects on ALZHEIMER'S DISEASE patients with mild to severe memory problems, and older people with age-related memory impairment.

premotor cortex A part of the brain found in the FRONTAL LOBE closely associated with the MOTOR CORTEX that is connected to the RETICULAR FORMATION of the BRAINSTEM. Specifically, the premotor cortex is responsible for identifying objects in space, choosing strategies of action, and programming movement; it also sends output fibers to those reticular NEURONS that influence the muscles of the back, hips, shoulders, and thighs and appears to help regulate POSTURE and stabilize the trunk and limbs during complex movements.

primary visual cortex Signals from the eyes are fed into this region of the brain from the lateral geniculate bodies, and this is where information from both eyes is first combined.

prions This "proteinaceous infectious particle" is a new kind of infectious agent that is basically a protein, capable of causing scrapie and other types of brain diseases, such as CREUTZFELDT-JAKOB DISEASE, FATAL FAMILIAL INSOMNIA, etc.

The term was invented in 1982 by Stanley B. Prusiner, a researcher at the University of California, San Francisco School of Medicine.

About 60 years ago scientists discovered that sheep were catching a disease (scrapie) that transformed their brains into pitted sponges, but researchers could never zero in on the virus. Then neurobiologists discovered a strange movement disorder among New Guinea tribesmen. Both, it turned out, were caused by prions.

Physicians have traced about 40 cases of a prion disease in adults to injections of infected growth hormone administered during childhood. A few others have caught prion diseases after receiving transplanted brain tissue or corneas from infected donors.

Called the *prion protein molecule (PrP)*, this protein arises from cells it may one day destroy. Normally, it can be found harmlessly sitting on the surfaces of NERVE CELLS until something induces it to infect a new cell and replicate by transforming the cell's normal PrP into another version of the mutant PrP.

About 10 percent of prion diseases are hereditary; that is, the gene for PrP mutates, which leads to substitutions or alterations among the 253 AMINO ACIDS that make up PrP. Somehow, these slight differences induce the protein to switch its shape. Different diseases will result depending on the makeup of the rest of the gene.

Some scientists think that accumulation of toxic forms of PrP causes cellular destruction. But others believe that imbalances in normal PrP concentrations can hurt cells.

Some scientists suspect that the loss of functional PrP can lead to the disintegration of the brain. They also believe that normal PrP helps produce SYNAPSES, without which nerve cells cannot communicate.

protein kinase C (PKC) A molecule found on the surface membrane of NERVE CELLS existing in all animal cells, where it plays a role in growth, blood clotting, and the action of hormones. It was first discovered in the early 1970s by a Japanese scientist.

PKC acts by attaching a phosphate group onto specific sites on the other molecules, changing the function of those molecules, increasing or decreasing their level of activity.

Scientists first realized the potential of PKC in 1986 when Princeton University researchers noted that the protein mimicked cellular changes that occur during learning. Scientists already knew that the electrochemical action in NEURONS changes as an animal learns, and that a protein requiring calcium is involved.

When researchers realized that a single molecule was responsible for learning and memory, they reasoned that its appearance should coincide with learning and its disappearance, with forgetting. Research suggests that PKC orchestrates neuronal functions necessary for learning and memory.

Researchers have also discovered that chemicals that block PKC prevent short-term (but not long-term) memory in snails, suggesting that other mechanisms might be responsible for memories that last more than a few minutes.

Scientists are also investigating the role of PKC in memory disorders such as ALZHEIMER'S DISEASE. One recent study at the University of California/San Diego found that the brains of 11 Alzheimer's victims contained only half as much PKC as the brains of seven people who had died of natural causes.

pseudodementia A disorder that mimics DEMENTIA but that includes no evidence of brain dysfunction; nearly 1 out of 10 of those thought to be suffering from true dementia in fact have a depressive illness. Unlike dementia, DEPRESSION is treatable; many people respond well to antidepressant drugs. Not surprisingly, pseudodementia is found most often in elderly patients.

Pseudodementia is believed to be a way of avoiding depression or asking for help; when it occurs after a minor BRAIN INJURY it is often linked to the patient's desire to avoid an unpleasant experience. Pseudodementia can also be found among those who have experienced a minor organic brain injury, which after recovery appears to produce a degree of impairment in excess of what would be expected.

psychedelic drugs Another term for HALLUCINOGENS that was coined in the 1960s from the Greek word for "mind-manifesting" by psychiatrist Humphrey Osmond.

psychic blindness The inability to recognize objects despite normal vision.

psychopharmacology The branch of pharmacology concerned with the effects of drugs on mental processes and behavior. Drugs have been used for hundreds of years to induce sleep and lessen pain, but it wasn't until the midtwentieth century that psychotropic and neuroleptic drugs were introduced.

The term *psychotropic* (from the Greek *psyche* for "mind" and *tropikos* for "turning") describes drugs that affect mood, including antidepressants, sedatives, stimulants, and tranquilizers. *Neuroleptic* (from the Greek *neuro* for "nerve" and *lepsis* for "taking hold") refers to one of a group of drugs used to modify the manifestation of psychosis. They are also known as "major tranquilizers" or "antipsychotics."

Psychopharmacologic drugs include the following drug classes: antipsychotics, antineurotics (or antianxiety drugs), and antidepressants.

psychosurgery Any brain operation performed to treat mental symptoms as a last resort in cases which have not responded to any other treatment. While psychosurgery was first practiced as long as 2,000 B.C., the first widespread use of this form of treatment was not until the 1930s; it reached its peak in the 1960s and began to decline in the 1970s.

In the first half of this century, prefrontal LOBOTOMY was once the most common type of psychosurgery, but it has been replaced by other safer operations because of its harmful side effects.

The most effective targets for this type of surgery were the FRONTAL LOBES; other regions included the cingulum, the AMYGDALA, several areas in the THALAMUS, and the HYPOTHALAMUS.

The most common type of psychosurgery today is STEREOTAXIC SURGERY in which a scalpel or probe is inserted into a small drilled hole in the skull above one temple. Under X-RAY control, the probe is guided to a specific brain area where the surgeon makes small cuts in nerve fibers. This type of surgery is used to treat severe DEPRESSION, ANXIETY, or severe obsessive-compulsive disorder.

Other psychosurgical techniques include more complex operations in which the brain is exposed by cutting away a portion of the skull; parts of the brain are then removed. TEMPORAL LOBE EPILEPSY is treated this way by removing parts of the temporal lobe; rarely, complete lobes are removed to treat violent or aggressive behavior.

Psychosurgery remains a controversial treatment because, while benefiting some subjects, it involves destroying perfectly healthy brain tissue, it may have unpredictable results and may cause negative changes in intellect or personality. Critics of the procedure liken it to the abuses of human subjects during biomedical experiments in Germany during World War II. Proponents argue that prohibiting psychosurgery deprive patients of their right to effective medical treatment.

punch drunk syndrome A problem resulting from multiple repeated blows to the head (such as those experienced by boxers or football players) that can result in a short-term memory problem and other abnormal findings on neuropsychological tests.

The condition was first described in 1928 when it was noted that the brain under microscope showed many signs in common with ALZHEIMER'S DISEASE: widespread NEUROFIBRILLARY TANGLES and neural scarring. It is believed that the BRAIN DAMAGE and resulting memory loss is caused by rapid movements of the head, causing HEMORRHAGES and damaged BRAIN CELLS. In particular, the brains of boxers often exhibit nerve degeneration and loss of nerve fibers in the HIPPOCAMPUS to a degree far exceeding the brains of Alzheimer's disease patients.

Purkinje, Jan Evangelista (1787–1869) A pioneer Czech experimental physiologist helped create a modern understanding of the brain, among other organs. He is best known for the discovery of large NERVE CELLS in the CORTEX of the CEREBELLUM (named Purkinje cells in 1837). A graduate of the University of Prague, he later taught physiology there, moving on to the University of Breslau in Prussia, where he established the world's first independent department of physiology and the first official physiology lab.

pyramidal cells Cortical cell type involved in motor activity; the neurons are named for their pyramidal shape.

pyroglutamate (2-oxo-pyrrolidone carboxylic acid, or PCA) This AMINO ACID is an important flavor enhancer found naturally in a wide variety of fruits and vegetables, dairy products and meat; it is found in large amounts in the brain, CEREBROSPINAL FLUID, and blood. It is also a suspected enhancer of cognitive ability.

PCA is able to penetrate the BLOOD-BRAIN BARRIER, where some researchers believe it stimulates cognitive function, improving memory and learning in rats. At least one study has shown it is effective in alcohol-induced memory deficits in humans and in patients suffering from MULTI-INFARCT DEMENTIA. Administration of this amino acid increased attention and improved short- and long-term retrieval and long-term memory storage.

When compared with a placebo in studies of memory deficits in 40 aged patients, results indicated that PCA improved verbal memory functions in those who were already affected by an age-related memory decline.

One form of the substance is already being used in Italy to treat SENILITY, MENTAL RETARDATION, and alcoholism. It is found in health food and vitamin stores in a variety of preparations under several names.

See also MEMORY ENHANCEMENT.

pyrrolidone derivatives A class of NOOTROPIC drugs including PIRACETAM and its analogues OXIRACETAM, PRAMIRACETAM, ANIRACETAM and others. The mechanism behind their memory-enhancing properties seems to be the increase in transmissions at all synapses; most research suggests that the drugs affect the cholinergic system and the adrenal cortex in the brain.

Pythagoras (c. 580 B.C.–c. 500 B.C.)   Greek philosopher who suggested that the mind was located in the brain and that the brain was the home of the soul.

R

rabies Known popularly as *hydrophobia,* this is an acute viral disease of the CENTRAL NERVOUS SYSTEM that affects all warm-blooded animals, causing severe BRAINSTEM ENCEPHALITIS with a high death rate. It is usually transmitted to man by the bite of an infected animal.

While the usual incubation period is between one and two months for bites on the extremities, incubation periods ranging from 10 days to more than a year have been reported. Bites on the face or neck can have an incubation period as short as two weeks.

Symptoms Symptoms usually begin with personality changes and periods of excitement. This is followed by malaise, fever, breathing problems, salivation, and painful throat-muscle spasms induced by swallowing. Eventually, merely seeing water can induce convulsions and paralysis; death occurs after this stage within four to five days from respiratory failure or heart arrhythmia. This disease is nearly 100 percent fatal during the acute stage.

Treatment Rabies vaccine and antiserum should be administered to anyone with an animal bite sustained in an unprovoked attack. If a person is bitten by an infected animal, daily injections of rabies vaccine, together with an injection of rabies antiserum, may prevent the disease from developing. Foxes, bats, raccoons, and skunks are the major animal reservoirs in the United States, and a rabies epidemic in the 1990s among wild animals has been reported among certain areas in the northeast.

rapid-eye-movement sleep Also known as *paradoxical sleep,* this is one of two types of sleep characterized by an increase in electrical activity within the brain. (The other type of sleep is known as *NREM, or nonrapid eye movement sleep.*)

During REM sleep, the temperature and blood flow to the brain increases, and brain waves begin to resemble the active pattern of an awake person. Eyes move rapidly and dreaming occurs.

REM sleep usually begins about 90 to 100 minutes after a person first falls asleep. The first REM period lasts only about 10 minutes, but each period lasts longer and longer throughout the night; the last of a night's four or five REM periods may last as long as an hour. Babies spend about half of their sleeping time in REM sleep because REM is related to brain growth during development; adults spend about one-fifth of their time asleep in REM.

When REM sleep intrudes into wakefulness, this is known as NARCOLEPSY.

See also SLEEP AND THE BRAIN; SLEEP APNEA; SLEEP DISORDERS.

reading The ability to read is a complex process handled by an elaborate network of brain regions that handle visual information and make sense of the words it sees. While scientists do not agree on the precise process, some researchers suggest that the ability to read depends on specific brain structures. Critics of this view believe that reading is the result of more general brain activities, such as those responsible for sorting objects into meaningful groups.

Recent research has lent credence to the specific structure theory, finding that the FUSIFORM GYRUS showed distinctive electrical responses to patterns of letters. Researchers suspect that this activity takes place in a portion of the brain's visual system that specializes in word recognition.

While electrical activity during this process typically occurs on both the sides of the brain, other parts of the visual system on the side more heavily involved in language (usually the left) probably also contributes to word recognition. For example, recent BRAIN SCANS have found that reading both real and nonsense words increases blood flow in a visual area on the left side of the brain.

receptor A specialized component of a cell that is embedded in the membrane of NERVE CELLS and can detect mechanical changes in the environment, triggering impulses in the sensory NERVOUS SYSTEM. Certain receptors bind NEUROTRANSMITTERS. The neurotransmitters, through activation of the receptor, initiate electrochemical changes in neuronal functions. Receptors are generally found on the DENDRITES and cell bodies of NEURONS.

reflexes An automatic, predictable action that occurs in response to a particular stimulus over which the person has no voluntary control. While the brain controls most of the body's actions at any one moment, there are times when the body must react as quickly as possible without waiting for a response to reach the brain, which might be preoccupied elsewhere. These "emergency reactions" of reflexes take place without any conscious instruction from the brain.

The simplest sort of reflex involves a sensory NERVE CELL at the skin surface that reacts to a stimulus (such as touching a finger to a hot pan). The cell sends a signal along its nerve fiber to the SPINAL CORD; messages are conveyed to neurons in the central GRAY MATTER of the cord, where they split up and follow two paths. One path follows a short reflex loop through the spinal cord via relay NEURONS and back out along MOTOR NEURONS. Almost immediately muscles contract to pull the finger away. Some other messages travel the second path up the spinal cord to the brain; once in the brain, awareness of the stimulus dawns, but by this time the finger has already been pulled away.

The neurons involved in this circuit, encompassing the original sensation to the final action, are called a *reflex arc*.

One of the best-known reflexes is the simple knee-jerk reflex. When a rubber hammer taps the knee just below the knee cap, it stretches a tendon of one of the thigh muscles; a signal passes via a sensory neuron to the spinal cord, which activates a pool of motor neurons; these neurons cause the muscle to contract, jerking the lower leg.

Many reflexes are present at birth, including those that control basic body functions, such as shivering in response to cold or breathing faster when the level of carbon dioxide rises in the blood. The part of the NERVOUS SYSTEM concerned with these processes is the AUTONOMIC NERVOUS SYSTEM, and parts of the BRAINSTEM and the HYPOTHALAMUS help process information for this system. Some autonomic system reflexes can be controlled to a degree—it's possible to stop emptying the bladder voluntarily—but ultimately, reflex is stronger than voluntary will.

On the other hand, some inborn reflexes are found only among infants, and disappear later in life; these include the grasp reflex that causes an infant to grasp a finger that is placed in its palm.

NEUROLOGICAL EXAMINATIONS typically include testing of some simple inborn reflexes, such as the knee jerk, pupil constriction in the presence of light, and the plantar reflex (curling toes in when the sole of the foot is irritated). Abnormal reflex reactions may be a symptom of a malfunctioning nervous system. The examination of vital reflexes controlled by the brainstem is the basis for diagnosing BRAIN DEATH.

Reflexes that are not inborn but that are learned as a result of experience are called *conditioned reflexes*. They occur as a result of *conditioning*—when new pathways and connections within the nervous system are formed as a result of learning. Operant conditioning is an especially important part of learning; once an acceptable response to a new situation has been discovered and repeated several times, it is then automatically elicited by that stimulus and becomes a reflex. For example, a person who drives to work every day can make the same drive without consciously making the effort to follow the route.

Primitive reflexes, as opposed to inborn reflexes, are automatic movements present at birth that occur in response to a stimulus but that disappear during the first few months of life. They are believed to represent actions that might have been an important survival tactic during earlier stages of evolution.

Examples of these primitive reflexes include:

- *grasp reflex*—For the first four months of life, an infant will firmly grasp any object placed in its palm.
- *Moro's reflex*—If a baby's head is momentarily unsupported, arms will be swung outward and brought together in an embracing movement while legs are extended and the baby cries. This reflex lasts for the first three or four months of life.
- *tonic neck reflex*—During the first week of life when a baby turns its head to one side, the arm and leg on that side are stretched out, while the arm and leg on the opposite side flex.
- *walking or stepping reflex*—When a baby is held upright with the feet touching the ground a forward-stepping movement is made by each leg as the weight is placed on the other foot. This reflex is present for the first two months of life and then returns at about the age of six months.
- *rooting reflex*—Touching a baby's cheek with the fingertip near the corner of the mouth will cause the head to turn so that the finger enters the mouth; this reflex enables the baby to find the nipple.

REM See RAPID-EYE-MOVEMENT SLEEP.

reticular activating system A system of nerve pathways in the brain concerned with the level of consciousness (from states of sleep, drowsiness, and relaxation to full attention). The system combines information from all of the senses and from the CEREBRUM and CEREBELLUM and determines the activity of the brain and the AUTONOMIC NERVOUS SYSTEM.

The diffuse pathways extends from the caudal medulla to the MIDBRAIN. The ascending and descending long tracts of the BRAINSTEM pass through and around the RETICULAR FORMATION. Because its NEURONS tend to have long AXONS, the system can have profound effects on overall brain and SPINAL-CORD activity.

reticular formation A network of nerves deep in the brain from the MEDULLA OBLONGATA to the MIDBRAIN. This structure (*reticular* is derived from the Latin word for "net") receives information from all over the body, sending it to cells in the HYPOTHALAMUS, CEREBRAL CORTEX, CEREBELLUM, and SPINAL CORD. In this way, the reticular formation controls the activity level of the entire nervous system and plays a role in movements that don't call for conscious attention; it is also involved in sending or inhibiting sensations of pain, temperature, and touch.

The reticular formation, in conjunction with neurons in the THALAMUS and others from various sensory systems of the brain, make up the RETICULAR ACTIVATING SYSTEM—the basic process that allows people to maintain consciousness.

It is the reticular activating system that allows a person to focus, excluding background information and "tuning out" distractions. It also serves as an effective filter for the continuous stimuli bombarding a person's nervous system; it is this filtering that allows a person to nap while riding in the car but to suddenly snap to attention when the sound of the car's engine changes as it slows down to a stop.

retinoblastoma A rare malignant tumor of the retina found in infants, a tendency that is often inherited and occurs once in every 20,000 births. First appearing as a white color in the pupil, the affected eye may be blind with strabismus (squint). Retinoblastoma can spread from the eye, along the OPTIC NERVE to the brain.

Treatment Removal or radiation therapy of the affected eye; if both eyes are affected, the eye with the larger tumor may be removed and the other given radiation therapy.

retrograde amnesia (RA) A type of AMNESIA that is principally a deficit of recall and recognition of information in which the patient has a gap in memory extending back for some time from the moment of damage to the brain. The memory gap usually shrinks over time. In addition, RA usually causes an inability to remember personal and public events instead of loss of language, conceptual knowledge, or basic cognitive skills.

Retrograde amnesia appears to be most pronounced for the period immediately before the trauma, with less disruption of more remote memories. This means that older patients with retrograde amnesia can probably describe their graduation days but would have trouble talking about what happened the day before the trauma.

Cause Retrograde amnesia may occur following STROKE, HEAD INJURY, administration of electroconvulsive therapy, or in cases of psychogenic amnesia.

Diagnosis Psychologists have developed tests for RA that can measure a patient's memory for events. By compiling a life history of the patient from relatives and friends, the tester can compile a series of questions about each period of a patient's life with which to test the patient. Examiners can also use an autobiographical cueing procedure involving the recall of personal events in response to specific words. This test can uncover retrograde amnesia if the patient can recall events only from certain periods of his or her life. However, this procedure may be unreliable because it is hard to determine whether the patient's memories are accurate. Retrograde amnesia may also be tested by measuring a patient's ability to remember public events because it is assumed that memory for public and personal events have a common basis.

The most extensive test for retrograde amnesia is the Boston Remote Memory Battery, which has three parts with easy and difficult questions. The easy questions may be answered on the basis of general knowledge, while the difficult questions reflect information requiring a particular time period. Unfortunately, this test is culture specific and cannot be used effectively outside the United States without being reformatted.

Generally, retrograde amnesia is less of a problem for patients with memory deficits than is anterograde amnesia (problems acquiring new information after trauma or an illness).

See also AMNESIA; SHRINKING RETROGRADE AMNESIA; TEMPORAL LOBECTOMY.

Rett syndrome A recently recognized brain disorder that affects only girls between 7 to 18 months of age, striking about one in every 15,000 female babies.

The syndrome was discovered by Dr. Andreas Rett of Vienna, who described it in 1966; it has become widely recognized by physicians only since the 1980s.

Symptoms An apparently normal baby begins to show symptoms shortly before or after the first birthday when autisticlike withdrawal sets in. Although this symptom eases in time, higher brain function continues to deteriorate, leading to severe MENTAL RETARDATION. Skills such as walking and talking gradually fade away, and the girl becomes more and more handicapped and emits inappropriate cries and laughter. The child also loses purposeful use of her hands, wringing them in a constant "hand-washing" movement in front of the face or chest.

Cause While scientists don't know yet what causes this syndrome, because it affects only girls it is likely that the condition has a genetic origin in some defect of the X chromosome.

Treatment There is no cure, and patients need constant attention because of the severity of the handicap.

See also APPENDIX A; ASSOCIATION FOR CHILDREN WITH DOWN SYNDROME; ASSOCIATION FOR CHILDREN WITH RETARDED MENTAL DEVELOPMENT; CENTER FOR FAMILY SUPPORT; FEDERATION FOR CHILDREN WITH SPECIAL NEEDS; INTERNATIONAL RETT SYNDROME ASSOCIATION; JARC; MENTAL RETARDATION ASSOCIATION OF AMERICA; NATIONAL ASSOCIATION OF DEVELOPMENTAL DISABILITIES COUNCILS; NATIONAL DOWN SYNDROME CONGRESS; NATIONAL DOWN SYNDROME SOCIETY; PARENTS OF CHILDREN WITH DOWN SYNDROME; PILOT PARENTS; VOICE OF THE RETARDED; YOUNG ADULT INSTITUTE AND WORKSHOP.

Reye's syndrome A rare condition, nearly exclusive to children under age 15, characterized by BRAIN DAMAGE following chicken pox, influenza, or an upper respiratory infection. Because it has been associated with the administration of aspirin, physicians recommend that children never be given aspirin for viral infections or fever of unknown cause. Reye's syndrome is a leading cause of death among children beyond infancy; survivors often suffer brain damage.

The death rate from this condition has dropped dramatically from 60 percent to 10 percent as scientists begin to understand the disorder. The chances for recovery are not as good for those who have reached stages of deep COMA, and SEIZURES. Severe attacks carry the risk of lasting brain damage.

See also NATIONAL REYE'S SYNDROME FOUNDATION (for address, see Appendix A).

Symptoms About a week into the viral illness, signs of Reye's syndrome are vomiting, confusion, lethargy, disorientation, and jaundice. As the brain swells, it may trigger seizures, coma, heart disturbances, and breathing problems.

Treatment There is no specific treatment; corticosteroid drugs and mannitol infusions control brain swelling; dialysis or blood transfusions may correct blood chemistry changes; a ventilator may assist breathing. This type of supportive care has reduced the death rate in the most severe cases from 80 percent to below 50 percent and in milder cases down to 10 or 20 percent.

right brain The right CEREBRAL HEMISPHERE, linked with spatial skill. See HANDEDNESS; SPLIT-BRAIN RESEARCH.

Ritalin A CENTRAL-NERVOUS-SYSTEM stimulant that increases nerve activity in the brain by triggering the release of the NEUROTRANSMITTER NOREPINEPHRINE. This drug reduces drowsiness and increases alertness by its action on the RETICULAR ACTIVATING SYSTEM in the BRAINSTEM and midbrain. While Ritalin is a stimulant, paradoxically it is given to treat hyperactivity in children. It is given as part of a treatment program for various attention deficit disorders in children. In general, it is a safe drug.

Adverse effects Possible side effects include shaking, sweating, palpitations, nervousness, sleeping problems, HALLUCINATIONS, paranoid delusions, and SEIZURES. Long-term use may lead to drug tolerance and dependence.

S

Schilder's disease A rapidly progressive sheath-destructive disorder featuring widespread demyelination of the NEURONS in the CEREBRAL HEMISPHERES of the brain. This disease occurs most often in children and ends in death within a few years of onset.

schizophrenia The most common form of psychosis, affecting about one percent of the population, schizophrenia (or "fragmented mind") results in a break from reality involving bizarre delusions, illogical thinking, incoherence, and HALLUCINATIONS. Schizophrenia also interferes with the ability to concentrate on and think about incoming information, but it is unclear to what extent this depends on the subtype of the disorder and to what extent it reflects the patient's problems with paying attention to outside events.

Originally termed *dementia praecox* by German psychiatrist Emil Kraepelin, schizophrenia has eluded researchers who have spent a great deal of time searching for evidence of physical dysfunction in the brains of schizophrenia patients.

It appears that schizophrenia may be caused by a malfunctioning DOPAMINE system, and new research suggests that the roots of schizophrenia appear much earlier in brain development. In fact, considerable evidence suggests that malfunctioning fetal brain development may set the stage for later appearance of the disorder. It may be that aberrant organization of fetal BRAIN CELLS during development may combine intact and impaired NEURONS together in dysfunctional circuits. Some researchers suggest that viral infections during pregnancy (together with other prenatal or birth problems) may play a role in the development not just of schizophrenia, but also of AUTISM and DYSLEXIA. As evidence, researchers cite a Finnish study that found a higher rate of schizophrenia among children

of women exposed to a flu epidemic during the second trimester of pregnancy. Schizophrenia has also been linked to birth in the winter when viral infections are common.

Twin studies have also shown that some type of genetic mechanism strongly influences about half of all cases of schizophrenia.

Some researchers believe that many schizophrenia patients' brain development begins to break down in midpregnancy when many large neurons arrive at their final destination. In parts of the CORTEX (the brain's outer layer) and within deeper regions associated with emotion and memory, researchers have found disorganized ensembles of neurons.

By staining schizophrenics' brains after autopsy, scientists have also found missing or abnormally sized neurons and abnormal myelination of nerve fibers.

People with both a family history of schizophrenia and a second trimester exposure to viral infection may experience the greatest chance of developing schizophrenia themselves. Minor complications at birth or shortly thereafter may boost these odds even further, scientists suggest. Other scientists suggest that families with high percentages of schizophrenia may lack the genetic instructions that guide cortical neurons during development to their final destination in circuit formation.

More recent research suggests that the root of schizophrenia may lie in abnormalities in the THALAMUS and related structures; scientists have already suspected that the thalamus helps focus attention and process sensory information. When comparing brains of normal and schizophrenic patients, researchers at the University of Iowa Hospitals and Clinics in Iowa City found that the area of greatest difference in strength of signal during MAGNETIC RESONANCE IMAGING (MRI) was found in the thalamus and nearby tissue leading to the front of the cortex. Schizophrenic men also had a much smaller thalamus than normal men.

Malfunctions in the underlying function of the thalamus, which develops before or shortly after birth, may be the root of the problem that underlies the various symptoms of schizophrenia.

Treatment Since the 1950s, doctors have used the phenothiazines (especially CHLOROPROMAZINE) to tame the symptoms of schizophrenia. More recently, haloperidol has also been helpful in controlling some of the most problematic symptoms; neither drug offers a complete cure.

Recent Swiss research suggests that training to improve attention, memory and basic reasoning skills may play a role in treating many cases of the disease. Their approach of cognitive rehabilitation differs from other more traditional programs, which focus on teaching social skills. In studies at the University of Bern, researchers emphasize thinking abilities by having patients sort cards containing geometric shapes, colors, and days of the week. Training then advances to word problems and interpreting the meaning of social interactions and other complete social skills. As many as 18 months after the program, participants showed substantial improvement on tests measuring attention and overall mental condition. However, these patients are still not capable of complex thought and social skills.

In addition, schizophrenic children suffer from attention and memory problems that undermine their ability to communicate with others. In recent studies at UCLA, while motor and perceptual skills remain intact, these youngsters fail at tests of rapid mental activity and have significant problems copying a remembered shape. In addition, tasks that normally would spark an electrical surge in one or both brain hemispheres have no effect on schizophrenic youngsters.

scopolamine An antispasmodic drug that blocks neurotransmission of certain chemicals in the brain, including ACETYLCHOLINE, important in the normal function of memory. If given to normal subjects, the drug causes a severe memory loss which is reversed by the administration of physostigmine. Under the influence of scopolamine, retention remains intact, but effortful retrieval is impaired. Scopolamine appears to disrupt efficient encoding processes leading to a deficiency in effective retrieval of information. It has a more potent effect than sedatives or tranquilizers on human cognitive abilities, but the strength of the AMNESIA following scopolamine administration depends on the memory task used to define it.

Seasonal Affective Disorder (SAD) A syndrome of winter depression, SAD is specifically related to changes in the length of daylight across the seasons. While its exact cause is not known, the disorder has been linked to a malfunction in the brain's biological clock that controls temperature and hormone production.

As many as 12 million Americans may suffer from this disorder, and up to 35 million others may experience milder forms. It's at least four times as common among women, usually beginning in the 20s and 30s (although it has been reported in some children and teenagers). Other estimates suggest that as many as half of all women in northern states experience pronounced winter DEPRESSION, but very few receive the necessary treatment because their doctors don't know how to tell the difference between typical depressive symptoms and SAD.

The PINEAL GLAND appears to be particularly important in the development of SAD. Nestling near the center of the brain, the pineal gland processes information about light through special nerve pathways and releases the sleep-inducing hormone MELATONIN, also responsible for regulating CIRCADIAN

RHYTHMS. Melatonin is produced in the dark and peaks during the winter. Experts believe it may suppress mood and mental quickness. Interestingly, manic depressives are extremely sensitive to light, and their melatonin levels plummet when exposed to light.

The body is regulated by some sort of biological clock that sets the pace for everyday rhythms of sleep, activity, temperature, and cortisol and melatonin release. Most people maintain a certain flexibility in this system, allowing them to synchronize this biological clock to environmental changes. But experts suspect that some people—perhaps those prone to depression—don't synchronize their clocks so easily. It could be that their internal clock is out of step with the world's 24-hour rhythm so that melatonin is released too early (causing evening sleepiness and early morning awakening) or too late (causing insomnia and problems awakening).

Treatment While some cases eventually disappear in time, others persist for a lifetime. The best treatment for this disorder is phototherapy—exposure to additional special types of light during the winter—which will reverse this type of depression in most people.

Treatment is effective and inexpensive; patients must only be sure to get an accurate diagnosis and the right kind of light box to provide enough high-intensity light for a certain time each day. After a few days spent sitting for a few hours under special, bright fluorescent lights, symptoms subside; symptoms reappear if treatment stops. In general, patients must sit about 3 feet away from a bank of special lights of between six and eight fluorescent bulbs about three hours daily. Ordinary room light is not bright enough to affect SAD.

While researchers are still studying this treatment, many physicians recommend it for this type of depression. *Treatment should be under the supervision of an expert.* Experts believe that the treatment works by in-creasing the secretion of the hormonal chemical melatonin in the brain, helping to regulate the natural circadian rhythm.

Because light therapy may be only partly successful in eradicating symptoms, treatment may be bolstered by the use of antidepressants. Antidepressants alone may be used instead of light therapy for people with SAD, but often the two treatments are used together. Also, the two treatments together often means that lower doses of antidepressants can be used.

Many physicians adjust the dose of antidepressants with the changing seasons—increasing the dose as the days become shorter, decreasing it as the days lengthen.

More and more doctors are considering Prozac and the other SSRIs to be the drug of choice for SAD, primarily because the SEROTONIN system is believed to be part of the problem in this disorder. Desyrel has also been used successfully with SAD patients. Older antidepressants may also be beneficial, such as the tricyclics desipramine or imipramine. (Doctors often stay away from the more sedating tricyclics, such as amitriptyline and doxepin, because people with SAD tend to sleep too much as it is.)

sedatives Drugs that relieve anxiety and tension, including barbiturates, administered at lower doses than those needed for sleep. They have been generally replaced by tranquilizers, which are less likely to cause dependence.

See also CENTRAL NERVOUS-SYSTEM DEPRESSANTS.

seizure A sudden burst of abnormal electrical activity from some area in the brain caused by one of a number of different conditions. While all seizures used to be called *epilepsy,* today the more modern term is *seizure disorder.* Seizures that occur on a regular basis, however, are still termed *epileptic.*

See also SEIZURE, FEBRILE.

Cause Seizures may be caused by a wide variety of neurological or medical problems, including STROKE, heart disease, kidney problems, sinus infection, middle-ear disorders, injury, high fever, chemical abnormalities in the blood, acute alcoholic toxicity, drug poisoning, or old scar tissue from an injury. When a clear-cut cause cannot be found, doctors usually assume that a seizure is caused by a metabolic disorder or a birth injury.

Diagnosis In order to determine the cause of seizures, doctors need to assess an accurate description of the seizure, complete physical exam, blood tests, and ELECTROENCEPHALOGRAM (EEG), CAT SCAN or MAGNETIC RESONANCE IMAGING (MRI).

Symptoms A seizure that arises in only a small portion of the brain may set off a simple case of tingling in a small area of the body. Other symptoms may include HALLUCINATIONS, intense feelings of fear, or DÉJÀ VU. If the abnormal electrical activity spreads across the brain, the patient loses consciousness and experiences a GRAND MAL SEIZURE.

Treatment Seizures can be prevented in more than 90 percent of cases, especially if the cause has been identified. The most common antiseizure medication is valproic acid (Depakene). Alternatively, other antiseizure medications include PHENYTOIN (Dilantin), carbamazpine (Tegretol), or phenobarbital. Medication that works the best with the fewest side effects should be continued for at least five years after the last seizure.

seizure, febrile A common type of childhood seizure characterized by twitching limbs and loss of consciousness triggered by a rapidly escalating fever. About one in 20 children will have one or more febrile seizures, which tend to run in families and are not considered serious. They usually appear in children between six months and five years.

Most children who experience febrile seizures are completely normal; about 30 to 40 percent will experience another such seizure within the following six months. The chances of recurrent febrile seizures are increased if there are mental problems or a family history of EPILEPSY or if the first seizure was prolonged. Children with all three risk factors have a 10 percent chance of developing epilepsy. However, in healthy children the risk of developing epilepsy is small.

Cause The fever that triggers the seizure usually develops with an acute infectious illness such as an ear infection or tonsillitis. The seizures themselves are caused by a disturbance in the normal electrical activity of the brain.

Symptoms Loss of consciousness followed by uncontrollable twitching of arms or legs for several minutes.

Treatment During the seizure, the mouth should never be wedged open to prevent biting of the tongue, which rarely occurs anyway. If the child has not had previous seizures, a physician should be contacted. Any seizure that lasts longer than five minutes should be treated as an emergency. No other treatment is necessary for the seizure other than treatment of the underlying illness.

Prevention Seizures may be prevented by lowering the child's temperature by using acetaminophen at the first sign of fever. Bedclothes should be removed, and a fan pointed toward the child. While sponging the child with lukewarm water may be comforting, itwill most likely not help in reducing the temperature.

selective serotonin reuptake inhibitor (SSRI) A class of new antidepressants that prevent brain cells from reabsorbing SEROTONIN, thus effectively raising the levels of this NEUROTRANSMITTER. A malfunctioning serotonin system has been implicated in the development of DEPRESSION. The SSRIs include Prozac (fluoxetine), Zoloft (sertraline), and

Paxil (paroxetine). Two other new drugs also affect serotonin—Serzone (nefazadone) and Luvox (fluvoxamine).

In addition to depression, these new antidepressants—especially Prozac—appear to work for a wide range of other mood disorders in addition to depression, such as ANXIETY or panic disorders, posttraumatic stress, eating disorders, or obsessive-compulsive disorder.

These SSRIs have moved to the forefront of modern psychiatric treatment because they work as well as any of the older antidepressants while causing far less serious side effects. This lack of side effects is primarily due to the fact that they work so selectively in the brain, affecting just one neurotransmitter system (serotonin) instead of other neurotransmitter systems and RECEPTOR sites throughout the brain.

This is quite different than the shotgun approach of older antidepressants such as the MONOAMINE OXIDASE (MAO) INHIBITORS or TRICYCLICS, which interfere with neurotransmitters and receptor sites all over the brain.

When a drug blocks a specific neurotransmitter, it causes side effects; the more neurotransmitters that are blocked, the more variety of side effects will result. For example, blocking the reuptake of NOREPINEPHRINE can produce tremors, sexual dysfunction, and tachycardia. Blocking the reuptake of DOPAMINE can produce movement disorders and changes in the endocrine system. By specifically blocking serotonin alone, scientists can sidestep those problems (although patients may still experience stomach upset, insomnia, and anxiety).

The more receptors and neurotransmitters that are affected, the more side effects are produced. This is why a tricyclic antidepressant, which blocks the reuptake of norepinephrine and serotonin plus four different types of receptors, is associated with many more side effects than the SSRIs, which affect only one neurotransmitter and barely disturbs receptors at all.

Interestingly, it now appears that the serotonin neurotransmitter system may be far more complex than anyone had realized, linking areas throughout the brain in an interwoven tapestry of serotonin-producing connections. Not surprisingly, serotonin receptors are especially plentiful in the areas of the brain-controlling emotion. What's more, within the past decade scientists have realized there are at least six different receptor types in the serotonin system, each responsible for sending different signals to different parts of the brain. The next step is to find a drug that can affect just one of these receptor types and to develop a simple lab test that can identify specific serotonin malfunctions. While it's apparent that serotonin is of vital importance in the development of depression, scientists aren't so sure that it's a simple cause-and-effect relationship; the brain's biochemical pathways for emotion and mood are just too complex. While it *may* be true that scientists can directly relieve depression by increasing serotonin, it is also true that altering serotonin levels causes slight effects in other neurotransmitter systems and that *those* changes relieve depression.

self-hypnosis See HYPNOSIS.

senile dementia In the past, DEMENTIA was divided into two forms; presenile (affecting people under age 65) and senile (over age 65). These designations are no longer used today.

Senile dementia (or SENILITY) is a catchword that has been used for many years to label almost any eccentric behavior in the elderly. It has sometimes been equated with such terms as *chronic brain failure, chronic brain syndrome, organic brain syndrome,* or ALZHEIMER'S DISEASE.

Between 50 to 60 percent of older people with impaired memories have Alzheimer's; approximately 20 to 25 percent of brain impairment is caused by STROKE, and the remainder is the result of other causes, including normal aging.

There are a number of reasons for confusion, forgetfulness, and disorientation besides Alzheimer's disease. It could be caused by overmedication or medication interaction, chemical imbalances (lack of potassium, abnormal sugar, etc.), DEPRESSION, sudden illness, malnutrition and dehydration, or social isolation.

senility A term once referred to changes in mental ability caused by old age. However, the term *senile* simply means "old" and therefore, senility does not really describe a disease; it is considered by many people to be a derogatory or prejudicial term.

Most people over age 70 suffer from some amount of impaired memory and reduced ability to concentrate. As a person ages, the risk of DEMENTIA rises to affect about one of five over age 80. Depressive illness and confusion due to physical disease are also common.

The terms *chronic* ORGANIC BRAIN SYNDROME and *acute or reversible organic brain syndrome* have been used respectively to refer to those dementias that cannot be treated (chronic) and to those that respond to treatment (acute).

See also AGING AND MEMORY; ALZHEIMER'S DISEASE.

senses and the brain One of the chief responsibilities of the brain is the processing and interpretation of information picked up by the body's five senses: sight, smell, touch, sound, and taste. The primary receiving centers for the major sensory nerves is the THALAMUS, located in the MIDBRAIN next to the third ventricle and the BASAL GANGLIA. The thalamus integrates all the various sensory impulses (such as recognizing pain) and, like some giant traffic manager, sends all sensory stimuli to the CEREBRAL CORTEX, where the messages are received and translated in to a response. The thalamus is also responsible for the sense of movement and position and the ability to identify sizes and shapes of objects.

Sensory impulses travel on three major pathways depending on the type of sensation and typically involves three NEURON relays. Information about these paths is of crucial importance when making a neurological diagnosis and can help health-care workers pinpoint the location of BRAIN DAMAGE.

AXONS, which are responsible for carrying messages of heat, cold, and pain, make connections with the cells of secondary neurons in the SPINAL CORD. Temperature and pain fibers pass immediately to the opposite side of the spinal cord and travel upward to the thalamus.

Sensations of touch, light pressure, and limb localization travel for some distance before entering the gray column of the spinal cord, completing the connection.

Stimuli from muscles, joints, and bones (including the sense of position in space and vibration) travel uncrossed to the BRAINSTEM via the axon of the primary neuron.

In the MEDULLA, connections are made with secondary neuron cells whose axons then cross to the opposite side and travel to the thalamus.

Cutting a sensory nerve will cause the total loss of sensation in the area of the body it serves. Severing the spinal cord will therefore permanently anesthetize the area below the injury.

Assessment of the health of this system involves testing (with eyes closed) of tactile sensation, superficial pain (such as a pinprick), vibration, and proprioception (subjective sense of joint position). Tactile sensation is tested by lightly touching a cotton ball to the same areas on each side of the body; the sensitivity of different areas of the body is compared.

Because pain and temperature sensations are transmitted together, it is not usually necessary to test separately for temperature sensation. A patient's sensitivity to superficial pain can be evaluated asking the person to differentiate between the sharp and blunt ends of a broken wooden cotton swab stick or tongue depressor applied with equal intensity to both sides of the body. A safety pin should not be used because it can break the skin.

Vibration and proprioception are transmitted together, and the strength of these senses are often lost together. A person's sense of vibration is evaluated by having the patient report when he or she feels a low-frequency tuning fork stop vibrating when placed against a bony prominence of the body. Side-to-side comparisons are made.

A person's ability to sense his or her own body's position in space can be tested by having him or her close both eyes and describe the direction that he or her toes have been moved.

After all these peripheral sensations have been tested, it's also important to determine if the brain is correctly integrating these sensations. This can be tested by evaluating whether a patient can perceive how many objects he or she has touched when he or she touches two sharp objects at the same time. Similarly, a person should be able to tell when he or she is touched in two places on his or her body at the same time (with eyes closed).

sensory area Part of the CEREBRAL CORTEX that receives tactile sensory information from the skin, including pressure receptors, thermoreceptors, etc.

sensory cortex A part of the CEREBRAL CORTEX parallel to the MOTOR CORTEX that is responsible for awareness of body sensations such as hot or cold.

sensory deprivation The removal of a person's normal sights, sounds, and physical feelings. Studies have shown that sensory deprivation can produce a variety of mental changes and a slowing of brain activity. Volunteers who lay immobile in a darkened environment, wearing masks and gloves in a sound-proof room, reported feelings of unreality, concentration problems, and HALLUCINATIONS.

serotonin A chemical that is found in many tissues of the body. In the brain, serotonin acts as a NEUROTRANSMITTER (a chemical involved in transmitting nerve signals between NERVE CELLS) that is believed to be involved in mood states (especially DEPRESSION) and consciousness. The class of antidepressant drugs called SELECTIVE SEROTONIN REUPTAKE INHIBITORS (SSRI) (including Prozac, Zoloft, and Paxil) are used to treat depression by inhibiting the absorption of serotonin in the brain, effectively boosting the levels of the neurotransmitter.

sex differences in the brain See GENDER DIFFERENCES IN THE BRAIN.

sexuality and the brain While sexual activity appears to be a physical activity, it is the brain that is of profound importance in sexuality itself. Sexual activity is moderated by the LIMBIC-SYSTEM structures in the TEMPORAL LOBE; damage in this area has been linked to hypersexuality, an abnormal condition characterized by an increased sex drive and an indiscriminate choice of partners. In both men and women, the sex drive and sexual response appear to be triggered by the sense organs or HYPOTHALAMUS. Instinctual sexual behavior is genetically programmed in the hypothalamus and the limbic system and is triggered by sex hormones in these areas.

In most mammals, sexual arousal is linked to chemicals (pheromones) with distinctive odors that the female releases when she is in heat (the period of time when her eggs are ready to be fertilized). These pheromones stimulate males of the same species to try to mate with the female.

However, in humans there is no period when the female is in heat, although some women do feel more interested in sex after ovulation. Moreover, in humans, males seem fairly uninterested by pheromones, even though such chemicals do exist to stimulate the human male sex drive.

sexual orientation and the brain The process that makes a person male or female in orientation is quite complex. A child's outward sexual characteristics—his or her gender—is determined at conception by the X or Y chromosome present in the fertilizing sperm. This sets off a series of hormonal events culminating in the development of characteristically male or female genitals and gonads.

While the bodies of both boys and girls in early childhood (other than genitals) appear to be identical, by the teenage years hormonal activity begins to influence the development of adult sex differences. But hormonal activity appears to be most important in infancy because research has suggested that hormonal activity at birth affects the physiological makeup of the infant's brain, affecting personality traits.

Research has shown that natural or artificially induced hormone imbalances can produce "male" changes in female brains and vice versa, together with related personality changes—girls exhibit more aggression, and boys become gentler. These results suggest that sex roles may be as much a result of brain development as social conditioning. Research suggests that the brain's exposure to sex hormones at a specific critical phase in very early life determines sexual behavior for the rest of life, no matter what a person's outward sexual characteristics. In rat experiments, females given male hormones for a few days just after birth fail to mate as females should and cannot ovulate. In addition, the preoptic part of their hypothalami shows a more characteristic male, not female, brain-cell pattern.

Moreover, in 1991 researchers discovered that the brains of homosexual men were anatomically different from those of heterosexual men. In homosexual men, a tiny node in the front of the HYPOTHALAMUS (an area of the brain concerned with sexual behavior) was only about a third of the size of the node in heterosexual men; this node was roughly the same size as in heterosexual women. Researcher Simon LeVay of the Salk Institute in San Diego emphasized that his findings did not prove that the brain variation caused homosexuality, nor did he know when the brain abnormality appeared. LeVay's study was based on autopsies of 19 homosexual men, and 16 men, and 6 women believed to be heterosexual. (The researchers could not obtain the brains of lesbian women because these women rarely die of sexually transmitted diseases and, therefore, their sexual orientation was not often noted on medical charts.) While the brains of all subjects were fairly young (about age 40), more than half had died from AIDS. This prompted critics to attribute the differences in the brains to the disease and not to sexual preference.

Other researchers have found a second difference between the brains of homosexual and heterosexual men. A pair of researchers at the University of California at Los Angeles discovered a difference in the anterior commissure, a pencil-sized bundle of nerves that may carry sensory information between the lobes of the brain. The brain structure in gay men was 34 percent larger than in heterosexual men and 18 percent larger than in heterosexual women. Researchers concluded that the difference could mean homosexual men may process information differently.

In their study, they examined brain tissue from the autopsies of 34 men listed as gay and 75 men and 84 women presumed to be heterosexual. While none had neurological diseases, 24 of the gay men and six of the heterosexual men had died of AIDS. Because this disease is known to cause brain and nerve damage, critics suggested the brain differences could be related to disease. On the other hand, researchers pointed out that AIDS causes brain atrophy, which would mean that the front commissure should be smaller instead of larger than in those with healthy brains.

shaken baby syndrome A type of brain damage caused by violent shaking of a child that often results in hemorrhages and swelling of the brain. Shaken-baby syndrome is common in cases of child abuse and neglect.

shrinking retrograde amnesia The gradual recovery from RETROGRADE AMNESIA, with older memories returning first. The existence of the phenomenon of shrinking retrograde amnesia is not surprising, considering that earlier memories can be derived from a different source from that needed to recall more recent experiences.

As recovery occurs, more and more of the episodic record becomes available and more recent memories can be recalled. It is believed that older experiences are more broadly distributed than newer events and that a gradual recovery process will restore some component of older memories before it restores more narrowly distributed newer memories.

shunt, brain A procedure in which a narrow piece of tubing is inserted into the brain to receive excess intracranial pressure. In the technique, the shunt is inserted into the back portion of the lateral ventricle and then threaded under the scalp toward the neck; still under the skin, the tubing is threaded to another body cavity, where the SPINAL FLUID is drained and absorbed.

sight See VISION.

sleep and the brain In order to function with peak skills, it is essential to get enough sleep and rest the brain, which can be taxed by too much work during the day and poor sleeping at night. In fact, sleep is an active process of the nervous system. Most people spend about a third of their lives sleeping, although the amount of sleep we need varies at any one time. Babies sleep for about 16 hours a day in several periods; at age 5 most children sleep 10 or 11 hours at night. Adults need between 7 or 8 hours of sleep to stay healthy and alert, although illness, exertion, and pregnancy increase the need for sleep. A few people are known as *nonsomniacs* and need only one or two hours of sleep each night.

As evening wears on and darkness falls, the eyes register the fading light with the brain's biological clock—the PINEAL GLAND, found deep within the brain. This gland then secretes MELATONIN, a sleep-related hormone that affects BRAIN CELLS that use SEROTONIN. Melatonin is concentrated in the raphe nuclei found along the BRAINSTEM behind the RETICULAR ACTIVATING SYSTEM—the part of the brain responsible for consciousness itself.

During sleep, the sensory input to the reticular activating system drops, and the electrical activity up through the CEREBRAL CORTEX drops. This doesn't mean that a sleeping brain is completely switched off, however. In sleep, the brain undergoes repeated activity cycles marked by several distinct stages.

Stage I sleep is characterized by relaxation as the person drifts in and out of sleep; heartbeat and breathing slow down, muscles relax and a slight noise would awaken the sleeper. After a few minutes, sleepers pass into *Stage II*, a stage of light sleep where the eyes roll slowly from side to side. The EEG will show "sleep spindles," and sleepers won't awaken unless the noise is much louder. As the body grows still more relaxed, the person enters *Stage III* sleep, wherein the long, slow DELTA WAVES appear. Heartbeat, breathing, body temperature, and blood pressure fall further, and muscles become more relaxed. About 20 to 30 minutes after sleep begins, the person enters *Stage IV*—deep sleep. At this point, EEG tracings show primarily delta waves; some sleepers may talk or sleepwalk in this stage. Then the cycle slowly reverses itself over the next 30 to 40 minutes, and the person slowly surfaces from Stage III to II. But instead of going on to experience Stage I again, the sleeper enters the first of several phases of REM SLEEP as the eyes suddenly start to flicker back and forth while breathing and heartbeat becomes irregular. Sleepers awakened during this stage report dreams.

During REM, noradrenalin-producing cells in the PONS (the middle section of the brainstem) triggers a burst of signals that spread to nearby cells, eventually affecting the entire cerebral cortex. Some scientists believe that the cortex then draws on its memory banks to construct a pattern of these signals—resulting in a dream. While this is going on, the brain electrically "freezes" motor neurons that control the large muscles; this prevents violent movements of arms and legs that would be harmful during REM sleep.

Periods of REM sleep alternate with NREM (non-REM) sleep in about a 90-minute cycle; the REM portion becomes longer each time as the NREM shortens. The fourth or fifth period of REM sleep may last as long as an hour. Eventually, sleep becomes shallower and the sleeper awakens.

Each sleep cycle lasts about 90 minutes, and there are about four or five cycles per night. During sleep, the brain revises, manipulates, and stores information. Of course, sleep is not a continuous process throughout the night. Instead, according to researchers at France's National Center for Scientific Research, the brain processes, reviews, consolidates, and stores information during "paradoxical sleep," (REM) which lasts for just about 20 minutes and occurs every 90 minutes in humans. During this portion of sleep,

all the senses are put on hold, disconnecting the brain from the outside world.

Sleep learning Despite popular ideas to the contrary, it's not possible to learn while asleep, even though some people can't learn effectively *without* sleep. Because both the conscious and subconscious play a role in the memory process, one can't work without the other.

Insomnia The inability to sleep deprives a person not just of valuable memory consolidation during rest but also interferes with learning during waking hours. This problem particularly affects the elderly, who often have more sleep problems and get very little fourth-stage, or "deep," sleep, during which the brain recharges itself. After a while, the person lives in a chronic state of fatigue and finds it difficult to pay attention.

sleep apnea Episodes of failure to breathe during sleep that may last for 10 seconds or longer may be caused either by a failure of the brain's regulation of breathing during sleep or by excessive muscular relaxation.

In central sleep apnea, the patient's airway stays open, but the diaphragm and chest muscles don't work because of a disturbance in the brain's regulation of breathing during sleep.

Obstructive sleep apnea, on the other hand, is more common and is caused by excessive relaxation during sleep of the muscles of the sort palate at the base of the throat and the uvula. These muscles block the airway, making breathing labored and causing loud snoring. A complete blockage will halt breathing, making the sleeper stop snoring. As the pressure to breathe makes muscles of the diaphragm and chest work harder, the blockage is opened and the patient gasps and briefly wakes. This type of sleep apnea may also be caused by enlarged tonsils and adenoids, a large tongue, or a small airway.

Often, people experience both central and obstructive sleep apnea (called *mixed apnea*), which is characterized by a brief period of central apnea followed by a longer period of obstructive apnea. Snoring is common in this condition.

The periods of arousal during the night are brief and aren't usually remembered; people who experience them will often complain of being sleepy during the day. Severe sleep apnea may lead to high blood pressure, heart failure, heart attack, or STROKE.

Obstructive sleep apnea affects one in every 100 men between the ages of 30 and 50, especially if they snore and are overweight. However, the condition may be found in women as well and in all ages. Some experts suggest that some cases of sudden infant death syndrome (SIDS) may be caused by sleep apnea; it becomes more and more common as a person ages.

Treatment Because most people with severe sleep apnea are overweight, the condition is eased with weight loss. In addition, people subject to sleep apnea should not drink alcohol within two hours of going to sleep and should not take sleeping pills. (Both substances slow down the breathing muscle activity and may worsen the condition.)

More and more patients are finding relief with "continuous positive airway pressure" — a mask that is worn over the nose and mouth during sleep, forcing oxygen into both nasal passages and the airway to keep them open.

Protriptyline and supplemental oxygen may help some people; surgery to remove excess tissue at the back of the throat may be helpful in some cases. Some may find relief with a tracheostomy (an opening in the windpipe), which bypasses the obstructed airway, allowing air to flow directly to the lungs during sleep.

sleep disorders One in three adults in the United States suffer from one of the more than 100 disorders of sleeping and waking. The disorders are divided into four main categories: the insomnias (problems in falling or staying asleep), problems staying awake, problems adhering to a consistent sleep/wake schedule, and problems with sleep-disruptive behaviors.

Insomnias are classified as transient (lasting just a few nights, usually due to excitement or minor stress), short-term (lasting up to three weeks due to major stress or illness), and chronic (continued poor sleep that may be caused by physical illness, psychological issues, poor sleeping environment, or lifestyle). While insomnias are not considered a disease, they are a symptom that can benefit from medical treatment.

Problems in staying awake are the usual reasons that drive people to seek help at one of the more than 200 sleep-disorder centers in this country. These problems are usually the result of SLEEP APNEA (a potentially fatal disorder in which breathing stops intermittently during sleep) and NARCOLEPSY (a disorder causing daytime sleep attacks).

Those people who have problems maintaining a consistent sleep/wake cycle usually have disruptions in their internal sleep center in the brain controlling sleeping and waking. A common example of this problems is JET LAG, in which the body's internal clock is upset by rapid travel across time zones (especially west to east). A form of this type of jet lag occurs among employees who must work rotating shifts, constantly changing their hours for waking and sleeping. Those who work night shifts also complain of more problems with poor sleep and daytime drowsiness.

sleeping sickness A serious infectious disease of tropical Africa spread by the bite of the tsetse fly, which transmits the protozoa *Trypanosoma brucei* to humans and animals. The protozoa multiply and spread to the bloodstream and eventually the brain, when it induces the strange lethargy from which the disease gets its name.

There are two forms of the disease: sleeping sickness of western and central Africa is spread primarily from person to person, while the east African version primarily affects wild animals, although it is occasionally transmitted to humans.

While sleeping sickness can be controlled by eradicating the tsetse fly, many thousands of Africans (and some tourists) still contract the disease each year.

Symptoms First, a painful nodule develops at the bite site; the West African version then slowly proceeds with fever and lymph-gland enlargement until the protozoa migrate to the brain, setting off HEADACHES, confusion, and severe lassitude with eventual complete inactivity, drooping eyelids, and a vacant expression. Untreated, the disease is fatal.

The East African form of the disease runs a faster course, beginning with a high fever a few weeks after infection. If the disease is not at first fatal from attacking the heart, the protozoan will continue to affect the brain.

Treatment Drug treatment will cure the disease, although the drugs can cause serious side effects. If the infection has already spread to the brain, it can cause brain damage.

Prevention Tourists should protect themselves against the bite of the tsetse fly in order to avoid the disease.

slow viruses of the brain

A group of viruses of the CENTRAL NERVOUS SYSTEM (including the brain) that cause symptoms of memory loss and DEMENTIA 10 or 20 years after the initial infection. The diseases take a slow course, the end of which is usually fatal. Included among diseases *suspected* to be caused by such a slow virus may be at least one type of ALZHEIMER'S DISEASE, KURU, CREUTZFELDT-JAKOB DISEASE, a rare complication of measles called subacute sclerosing panencephalitis and MULTIPLE SCLEROSIS.

smell, sense of

One of the five senses, it enables a human being to distinguish several thousand different odors, although scientists aren't sure of the exact mechanism by which this is possible.

A person is able to smell when odors travel up the nasal cavity to the OLFACTORY NERVES, which send electrical signals to the brain where the interpretation of smell occurs. Any glitch along this path will interfere with a person's ability to detect or identify odors.

The sense of smell is made possible because of the presence of smell RECEPTORS (specialized NERVE-CELL endings) in a small area of mucous membrane lining the roof of the nose. These receptors cells have cilia that reach down to the surface of the mucous membrane, and are stimulated by odor molecules. Odor molecules must dissolve in mucus before they can stimulate receptors, which is why this area must be kept moist.

When the molecule "keys" fit into the receptor "locks," the process triggers nerve impulses in the olfactory nerve that are transmitted to the brain, where they are translated in parts of the LIMBIC SYSTEM and FRONTAL LOBES. The system is exquisitely sensitive; as little as four molecules will give a recognizable smell.

Disorders of smell A person may either lose the sense of smell (anosmia) or experience distortions in this sense (dysosmia). Because the senses of smell and taste are so intimately intertwined, problems in smell usually affect the ability to taste as well; this is why elderly people often complain that food has lost its taste. Temporary problems with smell may occur when the mucous membrane in the nose becomes inflamed, such as with a cold, flu, or rhinitis. Cigarette smoking may also inflame the nose and interfere with the sense of smell. Overgrowth of the adenoids or a deviated septum will

MEDICATIONS THAT CAN AFFECT SENSE OF SMELL

Antibiotics
Anticoagulants (anti-blood-clotting drugs)
Antihistamines
Blood pressure medicine
Chemotherapy drugs
Dietary supplements
Nose drops
Oil of peppermint
Toothpaste
Vitamin D (high doses)

block airflow and interfere with the sense of smell. In rare cases, a person may lose the ability to smell because of a MENINGIOMA (tumor of the MENINGES, the membranes surrounding the brain) or a tumor behind the nose.

In addition, the olfactory nerves can be damaged during HEAD INJURY; if both nerves are completely torn, the person will permanently lose the ability to smell. Less severe damage may result in temporary smell distortions as the nerves heal. Between 5 and 10 percent of all major head injuries result in some malfunction in the sense of smell.

Fleeting unpleasant odors (cacosmia) may occur as a result of DEPRESSION or SCHIZOPHRENIA, in some forms of EPILEPSY and during recovery from severe alcoholism. Sometimes, a person with dysosmia may be convinced that the smell originates in the person's own body and may begin to wash compulsively.

Many diseases, including neurological problems, endocrine diseases, hereditary disease, cirrhosis, or kidney failure, may also interfere with the sense of smell. Damage to brain tissue caused by STROKE or toxic chemicals may alter the sense of smell, as can dietary deficiencies (especially in vitamin A, vitamin B_{12}, or zinc).

Smell may also be altered as a side effect of

medications, dietary supplements, and nose drops, or radiation therapy to the head.

See also OLFACTORY FATIGUE.

Smith, Edwin, surgical papyrus of An ancient Egyptian medical treatise that describes how a HEAD INJURY can have effects throughout the body. The papyrus, written between 2,500 and 3,000 years ago, contains information about 48 cases, in which 8 describe head injuries that affect other parts of the body.

Apparently intended as a textbook on surgery, it begins with the clinical cases of head injuries and works its way down the body, describing in detail the examination, diagnosis, treatment, and prognosis in each case.

The papyrus was acquired in Luxor in 1862 by the American egyptologist Edwin Smith, a pioneer in the study of Egyptian science. After his death in 1906, the papyrus was given to the New-York Historical Society, who turned it over for study to Egyptologist James Henry Breasted in 1920. He published a translation, transliteration, and discussion in two volumes in 1930.

smoking and the brain See ADDICTIONS; NICOTINE; STIMULANTS AND THE BRAIN.

Society for Children with Craniosynostosis A national support group for parents of children with CRANIOSYNOSTOSIS; the organization provides support, offers information and referrals, supports research, and publishes a newsletter. For address, see Appendix A.

Society of Neurosurgical Anesthesia and Critical Care (SNACC) A professional association for neurosurgeons and anesthesiologists interested in the care of patients with neurological disorders; the group sponsors continuing medical education and research in the care of neurosurgical patients and bestows an annual research essay award to a resident physician.

Founded in 1973, the society has 613 members and sponsors an annual convention in conjunction with the American Society of Anesthesiologists as well as an annual meeting. Its publications include the *Annual Summary of Society Meeting Proceedings*; the semiannual *Comprehensive Bibliography in Neuroanesthesia*; the annual *Course Book*; and its *Newsletter*. For the address, see Appendix B.

sodium pentothol See TRUTH DRUGS.

somatic nervous system The somatic ("bodily") nervous system features motor and sensory nerves; motor nerves branch from the CENTRAL NERVOUS SYSTEM and trigger muscle action on orders from the brain or SPINAL CORD, whereas sensory nerves bring information from sensory receptors in skin, tongue, eyes, nostrils, joints, and muscles. The information from these two groups of nerves is used by the body to control how we move and hold our body erect. Together, the AUTONOMIC NERVOUS SYSTEMS and the somatic nervous system make up the PERIPHERAL NERVOUS SYSTEM.

SPECT (single-photon emission computerized tomography) A type of brain scan that tracks blood flow and measures brain activity. Less expensive than PET (POSITRON EMISSION TOMOGRAPHY) SCANS, SPECTS may be used to identify the subtle injury following mild head trauma.

SPECT is a type of radionuclide scanning, a diagnostic technique based on the detection of radiation emitted by radioactive substances introduced into the body. Different radioactive substances (radionuclides) are taken up in greater concentrations by dif-

ferent types of tissue; this gives a clearer picture of organ *function* than other systems.

The radioactive substance is swallowed or injected into the bloodstream, where it accumulates in the brain. Gamma radiation (similar but shorter than X-RAYS) are emitted from the brain, detected by a gamma camera, which emits light, used to produce an image that can be displayed on a screen; using a principle similar to CS scanning, cross-sectional images can be constructed by a computer from radiation detected by a gamma camera that rotates around the patient. It's also possible to create moving images by using a computer to record a series of images right after the administration of the radionuclide.

Radionuclide is a safe procedure requiring only tiny doses of radiation. Because the radioactive substance is ingested or injected, it avoids the risks of some X-ray procedures in which a radiopaque dye is inserted through a catheter into the organ (as in ANGIOGRAPHY), and unlike radiopaque dyes, radionuclides carry almost no risk of toxicity or allergy.

speech The intrinsic ability to speak is hardwired into the brain at birth and usually starts with vocalized vowels at about seven weeks of age. Learning how to speak involves the ability to make and monitor sounds. It occurs when the brain activates MOTOR NERVES, sending signals to operate larynx, vocal cords, pharynx, soft palate, tongue, and lips. Sensory nerves bring the brain signals from speech muscles and from the ears, which pick up sound waves made by the voice. With this type of feedback system, a child can learn how to modify sounds to match words he hears. This is why a child who is deaf will not learn to speak on his own.

Infants learn first how to babble, and the responses of adults around them help them select sounds to reproduce. By the time a child is 16 weeks old, he or she can make consonant sounds and by 20 weeks can utter some syllables. The first meaningful word usually appears before the first year. By 21 to 24 months, a child is using two-word phrases, and by the age of three, most children speak constantly.

In an English-speaking country, a child will speak the *a* and other vowels, followed by 16 weeks with *m, b, g, k,* and *p*. By 32 weeks most children can say *t, d,* and *w*. The sounds of *s, f, h, r,* and *th* come later.

Speech disorders may be due to problems of articulation (anarthria or dysarthria) of LANGUAGE function (aphasia or dysphasia), problems in the production of voice sounds (aphonia or dysphonia), or to mental illness.

spina bifida   A general name for congenital abnormalities caused by the failure to close of an embryo's membrane-and-tissue-covered tube housing the CENTRAL NERVOUS SYSTEM. Literally meaning "spine in two parts," spina bifida is also known medically as a NEURAL TUBE DEFECT.

While defects can be found anywhere on the spine, they are generally found on the lower back.

Cause The precise cause is not clear, but there appears to be both environmental and genetic causes.

Types There are several types of spina bifida, including SPINA BIFIDA OCCULTA, MENINGO-CELE, MYELOMENINGOCELE, encephalocele, and ANENCEPHALY.

In *spina bifida occulta*, there is a small, incomplete closure but no obvious damage to the SPINAL CORD. Found in 20 percent or more of the population, the damage is so minor that many people don't know they have it (hence the name, *occulta*, or "hidden"). The site may be marked by a dimple, hair tuft or telangiectasia (red skin caused by expanded blood vessels). It may be associated with urinary or bowel problems, together with weakness or poor circulation in the legs that appears in adulthood.

Meningocele is characterized by the appearance of the MENINGES (the membrane covering the spinal cord) pushing out through an abnormal opening in the vertebrae, forming a sac (-cele) that looks like a bulge. The spinal cord itself is not damaged, and the sac is covered by skin. This defect can be easily repaired by surgery during the first few days of life.

The most severe form of spina bifida is myelomeningocele, which is what most people think of when they hear the term *spina bifida*. This abnormality is characterized by the protrusion of nerve and tissue from the spinal cord into a sac, which may or may not be covered by skin on the outside. Symptoms include muscle weakness, loss of sensation, paralysis below the defect, and incontinence. In addition, a malformation at the base of the BRAINSTEM can lead to a HYDROCEPHALUS (a buildup of CEREBROSPINAL FLUID) which must be relieved via a SHUNT to avoid BRAIN DAMAGE, including blindness, deafness, SEIZURES, and LEARNING DISABILITIES.

ANENCEPHALY is the medical term for the absence of the brain or spinal cord—the skull does not close and only a groove appears where the spine should be. There is no medical treatment that can save these infants, most of whom will die during the first few hours of life.

Diagnoses Genetic screening tests (including alpha fetoprotein, ULTRASOUND, and amniocentesis). Those with any such defects in their family may want to seek genetic counseling.

Outlook In the past, most children with the most severe cases of spina bifida (myelomeningocele) died soon after birth, but today immediate surgery saves the lives of most of these children. They usually must have a series of operations as they grow and usually need special devices to help them get around. With this treatment, about 80 percent of these children can walk by the time they enter school. Most need special training (such as how to insert catheters) to manage bowels and bladder and prevent serious bladder infections and kidney problems. Special diets and schedules allow many children to achieve bowel continence, especially when started in the preschool years.

These children may also experience lack of feeling, pressure sores, spinal disorders, eye problems, excess weight, MENTAL RETARDATION, or learning disability.

As adults, many can function sexually although some (especially males) may have some problems due to nerve damage. A woman with spina bifida can give birth, but she has a 4 to 5 percent chance of bearing a child with the same problem.

For more information, contact the SPINA BIFIDA ASSOCIATION OF AMERICA (see Appendix A for address).

Spina Bifida Adoption Referral Program

A national program that facilitates adoption of children with SPINA BIFIDA and that works through agencies and directly with birth parents and adoptive parents.

See also SPINA BIFIDA ASSOCIATION OF AMERICA.

Spina Bifida Association of America
A support group for individuals with SPINA BIFIDA, their parents, their relatives and friends, and concerned professionals. The association supports research, provides education and job training, monitors legislation, helps arrange adoption of spina-bifida children in special circumstances, and publishes materials.

Founded in 1972, the group has 90 local groups and publishes the bimonthly newsletter *Spina Bifida Insights*. For address, see Appendix A.

See also SPINA BIFIDA ADOPTION REFERRAL PROGRAM.

spinal accessory nerve   Also known as the eleventh cranial nerve, this nerve is responsible for movements of neck and back muscles.

See also CRANIAL NERVES.

spinal cord   The very center of the NERVOUS SYSTEM, the spinal cord is a long bundle of nerves extending from the base of the brain running along the inside of the spine (backbone). The spinal cord is the main link between the body and the brain, merging with the base of the brain; the lower end is about two-thirds of the way down the spine. Below this, the spinal cord splits to form several main nerves that continue within the spine, ending up at the legs and feet.

Like the brain, the spinal cord contains both GRAY and WHITE MATTER. The gray matter lies in the center of the cord and consists of thousands of the cell bodies of the MOTOR NEURONS that pass signals to body muscles. A thick layer of white matter surrounds thegray matter; white matter is made up primarily of AXONS (long, thin, wiry extensions of the cells) and contains the nerve fibers that pass signals to and from the brain.

The spinal cord is almost totally enclosed by the spinal bones; 31 pairs of large nerves called spinal nerves branch off the spinal cord at regular intervals and pass through the narrow gaps between the spinal bones. Each spinal nerve contains both sensory and motor neurons. Spinal nerves in the neck handle signals to and from the head, arms, and hands; nerves in the chest lead to the chest muscles, skin, and other organs (such as lungs and heart). Nerves from the lower end of the cord branch out through the stomach area, down into the legs and feet.

Some parts of the nerves carry information to the spinal cord, which relays the messages to the brain; these include nerve messages from the skin detailing touch, temperature, and pain, and messages from internal organs and muscles. Nerves carrying incoming messages are called sensory nerves.

Motor nerves carry outgoing information—signals from the brain traveling down the spinal cord that activate muscles and control the movements of the body.

The spinal cord, like the brain, is wrapped in three layers of MENINGES, and cushioned from shock by the fluid between the arachnoid and PIA-MATER layers. It is also possible to have an INFECTION here, called MENINGITIS; in some cases, the inflamed meninges may press on the brain or spinal cord and cause damage or even death.

See also LUMBAR PUNCTURE; SPINAL CORD SOCIETY.

Spinal Cord Society A national support group for SPINAL-CORD injury-patients and their families, health-care professionals, and others; it also promotes research and increases public awareness of the potential for a cure for the paralysis after a spinal-cord injury.

The group focuses on a cure rather than rehabilitation of paralysis due to spinal injury and promotes funding for reversal-oriented pure and applied medical research. The group also encourages establishment of spinal-injury centers in conjunction with existing hospitals and medical centers, maintains a data bank of chronic spinal-cord-injury case histories, and continuously monitors improving treatment. The society also guides research and screens patients for referral to other physicians or to a spinal-cord-injury center. Finally, it maintains a medical center in Minneapolis, Minnesota, that applies state-of-the-art treatment to paralysis victims.

Founded in 1978, the society has 9,000 members and publishes a monthly newsletter. For address, see Appendix A.

spinal tap See LUMBAR PUNCTURE.

split-brain research Research that slits a brain surgically into right and left halves so that each half can be trained and tested independently.

While the two CEREBRAL HEMISPHERES may appear almost as two separate brains, in fact they are joined by the CORPUS CALLOSUM'S—a bundle of 300 million nerve fibers. The left hemisphere in most people is dominant—it's responsible for writing, computing, speaking, and thinking logically. The right (or secondary) hemispheres handles spatial recognition that helps travelers find their way. The right brain is concerned with creative activities such as art and music, while the left is more analytical and logical. In general, the primary (left) hemisphere deals with analysis, while the secondary (right) hemisphere deals with synthesis.

In the 1950s, scientists successfully treated severe EPILEPSY by severing the nerve fibers connecting the two hemispheres. Despite common fears at the time, the mind did not split in two. While these patients appeared quite normal, a few quirks did exist. For example, a patient with severed hemispheres can describe an unseen object in the right hand but not in the left.

Scientists studying ELECTROENCEPHALOGRAMS have concluded that language dominance is found in the left hemisphere in most people, no matter whether they are right- or left-handed. Speech centers in some people are found in both hemispheres and a few others in the right hemisphere. In young children, the potential for speech can be found in both hemispheres; if the left is damaged, speech will develop in the right. By age 10, speech dominance is usually solidified.

spongiform encephalopathies A group of rare diseases (including KURU and CREUTZFELDT-JAKOB DISEASE) that are characterized by spongy appearance of the CORTEX, diffuse degeneration of NEURONS in the CEREBRUM, BASAL GANGLION, and SPINAL CORD, and the proliferation of GLIAL CELLS.

The diseases cause a rapid, progressive DEMENTIA similar to ALZHEIMER'S DISEASE but also accompanied by striking rigidity, weakness, and muscle spasms. In addition, there is usually a characteristic EEG pattern.

Treatment There are no specific treatments; the muscle spasms may respond to benzodiazepines such as clonazepam and diazepam.

SQUID (superconducting quantum interference device) A type of brain-scanning device that senses tiny changes in magnetic fields. When brain cells fire, they create electric current; electric fields induce magnetic fields, so magnetic changes indicate neural activity.

Stanford-Binet test (4th edition) This intelligence test is appropriate for those aged 2 to adulthood and yields a mental age (MA) and intelligence quotient (IQ). It is heavily weighted toward verbal performance and thus may underestimate the intelligence of children with specific communication disorders or who have been raised in environments that have not stimulated their verbal development.

See also WECHSLER INTELLIGENCE SCALE FOR CHILDREN REVISED (WISC-R).

stars, seeing What appears as random bursts of light when people hit their heads is actually caused by a jolt to the BRAIN CELLS responsible for vision. Normally, these cells respond to the electrical messages sent by the eyes, interpreting the signals as faces, objects, or whatever people are looking at. But a sudden blow to the head can also trigger activity in visual cells unrelated to, or less active during, the given visual scenario. This overactivity of visual processing cells is a burst of electricity that the brain interprets as bursts of light.

Stars most often appear following a blow to the back of the head because that is the location of the visual CORTEX. In fact, stimulating the cells in this part of the brain with a probe can also set off a twinkling-star show. Scientists also believe that the pulsing star-like visual HALLUCINATIONS often seen by MIGRAINE sufferers is caused by spontaneous electrical signaling in the visual cortex.

While stars don't normally appear unless the head has received a strong blow, the twinkling stars don't usually signal serious problems. On the other hand, the appearance of twinkling lights after only a slight blow—or none at all—should indicate a visit to the physician. Showers of lights or snake-shaped streams of light may signal a torn retina (nerve cells blanketing the back of the eye). A torn retina may be repaired with a laser, but if left untreated the retina may completely detach, causing partial or total blindness.

status epilepticus Repeated or prolonged attacks of epileptic SEIZURES without regaining consciousness between seizures. This medical emergency may be fatal if not treated quickly. This condition is most likely to occur if anticonvulsant drugs are suddenly stopped or taken inconsistently.

stereogram Two pictures each viewed by one eye, which when combined by the brain give the illusion of a three-dimensional shape.

stereotactic radiosurgery Also known as *gamma knife surgery*, this is a new technique of tightly focused radiation now being used for patients with inoperable BRAIN TUMORS. The procedure was pioneered in the late 1960s by Lars Leksell, M.D., a Swedish neurosurgeon at the Karolinska Institute in Stockholm. Since then, some 18,000 patients around the world have undergone the procedure to destroy tumors or correct life-threatening blood-vessel problems, with no reported deaths or complications from the procedure.

In the technique, the surgeon uses a small directed beam of radiation to treat areas that may be inaccessible by conventional surgery or for patients who may not be able to withstand an operation. The one-time application is an outpatient procedure that may serve as a substitute for the 20 to 30 radiation treatments normally required. Using the precisely directed beams of radiation, surgeons can focus on and destroy the diseased tissue and spare nearly all of the surrounding healthy tissue.

The key is to locate the disease tissue and program those coordinates into a linear accelerator—the unit that emits the radiation beam. The accelerator is rotated around the target area in the patient's brain, allowing high doses of radiation to be given directly to the designated site. The procedure usually takes an entire day and is performed with a local anesthetic. A CAT SCAN is used to determine the exact coordinates of the diseased tissue; with that information, doctors then affix a metal ring to the head, which helps the linear accelerator focus on the target area.

At present, this type of radiation is being used for patients with various types of brain tumors, as well as brain tumors that have not responded to conventional radiation therapy. It can also be used to treat malformed blood vessels in the brain that can cause seizures and are usually inoperable under normal situations.

The technique is also used to obtain a brain biopsy, to insert a permanent stimulating wire to control intractable pain, and to destroy areas of the brain to treat disabling neurological disorders.

Although the technique often costs less than traditional neurosurgery, it is still not widely practiced, and treatment is not always easy to find. For information on the technique, contact Elekta, 8 Executive Park West, Atlanta, GA 30329; (800) 535-7355. For more information about brain tumor support groups, see Appendix A.

stimulants and the brain A class of drugs that increase nerve activity in the brain by triggering the release of NOREPINEPHRINE. These drugs include NICOTINE, CAFFEINE, AMPHETAMINES, and COCAINE. There are two main types of stimulant drugs—those that stimulate the nerves of the central nervous system (including the amphetamines) and those that affect the respiratory system. CENTRAL-NERVOUS-SYSTEM stimulants reduce drowsiness and increase alertness by their action on the RETICULAR ACTIVATING SYSTEM in the BRAINSTEM. Respiratory stimulants act on the respiratory center in the brainstem.

Nerve stimulants include caffeine, dextroamphetamine, and methylphenidate; respiratory stimulants include doxapram and nikethamide.

Caffeine boosts the brain's flow of thoughts and output of motor signals to the muscles. Too much caffeine can cause heartbeat and respiration to increase and bring on insomnia. Amphetamine is a synthetic product resembling ephedrine available as tablets, powder, or ampules for injection. Amphetamines are chemically similar to the natural neurotransmitter NORADRENALIN, and amphetamines enhance the activity of noradrenalin in the brain by releasing quantities of noradrenalin stored in NERVE CELLS and preventing its reabsorption by blocking MAO. Amphetamine also may act on the RECEPTORS of certain cells.

Nerve stimulants can be given to treat NARCOLEPSY (a disorder characterized by excess sleepiness); they are also effective in the treatment of hyperactivity in children. They may also suppress appetite, but their adverse effects make these drugs a poor choice in the treatment of obesity.

stimulus Any sensory event (such as a flashing light or the touch of a feather) that causes the brain to become active.

stimulus-response memory The kind of memory involved when a dinner gong triggers a trained dog to salivate. This type of memory takes place in the brain below the outer CORTEX and survives damage to regions of the brain that is essential for other types of memory.

Stokes-Adams syndrome Insufficient flow of blood to the brain caused by heart problems that result in recurrent, temporary loss of consciousness. In most cases, the heart begins beating regularly again, the skin reddens and the person wakes up.

Symptoms Sudden attacks of fainting followed by a bluish tinge to the skin if the person does not regain consciousness quickly. There is a rapid breathing rate and slow pulse; seizures may occur due to lack of oxygen to the brain.

Treatment None needed if the patient wakes up. If consciousness does not return, prompt cardiopulmonary resuscitation may be needed to prevent brain damage. Most patients with this problem wear a pacemaker to regulate their heart rhythm and prevent future attacks.

stress and the brain The limbic system produces emotional arousal and the CORTEX monitors and modulates that arousal, but if more stressors accumulate, the balance in the brain may be disturbed. ANXIETY may represent tension between limbic and cortical impulses.

Social stress may intensify the damage from STROKE, SEIZURES, or the aging process in key brain structures, according to research.

Stress and memory Intense emotions triggered by a stressful or emotional event helps preserve memories of that experience primarily by activating a class of stress hormones (including cortisol) responsible for storing emotionally laden information, according to scientists at the University of California at Irvine. Drugs used to treat high blood pressure block these hormones and apparently worsen memories of emotional and exciting events. In general, the stronger the emotional experience, the stronger and more reliable the memory of that experience. The scientists explain that emotional experiences trigger the release of adrenergic hormones, which strengthen memories of events. The process may foster the intrusive memories that haunt people suffering from posttraumatic stress disorder.

On the other hand, while people with high concentrations of cortisol in the blood remember what they learned long ago, they may forget things they have just been told. In a McGill University study, researchers checked the cognitive skills and the concentration of cortisol in the blood of 130 volunteers aged 55 to 87. High amounts of cortisol correlated with subtle memory and attention problems. This subtle memory loss resembles what happens when the HIPPOCAMPUS is damaged.

striate cortex The primary VISUAL CORTEX.

striatum A term used for the combined entity of the caudate nucleus and the putamen; it is one of the four separate nuclei in the BASAL GANGLIA. The striatum (Latin for "striped") receives information including all forms of sensory information and data about the state of activity in the motor system from almost all parts of the CEREBRAL CORTEX. Its so-called stripes are made up of heavily myelinated AXONS of the connections from the motor and sensory cerebral cortices.

Recordings in the striatum shows that the neurons' activity starts just before and during a particular movement.

stroke Also called a *cerebral vascular accident*, a stroke is an interruption of blood supply to the brain or leakage of blood outside of vessel walls. Any area in the brain damaged by the stroke will affect brain function. Any area in the brain damaged by the stroke will affect further brain function, including sensation, movement, and memory. Strokes are fatal in about one-third of cases, and are a leading cause of death in developed countries. In the United States, stroke will occur in about 200 out of every 100,000 people each year; incidence rises quickly with age, and is higher in men than women.

While about half of patients recover more or less completely from their first stroke, any intellectual impairment and memory loss is usually permanent.

Warning signs Ominously, a 1991 Gallup poll found that 97 percent of respondents could not recognize a stroke's warning signs. While most stroke victims are elderly, a third of all stroke victims are under age 65.

Cause A stroke may be caused by any of three mechanisms: CEREBRAL THROMBOSIS (clot), cerebral embolism, or HEMORRHAGE. *Cerebral thrombosis* is a blockage by a clot that has built up on the wall of a brain artery, depriving the brain of blood; it is responsible for almost half of all strokes.

Cerebral embolism is a blockage by material that is swept into an artery in the brain from somewhere else in the body, depriving the brain of oxygen; it accounts for 30 to 35 percent of strokes.

Less common is *cerebral hemorrhage*, the most serious form of stroke, caused by the rupture of a blood vessel and bleeding within or over the surface of the brain. Hemorrhages account for about a quarter of all strokes. The hemorrhage is usually from a vessel at the base of the brain, where blood leaks into the brain substance itself, often resulting in COMA and paralysis. Death is almost inevitable if the hemorrhage is large.

Symptoms A stroke that affects the dominant of the two CEREBRAL HEMISPHERES in the brain (usually the left) may cause disturbance of language and speech. Symptoms that last for less than 24 hours followed by full recovery are known as TRANSIENT ISCHEMIC ATTACKS (TIAS); such an attack is a warning that a sufficient supply of blood is not reaching part of the brain. If circulation through smaller vessels is inadequate, brain tissue may die.

Blockage of the anterior cerebral artery on one side of the brain usually causes paralysis and sensory loss in the limb on the opposite side. If the artery of the dominant hemisphere (almost always left) is affected, mental confusion and speech impairment (APHASIA) may also occur.

A blockage of the main branch of the middle cerebral artery on one side produces paralysis and sensory loss on the opposite side, mainly affecting the face and arm. Aphasia can also occur when the area is in the dominant hemisphere. Blockage of smaller vessels of the middle cerebral artery produces one-sided blindness, inability to read (ALEXIA) or to recognize sensory stimuli (agnosia) or to perform skilled movements (apraxia) in combinations or as isolated symptoms.

Blockage of the main part of the posterior cerebral artery on one side causes damage to the THALAMUS and the VISUAL (OCCIPITAL) CORTEX, with occasional muscular weakness and sensory loss accompanied by burning pains, and ataxia.

Blocking the basilar artery on the underside of the brain is serious, often causing paralysis and sensory loss in all extremities and in the muscles supplied by the BRAINSTEM (cranial) nuclei. Blockage of the vertebral artery that runs toward the SPINAL CORD is not usually fatal, although symptoms can be disabling.

A brain hemorrhage of any size is likely to be fatal, whereas the majority of patients with a clot are likely to recover from the initial damage. A number of patients do die in the first weeks after a stroke from complications, such as pneumonia, heart problems, or kidney malfunction.

Stroke survivors find their brain problems gradually improve over months following a stroke.

Treatment Unconscious or semiconscious hospital patients require a clear airway, tube feeding, and regular changing of position. Any fluid accumulation in the brain may be treated with corticosteroid drugs or diuretics. A stroke caused by an embolism is treated with anticlotting drugs to help prevent recurrences. Long-term administration of these drugs also has been recommended for those with intermittent symptoms of stroke. Sometimes, aspirin or vascular surgery (cleaning out the vessels in the neck for patients with arteriosclerotic narrowing) has been tried with moderate success.

General care in the first stages following a stroke, such as physiotherapy and speech therapy are important to a patient's recovery.

Risk factors Certain things can increase the risk of stroke: *high blood pressure* that weakens the walls of arteries or ATHEROSCLEROSI (thickening of the lining of arterial walls). Stroke can also be caused by conditions that cause blood clots in the heart that may migrate to the brain: *irregular heartbeat* (atrial fibrillation), *damaged heart valves* or *heart attack.* Conditions that increase the risk of high blood pressure or atherosclerosis can also cause stroke, such as *hyperlipidemia* (fatty substances in the blood) or *polycythemia* (high level of red blood cells in the blood). *Diabetes mellitus* is a risk factor; people with diabetes are five times as likely to have a stroke as nondiabetics. However, the National Institutes of Health notes that diabetics who monitor their GLUCOSE levels closely and inject insulin have fewer diabetes-related complications, including stroke. In addition, smokers have a higher risk; one study found that those who smoke more than 25 cigarettes a day have 3 times higher risk of stroke from a clot, and 10 times higher risk of stroke from a burst blood vessel. But those who quit smoking can cut the risk to that of a nonsmoker in just two years.

Oral contraceptives also increase the risk of stroke in women under 50; however, the older high-dose pills were far more dangerous than today's low-dose versions. Several studies have suggested an increased risk for low-dose pills, but others have found a significant risk only in women who smoke as well as take the pill. Women who smoke, use birth-control pills, and have MIGRAINES appear to have an even greater chance of having a stroke.

Scientists don't yet understand why, but African Americans and Hispanics have a higher incidence of stroke; one reason could be that African Americans are more prone to high blood pressure.

Pregnancy is yet another risk factor; stroke is 13 times more common during the 9 months of pregnancy because of changes in blood consistency. Pregnancy-related high blood pressure may predispose a woman to stroke.

Finally, a history of untreated *transient ischemic attacks (TIAs),* is a risk factor of stroke; one third of those who have had a TIA will have a stroke within five years. Small doses of aspirin daily (as little as one-tenth of a tablet) may lessen that risk. The anticlotting drug Ticlid, which was recently approved by the U.S. Food and Drug Administration, is slightly more effective but has been associated with potentially serious side effects.

For more information, contact the NATIONAL STROKE ASSOCIATION or the NATIONAL INSTITUTE OF NEUROLOGICAL DISORDERS AND STROKE (for addresses, see Appendix A).

See also CEREBROVASCULAR ACCIDENT.

Stroke Clubs International A support group whose active members are stroke patients; associate members are those interested in the problems of stroke patients. The group is interested in uniting stroke patients to help each other, to teach them and their families about the nature of stroke and how to overcome problems, to help find jobs, and to provide hope and encouragement. The group maintains a list of more than 900 clubs throughout the United States. Founded in 1968, the club has 45,000 members and publishes the *Stroke Club International Bulletin.* For address, see Appendix A.

Sturge-Weber Foundation A support group for those with STURGE-WEBER SYNDROME and their families, concerned professionals, and supporters; the group serves as an information clearinghouse on the syndrome, which is a congenital neurological disorder characterized by facial port-wine stains, SEIZURES, glaucoma, and loss of motor control. The group also maintains a speakers' bureau, compiles statistics, and funds research. Founded in 1986, the group has 750 members and publishes a quarterly newsletter. For address, see Appendix A.

Sturge-Weber syndrome A rare congenital condition that affects the brain and the skin. A malformation of blood vessels in the brain may cause weakness on the opposite side of the body, MENTAL RETARDATION, and EPILEPSY. There is usually a large birthmark covering one side of the face.

subarachnoid hemorrhage A type of brain hemorrhage in which a blood vessel ruptures, spreading blood over the surface of the brain. This is a fairly unusual type of STROKE that usually affects a younger patient who is less likely to suffer from widespread CEREBROVASCULAR DISEASE.

About 8 percent of all stroke patients have this type of HEMORRHAGE, which is usually caused by the rupture of an intercranial aneurysm bleeding into the SUBARACHNOID SPACE around the brain. Common sites for these ruptures include the ANTERIOR COMMUNICATING ARTERY lying between the FRONTAL LOBES, the middle cerebral artery, and the posterior communicating artery.

Less commonly, the hemorrhage might be caused by a ruptured ANGIOMA (an abnormal proliferation of blood vessels within the brain).

This type of hemorrhage usually occurs spontaneously, and is not usually caused by any type of HEAD INJURY—but it may following on the heels of unaccustomed physical exertion.

A patient who loses consciousness after such a stroke may regain consciousness, but recurrent strokes are common and may be fatal.

The diagnosis is confirmed by CAT SCAN and large amounts of blood in the CEREBROSPINAL FLUID. An ANGIOGRAM may pinpoint the site of the burst blood vessel.

About one-third of patients recover; another one-sixth recover partially but have some disability (such as paralysis, mental problems, or epilepsy). Half of all patients die from the initial or subsequent strokes.

Incidence About 5 to 10 Americans per 100,000 suffer a subarachnoid hemorrhage each year. It is particularly common among patients between 35 and 60. Subarachnoid hemorrhages are slightly less common than an intracerebral hemorrhage (another form of stroke), characterized by bleeding within the brain itself.

Symptoms Immediate loss of consciousness or a sudden violent HEADACHE is usually the primary symptoms. Typically, the patient will experience symptoms similar to KORSAKOFF'S SYNDROME shortly after the hemorrhage—disorientation, confabulation, and memory problems. If the person remains awake, other symptoms may follow: photophobia (intolerance of bright light), nausea and vomiting, drowsiness, and neck stiffness.

Treatment Treatment is generally aimed at preventing future strokes, such as control of high blood pressure. A burst ANEURYSM or angioma may be surgically removed or obliterated.

subarachnoid space An area of the brain located between the arachnoid and the PIA MATER. Over the surface of the hemispheres, this cavity is low, but at the lower portions of the SULCI there are triangular spaces. The space has a spongy appearance and is filled with CEREBROSPINAL FLUID. The subarachnoid space is wider in the SPINAL CORD than in the brain, especially in the lower part of the vertebral canal.

subdural hemorrhage A large blood clot (HEMATOMA) that forms within the skull when blood seeps into the space between the DURA MATER, the tough outer layer of the MENINGES (covering of the brain) and the middle meningeal layer (arachnoid). The most common cause of this seeping blood is a torn vein on the inside of the dura mater resulting from a HEAD INJURY. Subdural hemorrhages are most common among the elderly or alcoholics who have fallen down.

The presence of such a hemorrhage is diagnosed by ANGIOGRAPHY and CAT SCANS. Following surgical treatment, most patients have a full recovery.

Symptoms Because the bleeding is very slow, months may pass before symptoms appear as a result of rising pressure inside the skull from the weight of the blood pressing on the brain. Fluctuating symptoms include HEADACHE, confusion, and drowsiness and the development of weakness and paralysis on one side. Because these symptoms are similar to STROKE, any recent head injury (within the past several months) should be reported.

Treatment Treatment include CRANIOTOMY (drilling burr holes in the skull), draining the blood and repairing damaged blood vessels.

subliminal learning Learning that takes place below the level of consciousness as contained in messages or information that is presented too quickly for normal awareness. The idea of subliminal learning is related to sleep learning, in which material to be learned is presented when the subject is asleep.

Subliminal advertising first reached public awareness during the 1950s, when some outdoor movie theatres reported huge concession sales following messages saying "eat popcorn" and "drink Coca-Cola" flashed on the screen during a six-week period. Popcorn business reportedly increased 50 percent, and soda sales rose 18 percent.

There is some research support to the notion that in a laboratory, subjects can process limited sensory information without conscious awareness if they are playing close attention to the task, but studies couldn't duplicate the subliminal effect reported during the 1950s. Scientists have concluded that it is unlikely anyone could learn or remember information if the person is not aware that it is being presented. Subliminal suggestion—if not learning—is relatively persuasive, however.

substance abuse Many scientists believe that the key to understanding substance abuse lies in the brain, particularly since the discovery that the brain has many RECEPTORS, not just for NEUROTRANSMITTERS but for many drugs such as NICOTINE, marijuana, HEROIN, and other OPIATES and BENZODIAZEPINES (such as Valium). Because scientists have discovered that certain drugs have specific actions in certain brain regions, they may be able to discover how to disrupt the effects of these drugs.

The problem is complex, however, because addiction involves not just the physical presence of receptors but also the psychological reality of motivation and pleasure that can lead to addiction. Addiction to harmful substances is related to the involvement of brain systems that control normal pleasurable activities associated with eating, drinking and socialization.

Scientists still don't fully understand either the location, organization, or chemistry of the brain system underlying positive emotions and pleasure, although they have found some interesting clues. They discovered that animals preferred cocaine to food and would ignore food completely in the presence of cocaine; however, this behavior would be completely reversed if the neurotransmitter DOPAMINE is removed from one particular area of the brain (the nucleus accumbens).

substance P A neuropeptide involved with the transmission of pain signals.

substantia gelatinosa The part of the brain where nerves for pain, temperature, and touch make the first contact with the SPINAL CORD.

substantia nigra A black-pigmented band of matter (its name means "black substance") located in the BASAL GANGLIA of the MIDBRAIN that produces the NEUROTRANSMITTER DOPAMINE. The absence of dopamine produces rigidity and tremor. In patients with PARKINSON'S DISEASE, the neurons in the substantia nigra that transmit dopamine die; the loss of these neurons is directly connected with the onset of symptoms. This loss of dopamine fibers is devastating to motor control, resulting in problems making voluntary movements and with uncontrollable tremors of the head, hands, and arms. However, patients can be successfully treated at first by boosting the stores of dopamine with the drug LEVODOPA. Eventually, Levodopa stops working.

sulci The valleys on the surface folds of the CEREBRAL CORTEX that become wider in cases of brain atrophy.

sumatriptan A MIGRAINE medication that appears to cancel pain from migraine and cluster HEADACHES. Although other migraine medications exist, sumatriptan was specifically created to take advantage of particular biochemical features of migraines. Sumatriptan was designed to block receptor binding of SEROTONIN, a NEUROTRANSMITTER whose role in headaches has long been suspected.

superior colliculus Nuclei within the THALAMUS that is most critical to carrying out the function of vision. This structure got its name by the way it looked to early scientists; the "colliculi" are two "pairs of hills" on top of the midbrain (brainstem), of which the highest (or "superior") two deal with vision.

supplementary motor area Found in the FRONTAL LOBE of the brain, this structure receives input fibers from the BASAL GANGLIA and sends output back to the basal ganglia, the RETICULAR FORMATION and the MOTOR CORTEX. The supplementary motor area is involved in planning and initiating movement. A malfunction in this area can interfere with voluntary movement and speech.

suprachiasmatic nucleus A pair of small cell clusters that receive and integrate visual information in the brain, the suprachiasmatic nucleus is found in the HYPOTHALAMUS and uses information about light intensity to coordinate internal rhythms. This brain structure gets its name from the Latin words for "above," because it lies just above the optic chiasm, where the nerve fibers from the eyes cross each other.

Each suprachiasmatic nucleus (there is one on either side of the hypothalamus) is made up of about 10,000 small, tightly packed cell bodies with sparsely branching DENDRITES. Researchers suspect that several different NEUROTRANSMITTERS might be released by NEURONS in these nuclei; however, SEROTONIN is the only neurotransmitter found there in high concentrations.

sylvian fissure A major crevice in the cerebrum separating the temporal and PARIETAL LOBES.

sympathetic nervous system A division of the AUTONOMIC NERVOUS SYSTEM that controls such activities as hormone secretion and heartbeat and consists of two chains of nerves passing from the SPINAL CORD throughout the body. Into these organs and other structures, the nerve endings release EPINEPHRINE and NOREPINEPHRINE. During the FIGHT-OR-FLIGHT RESPONSE, the sympathetic nervous system is elevated, increasing the heartbeat, dilating the airways, dilating the blood vessels in muscles, and constricting those in the skin and abdominal organs. This increases blood flow to the muscles and decreases the activity of the digestive system.

See also PARASYMPATHETIC NERVOUS SYSTEM.

synapse The point at which a nerve impulse passes from the AXON of one NEURON (NERVE CELL) to a DENDRITE of another. To send a signal, one neuron transmits an electrical signal to another by firing across the synapse gap between adjacent dendrites, which triggers the release of chemical messengers (NEUROTRANSMITTERS) that diffuse across the spaces between cells, attaching themselves to RECEPTORS on the neighboring nerve cell. The receiving dendrite has receptors that recognize the chemical transmitter and speeds the signal through the neuron.

The human brain contains about 10 billion neurons joined together by about 60 trillion synapses. For a long time, scientists have believed that change in the brain's synapses is the critical event in information storage. But researchers do not agree about how synaptic change actually represents information. One of the most widely held ideas is that the specificity of stored information is determined by the location of synaptic changes in the NERVOUS SYSTEM and by the pattern of altered neuronal interaction that these changes produce.

syphilis A sexually transmitted (or congenital) disease which can have devastating effects on the brain. Syphilis of the brain (*neurosyphilis*) can also cause paralysis in addition to DEMENTIA.

Cause Syphilis is caused by a type of bacterium called *Treponema pallidum*. Usually transmitted by sexual contact, the organism enters the body via minor cuts or abrasions in the skin or mucous membranes. It could also be transmitted by infected blood or from a mother to her unborn child during pregnancy. Neurosyphilis usually occurs 10 to 20 years after the initial infection, when it is considered to be in the tertiary (end) stage of the disease. Rarely seen today, it is encountered in elderly demented patients who were never properly treated for syphilis in their youth.

Symptoms Symptoms include subtle changes in personality, lack of attention, poor judgment, aggression, bizarre behavior, mood swings, and problems in concentration; some patients experience delusions of grandeur, but about 50 percent have a simple dementia.

Treatment Syphilis is not nearly as deadly as it once was, due to the introduction of penicillin; however, treatment at this late stage takes longer, and more than half of those treated suffer a severe reaction within 6 to 12 hours later because the body reacts to the sudden annihilation of large numbers of spirochetes (a type of bacteria). Brain damage already caused by the disease, however, cannot be reversed.

Prevention Infection can be avoided by maintaining monogamous relationships; condoms offer some measure of protection but not absolute protection. People infected with syphilis are infectious during the primary and secondary stages but not the tertiary stage.

T

tacrine See COGNEX.

tardive dyskinesia A type of movement disorder that occurs more than a year after continuous neuroleptic medication in as many as 20 percent of patients. Scientists believe that the disorder appears more often in those who have had acute reactions to neuroleptic drugs (such as chlorpromazine) and who have an underlying affective disorder.

See also TARDIVE DYSKINESIA/TARDIVE DYSTONIA NATIONAL ASSOCIATION; Appendix A.

Symptoms The dyskinesias include facial and limb movements, writhing or involuntary movements, and dystonia (posture disorder with spasm in the muscles of the shoulder, neck, and trunk). The involuntary movements are often restricted to the head and neck (such as chewing or tongue-thrusting). Symptoms may fluctuate, taking months or years to disappear after drug withdrawal. About half of the cases are reversible within five years, but some cases may never improve. The movements do not typically worsen once a plateau has been achieved.

Stopping and starting neuroleptic drugs is not effective and may even be associated with increased risk.

Treatment Treatment is difficult, and many medicines have been suggested, including tetrabenazine and reserpine. Other drugs that have been tried with varying success include baclofen, valproic acid, diazepam, alpha antagonists, amantadine, clonidine, and carbidopa-L-dopa.

Tardive Dyskinesia/Tardive Dystonia National Association A national support group for TARDIVE DYSKINESIA and TARDIVE DYSTONIA patients, relatives, and legal and health-care professionals. (Tardive dyskinesia and tardive dystonia are neuromuscular disorders of the face, trunk, and extremities that occur primarily as a side effect of certain psychotropic and neuroleptic drugs.)

The association is working to establish national legislation requiring that patients be warned of the potential for drug-induced movement disorders and that patients' informed consent be obtained before these drugs are administered. The association also encourages research into alternative treatments and the prevention and cure of the disorders. The group provides guidance, support networks, referral services, and assistance for afflicted patients and their families, operates a speakers' bureau, and compiles statistics.

Founded in 1985, the group has 510 members and publishes a semiannual newsletter and other informational brochures. For address, see Appendix A.

taste The sense of taste is far less acute than our sense of smell, partly because a person's taste CHEMORECEPTORS are far less sensitive than the olfactory receptors in the nose. A person would need 25,000 times more of a chemical compound to taste it than to smell it.

While a person's ability to taste is fairly crude (differentiating only sweet, sour, salty, and bitter), when added to temperature and touch, produce the variety of flavors a person can differentiate. But it is the sense of smell that can enable a person to distinguish the most flavors. In fact, the sense of smell is so important to the sense of taste that losing the ability to smell (such as during a cold) will interfere with a person's ability to taste anything.

The mechanism of taste depends on the translation of a chemical signal into an electrochemical one, and it begins in the taste buds on the tongue, palate, throat, and tonsils. Adults have about 9,000 of these taste buds, each containing groups of taste-sensitive cells containing taste-sensitive hairs. (Taste buds for sweetness lie at the tip of the tongue; sour is found on the left and right front sides; salt behind sour and bitter along the back of the tongue).

Substances must first dissolve in water or saliva to allow the molecules to bind to the surface of a taste bud; chemicals in food or drinks dissolve in saliva, flowing into the pores found in the protuberances of the tongue; around these pores are taste buds. The molecules produce an electrochemical change within the taste-bud receptor cell and stimulate hairs projecting from the taste-bud cells, triggering signals sent from the cells along nerves to taste centers in the brain via part of the seventh nerve (GLOSSOPHARYNGEAL NERVE) to centers in the lower BRAINSTEM, on to the thalamus, and then to the CEREBRAL CORTEX. Because olfactory nerves cross over in the MEDULLA, tastes from each side of the tongue are registered in the opposite BRAIN HEMISPHERE. Along the way, some of the NEURONS communicate with the LIMBIC SYSTEM.

Tay-Sachs disease A serious, inherited, and fatal brain disorder that is most commonly found among Ashkenazi Jews. It is caused by a deficiency of the enzyme hexosaminidase, a protein essential for regulating chemical reactions in the body. This deficiency causes an accumulation of a harmful substance in the brain.

The gene for Tay-Sachs is recessive; an Ashkenazi Jew has a 1 in 25 chance of carrying the gene; if two carriers marry, there is a one in four chance that they will have an affected child.

The disease is diagnosed through physical examination and family history and confirmed with an enzyme analysis of tissue samples.

Incidence The disease is found in one out of 2,500 Ashkenazi Jews, which is about 100 times higher than in any other ethnic group.

Symptoms Blindness, DEMENTIA, deafness, SEIZURES, and paralysis appear during the first six months of life. An extreme startle response to sound is one of the earliest symptoms. The disease progresses rapidly, usually killing affected children by age three.

Treatment There is no treatment. Prenatal screening can show that a fetus may be affected; the parents may choose to have an abortion. Carriers and those with an affected child or relative should receive genetic counseling before starting a family or planning another pregnancy.

tectum, midbrain Midbrain "roof," a term referring to the inferior and superior colliculi.

tegmentum The region of the MIDBRAIN below and in front of the cerebral aqueduct that contains the nuclei of several CRANIAL NERVES, the RETICULAR FORMATION and the pathways that link the FOREBRAIN and the SPINAL CORD.

telencephalon Also known as the endbrain, this is one of two subdivisions of the FOREBRAIN; telencephalic structures account for about 75 percent of the weight of the entire human CENTRAL NERVOUS SYSTEM. These structures include the two CEREBRAL HEMISPHERES that (while separated by a large fissure) are connected by a mass of crossing fiber tracts (corpus callosum).

temperature regulation The control of the body's temperature is of critical importance to proper function. It is believed to be controlled by the HYPOTHALAMUS, which acts like a type of thermostat and constantly monitors internal temperature, automatically activating mechanisms to compensate for changes.

The need to raise or lower internal temperature is monitored by the body's thermoreceptors. When the body's temperature falls, blood vessels in the skin are constricted, shunting blood away from the skin to deeper vessels to prevent excessive cooling. The hypothalamus also sends nerve impulses to stimulate shivering, which generates heat by making muscles work harder.

Conversely, when the body overheats, the hypothalamus triggers sweating, increases and dilates blood vessels in the skin, boosting blood flow in order to radiate heat away from the body. This is why the skin of an overheated individual appears to be quite red.

A whole variety of factors can disrupt the body's heat-regulating system, causing heat stroke, fever, or hypothermia. These factors could include thyroid disorders, infection, and overexposure to cold or extreme heat.

The average normal body temperature measured in the mouth is 98.6°F. (37°C.). However, normal body temperature by no means remains constant at this level; body temperature varies among individuals and also in the same person depending on exercise, sleep, eating, and drinking. Moreover, temperature fluctuates according to the time of day (lowest at about 3 A.M. and highest at about 6 P.M.) and also depends on the stage of the menstrual cycle (lowest during menstruation and highest at ovulation). In most people, temperature varies between 97.8°F. and 99°F.

Where the temperature is taken can also have an effect; temperature measurement is highest when taken rectally (rising by about 0.5°F. to 0.7°F.) and is lower when taken in the armpit by about 0.3°F.

temporal artery   A branch of the external CAROTID ARTERY that supplies blood mainly to the temple and the scalp.

temporal cortex   See TEMPORAL LOBE.

temporal lobe   The part of the brain that forms much of the lower side of each half of the CEREBRUM (the main mass of the brain).

The temporal lobes are concerned with smell, taste, hearing, visual associations, some aspects of memory, and a person's sense of self. Any interference in the normal function of the temporal lobes may cause peculiarities in any of these functions. A HEAD INJURY may cause direct and diffuse effects in the temporal lobe; there is some evidence that the tips and undersurface of the temporal lobe are particularly vulnerable to trauma.

A great deal of research has centered on the temporal lobe. Some scientists have spent time probing the lobes and recording the resulting effects in patients; others have studied the results of removing part or all of the temporal lobe.

During the 1950s, Canadian surgeon Wilder Penfield (see PENFIELD, WILDER) was the first to stimulate this part of the brain during surgery. He found that while stimulating various areas of the CORTEX produces a range of responses from patients, only stimulation of the temporal lobes elicits meaningful, integrated experiences (including sound, movement and color) that are far more detailed, accurate, and specific than normal recall. Interestingly, some of the memories that popped up during Penfield's stimulation were unremembered in the normal state, while stimulation of the same spot in the temporal lobe would elicit the exact same memory again and again.

Research also suggests that removing the left temporal lobe causes verbal memory deficits, while removal of the right lobe impairs nonverbal memory (such as memory for mazes, patterns, or faces).

Recent studies of gender differences in the brain has found that in cognitively normal men, a tiny region of the temporal lobe behind the eye has about 10 percent fewer NEURONS than it does in women. The neurons in this region are responsible for understanding language as well as melodies and speech tones.

See also TEMPORAL LOBECTOMY; LEUCOTOMY.

temporal lobectomy The surgical removal of both TEMPORAL LOBES is associated with severe AMNESIA, when the HIPPOCAMPUS is also removed. Amnesia does not develop following lesions involving the uncus or AMYGDALA as long as the hippocampus is not removed.

Removing one of the temporal lobes results in a material-specific memory deficit; that is, removing the left temporal lobe causes a verbal memory deficit, while those with right temporal lobectomies have more problems in remembering nonverbal material such as faces, patterns, and mazes. Left temporal lobectomies result in more problems in learning and retaining verbal material (such as paired associates, prose passages, or Hebb's recurring-digit sequences). In addition, stimulation of the left temporal lobe leads to a number of naming errors and impaired recall.

Interestingly, different areas within the left temporal lobe caused two different kinds of memory problems. Stimulating the anterior region caused an ANTEROGRADE AMNESIA; stimulating the posterior section caused a RETROGRADE AMNESIA.

Patients who have undergone removal of the right temporal lobe can usually perform verbal tasks but have problems with learning visual or tactile mazes or in figuring out whether or not they have seen a particular geometric shape before. They also have problems recognizing tonal patterns or faces. But those with right temporal lobectomies were impaired in maze learning only if there was extensive hippocampal lesions. The same was true for recognition of photographs.

In fact, researchers have found that the more extensive the section of hippocampus removed, the greater the memory deficit. Among those whose left temporal lobe was removed, those with extensive hippocampus involvement had more problems with short-term verbal memory than those with no or little involvement.

temporal-lobe epilepsy See EPILEPSY.

tension headaches See HEADACHES.

tetrahydroaminoacridine (THA) Also known as *tacrine* or its brand name, *Cognex*, this drug currently is being studied as a treatment for ALZHEIMER'S DISEASE. Early indications with the drug suggested that memory loss improved in those given the medication. It is believed that the drug works by increasing the level of ACETYLCHOLINE, which is deficient in the brains of Alzheimer's patients. Unfortunately, the drug does *not* stop the degeneration of brain tissue; therefore it cannot cure the disease. Although it has been found that THA can harm liver function during treatment, the risk of permanent damage from long-term treatment is not known.

THA, developed by the Warner-Lambert Co., was denied approval by an advisory committee to the Food and Drug Administration in 1991 because of its negative side effects on the livers of some patients. While the FDA acknowledged that THA did help Alzheimer's patients, it was concerned over reports of liver damage; the damage is reversible once detected, but frequent blood tests are required and THA must be stopped.

At present, there is no drug currently on the market to treat Alzheimer's disease, which affects 4 million Americans.

thalamus The crucial brain structure that first receives messages from the body about heat and cold, pain and pressure, smell and taste. Named for the Greek word for "chamber" or "inner room," the thalamus is important in the factual memory circuit and serves as the entrance chamber to the perceptual CORTEX. All sensory organs (except for smell) enter the cortex via the thalamus. It is the part of the brain that automatically responds to extremes in temperature and pain. It is critical to states of awareness and all sensorimotor function.

A bit smaller than the CEREBELLUM, the thalamus is found deep inside the HEMISPHERES of the CEREBRUM.

One of the main parts of the DIENCEPHALON, the thalamus is active during memory and is involved in many cases of memory disorder—particularly in WERNICKE-KORSAKOFF SYNDROME. One of the best-known cases of thalamic damage and memory problems is N.A., a man who was stabbed in the thalamic region at age 22 and who suffered significant memory problems. Other cases of memory problems involving the thalamus have been reported, primarily with tumors, which can lead to a rapidly developing DEMENTIA.

The thalamus also seems to regulate cycles of sleep and wakefulness and seems to direct the way a person sometimes feels well or poorly.

theta waves A type of brain wave commonly seen in children under five and usually in adults suffering from extreme mental illness.

thirst The urge to drink. Control of the body's fluid intake is one of the most crucial functions of the brain because the proper function of each and every cell depends on a proper fluid environment. Thirst is one way to control the amount of water in the body; the other way is by the volume of urine that is produced by the kidneys. Sufficient fluids are even more important in maintaining life than food.

The HYPOTHALAMUS controls fluid intake, partly by monitoring the amount of dissolved substances in the blood to assess how dilute the blood is and the total blood volume. The concentration of sugar, salt, or other substances in the blood rises when fluid intake drops; as this particle concentration rises, the concentrated blood passes through the hypothalamus in the brain. Here, special nerve RECEPTORS are stimulated, inducing the sensation of thirst.

When the body needs to boost its fluid intake (such as after a large loss of blood or during dehydration in hot weather), thirst increases; at the same time, the PITUITARY GLAND releases antidiuretic hormone (ADH) to retain water and decrease the urine volume.

Thirst is depressed when there is too much water in the blood; when this happens, urination increases and the need to drink disappears.

thought Mental activity involving problem solving, reasoning, and the formation of judgments. The hallmarks of thought are the substitution of symbols (words, numbers, or images) for objects, the formation of these symbols into ideas, and the arrangement of ideas in a certain order in the mind. Certain aspects of thought can be tested; these include speech and efficiency, idea content, and logical relationships between ideas.

In recent research, neuroscientists have recorded a visual representation of the chemical and electrical activity that characterized thinking in the brain cells. Using a technique called *optical imaging*, cameras recorded tiny differences in reflected light flashing across the surface of the brain as thinking occurred. Scientists don't know what causes the changes, which are too subtle to be seen by the naked eye. The procedure was used to help surgeons figure out which part of the brain to preserve during surgery to treat EPILEPSY. Before this technique was tried, information had to be obtained by scattering tiny electrodes across the brain's surface and mapping the trajectories of electrical impulses.

thought disorders Conditions that feature abnormalities in the structure or content of thought as evidenced by a person's speech, writing, or behavior. SCHIZOPHRENIA is one of the most common mental illnesses that is characterized by thought disorders. Patients can lose a logical connection to associations, jumping from one unrelated subject to another, or making indirect associations or "clang associations" (words that sound the same but don't connect logically).

Other thought disorders found in schizophrenia include neologisms (inventing new words), thought blocking (interrupted train of thought), auditory HALLUCINATIONS, and having the feeling that thoughts are being introduced or removed from the mind by an outside entity.

All types of confusion (such as DEMENTIA and DELIRIUM) feature an inability to think clearly; flight of ideas (rapidly switching from one idea to another) is characteristic of mania as a result of loosening of associations.

Recurrent ideas that seem to keep returning to a person's mind are characteristic of obsessive-compulsive disorder, while slowed thinking is a hallmark of clinical depression.

Finally, delusions (false beliefs) are a form of distorted thinking and are found in schizophrenia and other psychotic illnesses.

thyroid stimulating hormone (TSH) Also known as *thyrotropin*, this is a hormone that is synthesized and secreted by the anterior PITUITARY GLAND under the control of thyrotropin-releasing hormone and that stimulates activity of the thyroid gland. Defects in the production of this hormone may lead to an over- or under-production of thyroid hormones. TSH is also given in an injection to test thyroid-gland function.

TIA See TRANSIENT ISCHEMIC ATTACK.

tic douloureux See TRIGEMINAL NEURALGIA.

Time Out to Enjoy (TOTE) A national support group for learning-disabled adults, health professionals, and those involved with LD adults. This group defines a learning-disabled adult as a person with normal to above-average intelligence with a deficit in one or more learning skills. The group's purposes are to educate the public about LEARNING DISABILITIES and to provide support to and resources for LD adults. It collects and provides information on educational and employment services and provides referrals for LD adults with specific needs. The group also conducts in-services, workshops, and panels for teachers, social workers, psychologists, and other professionals, and parents. For address, see Appendix A.

See also NATIONAL NETWORKER; ORTON DYSLEXIA SOCIETY; NATIONAL CENTER FOR LEARNING DISABILITIES; LEARNING DISABILITIES ASSOCIATION OF AMERICA; COUNCIL FOR LEARNING DISABILITIES.

tomogram A photograph of a section of skull and brain made by a computer from CAT or PET SCANS.

tomography The process of scanning through a single section of tissue and bone using X rays or ultrasound. By producing a series of slices at different depths, a three-dimensional image of the body structure can be given.

topectomy A more conservative type of psychosurgery that destroys parts of the frontal CORTEX itself instead of the white fibers below it, as in LEUCOTOMY. The operation was designed to avoid the problems of HEMORRHAGE, memory loss, and vegetative states that often occurred after other more radical LOBOTOMY.

The procedure was developed by research scientist J. Lawrence Pool at Columbia University in 1947 and was performed on patients at the New Jersey State Hospital in Greystone Park, New Jersey.

See also MONIZ, EGAS.

Tourette's syndrome The common name for Gilles de la Tourette's syndrome, this multiple chronic-tic syndrome is usually first noticed in children between the ages of 2 and 13. In general, the tics worsen during the life of the person. The syndrome is more common in males.

Symptoms Involuntary grunts, whistles, coughs, repeating words or phrases, in about half the cases, uncontrolled use of offensive language (coprolalia) appears. It may be possible to voluntarily suppress tics in the early stages of the disease by concentrating on stopping the behavior.

Treatment The drug of choice is haloperidol (Haldol), although frequent side effects may interfere with successful treatment. (These side effects include sedation, low blood pressure, and Parkinsonlike movements.) See TARDIVE DYSKINESIA.

Other possible drug treatments: pimozide (Orap), a haloperidol-related drug that may work when Haldol fails, and clonidine (Catapres) which helps about half the patients who have a tic recurrence while on Haldol. Maximum improvement may not appear for six months on clonidine, and behavioral symptoms respond more to clonidine than do tics. Side effects of clonidine include sedation, fatigue, and low blood pressure on standing. The drug should not be quickly withdrawn because of the possibility of high blood pressure spikes.

Other drugs include tetrabenazine, which has been successful in young patients; nifedipine, flunarazine and verapamil, and botulinum toxin A (Botox).

Tourette Syndrome Association   An organization for people with TOURETTE'S SYNDROME and their families and friends, physicians, nurses, teachers, psychologists, social workers, and other professionals and organizations such as mental-health agencies.

The association disseminates educational materials, schedules professional meetings and seminars, and provides research support through the Tourette Research Brain Bank at Mt. Sinai Hospital in New York City. The group also informs members of rights, services, and benefits provided by the government and other groups, provides lists of doctors experienced in treating the disorder, operates support groups and other services to help those with TS and their families, and maintains advocacy-referral services for education, employment, and housing. The association also makes research grants.

Founded in 1972, the group has 30,000 members and 60 regional groups; it publishes the quarterly *Leadership Bulletins*; the annual *Medical Letter: Summary of the Recent Literature*; and the quarterly *Tourette Syndrome Association Newsletter*. For address, see Appendix A.

toxic encephalopathy   Encephalopathy (serious, generalized brain dysfunction) caused by NEUROTOXINS that is more serious than a TOXIC MOOD DISORDER and occurs after long-term exposure to toxic substances. Symptoms include personality changes, memory problems, and fuzzy thinking, listlessness, convulsions, COMA, and respiratory arrest. Recovery from this condition may take weeks, and some people may never recover.

toxic mood disorders   Personality and mood changes caused by exposure to NEUROTOXINS that damage the brain. There are a wide variety of substances that may cause mood or personality changes, but the most common sources are lead and mercury, some solvents and gases, and pesticides. The solvent carbon disulfide, used primarily in industrial uses, can cause a severe manic DEPRESSION. While regulations today require ventilation in the rayon and cellophane industries, which use this product, even regulated levels may cause toxic mood disorders and symptoms of depression, irritability, and insomnia.

See also TOXIC ENCEPHALOPATHY.

Symptoms The symptoms of a toxic mood disorder may be subtle or wrongly associated with depression; other symptoms may be obvious or subtle. They may include personality changes such as irritability, social withdrawal, and the inability to cope with even minor problems. Mental changes may include short-term memory loss, concentration problems, mental slowness, and difficulty in following instructions. Neurotoxins may also interfere with the hormones regulating sleep, causing some people to sleep too much and others to experience insomnia. Chronic fatigue caused by neurotoxic exposure will also have neuropsychiatric impairment that may show up only with specialized tests. Symptoms may also include problems in walking, muscle weakness, or diminished manual dexterity.

Diagnosis To identify whether a particular set of symptoms are toxic in nature, the patient should have a careful history and physical including a neuropsychological evaluation and standardized testing by a certified neuropsychologist, various lab tests, and specific toxicological assessments.

Treatment Once exposure has been eliminated, symptoms can fade away within days, but the symptoms may reappear and worsen if exposure continues.

tranquilizers See CENTRAL NERVOUS SYSTEM DEPRESSANTS; TRANQUILIZERS AND THE BRAIN.

tranquilizers and the brain Tranquilizers are divided into major tranquilizers (antipsychotics) and minor tranquilizers (antianxiety drugs).

Antipsychotic drugs work by blocking the action of DOPAMINE, a NEUROTRANSMITTER acting on the brain. LITHIUM is an antipsychotic drug that is thought to reduce the release of NOREPINEPHRINE, another neurotransmitter. They are used to treat psychoses, particularly SCHIZOPHRENIA and manic DEPRESSION. They are also used to calm or sedate those with other mental disorders, such as DEMENTIA, who have become agitated.

Antipsychotics include the phenothiazines (chlorpromazine, fluphenazine, perphenazine, thioridazine, trifluoperazine) and others, such as haloperidol and lithium.

Antianxiety drugs include benzodiazepines and beta-blockers. Benzodiazepines work by reducing nerve activity in the brain; beta-blockers reduce the physical symptoms of ANXIETY, such as shaking and palpitations. They are used to relieve symptoms of anxiety when it threatens a person's ability to cope in everyday life. They are also sometimes used to calm a person before surgery.

transient ischemic attack (TIA) A temporary impairment of the brain caused by an insufficient supply of blood, which can result in brief memory or speech problems, weakness, paralysis, dizziness, or nausea. Episodes usually last for a few minutes, but they may occur for up to a few hours. An attack that lasts for more than 24 hours is considered to be a STROKE.

Unlike a stroke, however, which may have the same symptoms but involve a lasting deficit, TIA symptoms fade without permanent damage. However, they should be regarded as a possible forerunner of stroke and should be reported to a physician. Stroke does occur in from one-fourth to one-third of all patients with TIAs.

Causes TIAs may be caused by a temporary block to an artery supplying the brain (EMBOLISM) or by a narrowed artery thick with fat deposits (ATHEROSCLEROSIS).

Symptoms A wide variety of symptoms may occur, depending on the site of the block and how long the blood flow is impaired. Symptoms may include weakness or numbness in legs or arms, disturbed speech (APHASIA), dizziness, or partial blindness. A TIA is always followed by complete recovery.

Symptoms of TIA may be confused with a BRAIN TUMOR or SUBDURAL HEMATOMA (blood-filled swelling); diagnosis may include BRAIN

SCANS and blood tests; ULTRASOUND, ANGIOGRA-PHY, or heart studies may be needed to pinpoint the problem.

Treatment Treatment is usually aimed at preventing stroke, via endarterectomy, ANTI-COAGULANT DRUGS, or aspirin.

tremor An involuntary, rhythmical alternating movement that may affect the muscles of any part of the body, although the hands, feet, jaw, tongue, and head are most often affected. Tremors are caused by the rapid alternating contraction and relaxation of muscles and are a common symptom of neurologic disease. Occasional tremors may be felt by almost everyone (usually during fear or excitement), triggered by the increased production of the stress hormone EPINEPHRINE.

Some tremors are unrelated to disease; these include the slight, persistent tremor common among the elderly. Another common tremor not associated with disease is *essential tremor*, a mild movement that runs in families and may sometimes be relieved by small doses of alcohol or by taking beta-blockers. Both of these types of tremor increase with movement of the affected part of the body.

More persistent tremors are caused by trauma, tumors, STROKE, or degenerative disease. Coarse tremors (four to five movements per second) that occur during rest, diminishing during movement, are a common sign of PARKINSON'S DISEASE. *Intention tremors* (tremors that worsen on movement) are a sign of CEREBELLUM disease. Tremors often accompany such diseases as MULTIPLE SCLEROSIS, WILSON'S DISEASE, mercury poisoning, thyrotoxicosis, and liver encephalopathy.

In addition, tremors may appear as a side effect of certain drugs (such as AMPHETAMINES, ANTIPSYCHOTICS, ANTIDEPRESSANTS, CAFFEINE, or LITHIUM) or as a sign of withdrawal. Alcohol withdrawal also may trigger tremors, indicating the presence of alcohol dependence. These "morning shakes" occur as the blood alcohol level falls; the tremors disappear when more alcohol is consumed.

See also INTERNATIONAL TREMOR FOUNDATION; Appendix A.

trephining The boring and scraping of the skull to release "evil spirits" conducted by prehistoric physicians, a treatment that usually relieved intracranial pressure caused by TUMORS, HEMORRHAGES, and skull fractures. CRANIOTOMY is an extension of trephining in which a flap of skull is entirely removed, exposing the MENINGES (brain covering) that covers the CEREBRAL CORTEX.

tricyclic antidepressants A class of antidepressants named for their three-ring chemical structure that have been used to treat DEPRESSION ever since the 1950s. Tricyclics include amitriptyline, amoxapine, clomipramine, despiramine, doxepin, imipramine, nortriptyline, and protriptyline and are sometimes used for other disorders in addition to depression, including obsessive compulsive disorder, panic disorder, and (in the case of imipramine) bedwetting.

The tricyclic antidepressants work by beefing up the brain's level of the NEUROTRANSMITTERS NOREPINEPHINE and SEROTONIN levels—chemicals that are abnormally low in depressed patients. The problem with cyclics is that they don't stop there. They go on to interfere with a range of other neurotransmitter systems and a variety of brain-cell *receptors*, slowing down nerve-cell communication all over the brain in the process. The more neurotransmitter systems and receptors that are affected, the more side effects a patient will have. Still, for some people the cyclics work better than any other drug there is.

Side effects Among other brain systems, the tricyclics act on histamine receptors, activating the body's FIGHT-OR-FLIGHT RESPONSE, speeding up the heart and shunting blood away from bodily functions, such as waste removal. The result is dry mouth, blurred vision, constipation, and urinary problems. These side effects may be especially annoying with amitriptyline, clomipramine, doxepin, imipramine, or protriptyline. Amoxapine (Asendin) or desipramine have the lowest risk for these side effects. Other side effects include weight gain, nausea, HEADACHES, inability to sweat, increased heart rate, drowsiness, sun sensitivity, decreased blood pressure, sexual function problems, or dizziness when standing up.

Like all antidepressants, tricyclics may be associated with a mild manic high or suicide attempts in some people. In one study of 231 nonsuicidal patients, about 3.5 percent taking the antidepressant drug Prozac became suicidal after beginning treatment, but about 6.5 percent taking both Prozac and a tricyclic became suicidal. In a retrospective study published in the British Medical Journal of 3065 patients with major depression, tricyclics worsened suicidal thinking slightly more than Prozac did (16.3 percent versus 15.3 percent). Actual suicidal acts were reported as 0.3 percent for Prozac and 0.4 percent for tricyclics.

In addition, tricyclics may affect a diabetic patient's blood-sugar levels or may cause dry eyes; this dryness may adversely affect contact lenses, coating them with deposits of thick secretions and making them feel gritty, itchy, or painful.

Patients who use clomipramine for too long run the risk of developing a group of symptoms called *neuroleptic malignant syndrome*, including fever, fast or irregular heartbeat, sweating, weakness, muscle stiffness, SEIZURES, or loss of bladder control.

Amoxapine causes a unique disorder, called TARDIVE DYSKINESIA, with speech or swallowing problems, lip smacking or puckering, loss of balance, cheek puffing, rapid or wormlike tongue movements, shakiness or trembling, shuffling walk, slow movements, arm or leg stiffness, uncontrolled chewing movements, and uncontrolled movements of hands, arms, or legs.

Some side effects may appear *after* treatment stops: headache, irritability, lip smacking or puckering, nausea or vomiting, diarrhea, abdominal pain, convulsions, puffing of cheeks or rapid wormlike tongue movements, restlessness, insomnia, vivid dreams, uncontrolled chewing movements, uncontrolled leg or arm movements, or unusual excitement. There may be rebound mild mania or mania in manic-depressive people not taking LITHIUM at the same time.

trigeminal nerve   Also known as the fifth cranial nerve, this nerve is responsible for facial sensation and jaw movements. This nerve arises from the PONS (part of the BRAINSTEM) and then branches into three parts, which then subdivide even further into a web of smaller nerves. These nerves supply sensations to the face, scalp, nose, teeth, mouth lining, upper eyelid, sinus, and front part of the tongue. They also control the amount of saliva and the amount of tears and are also involved in chewing.

Damage or disease in one area supplied by the trigeminal nerve may cause pain in a different area (such as tooth pain caused by inflamed sinuses).

See also CRANIAL NERVES; TRIGEMINAL NEURALGIA.

trigeminal neuralgia   A disorder of the fifth cranial nerve (TRIGEMINAL NERVE) that causes brief episodes of stabbing pain involving the cheek, lips, chin, or gums on one side. It usually begins in one particular "trigger" point and is often brought on by touching the face. Its nickname, *tic douloureux* ("painful twitch"), refers to the fact that the intense pain often causes wincing.

Trigeminal neuralgia is most often found in patients over age 50, but it also may be found in younger people with MULTIPLE SCLEROSIS. Attacks recur in clusters of brief episodes that may last for weeks; the recurrences tend to occur closer and closer together with time.

See also TRIGEMINAL NEURALGIA ASSOCIATION; Appendix A.

Treatment Carbamazepine may suppress the pain in most people, but others develop a resistance to the drug. If drug treatment is ineffective, surgery may be necessary.

Trigeminal Neuralgia Association A support group for those with TRIGEMINAL NEURALGIA, a neurological disorder characterized by sudden attacks of pain along one or more branches of the trigeminal nerve in the face and head. The group works to increase public and professional awareness and understanding of the disorder and coordinates the exchange of information among those with the disorder.

The group, founded in 1989, has 200 members and offers physician referrals. It is affiliated with the National Organization of Rare Disorders. For address, see Appendix A.

triple brain Paul MacLean's concept of the brain as having three layers, the R-complex that controls instinct, the paleomammalian (the limbic system) that controls emotion, and the neomammalian (the cerebrum) that controls thought.

triune brain See TRIPLE BRAIN.

trochlear nerve Also known as the fourth cranial nerve, this nerve (together with the third and sixth cranial nerves) is responsible for eye movements. It arises from the MIDBRAIN (part of the BRAINSTEM) and passes through the skull, entering the eye socket via a gap in the skull. This nerve supplies only one muscle of each eye; by contracting this superior oblique muscle, the eye rotates outward.

If this nerve is damaged, it may cause double vision.

See also CRANIAL NERVES.

truth drugs A group of drugs including sodium pentothal that are useful in psychiatry to help patients recall experiences and emotions they have tried to suppress. The drugs acts on the brain, lowering the inhibitory processes.

tryptophan An AMINO ACID converted by the brain into the NEUROTRANSMITTER SEROTONIN, linked to mood and sleepiness. Scientists have found that depressed patients often have low blood levels of tryptophan, and lowering the levels of this amino acid appears to worsen mood in healthy people. Some research appears to suggest that administering tryptophan may help ease DEPRESSION and boosts the effectiveness of certain antidepressants. However, tryptophan is no "happy pill"—giving it to people with normal mood does not make them even happier, most likely because their serotonin levels are not abnormal.

Several years ago the U.S. Food and Drug Administration banned the sale of tryptophan after 38 people died of a muscle-nerve disease associated with tryptophan pills; this disease was eventually traced to one batch of contaminated pills. Whether tryptophan is harmful at all has not been determined, although some scientists suspect that large doses of any amino acid may lead to eventual metabolic disturbances.

tuberous sclerosis A congenital inherited disorder in which the brain and other organs are studded with small plaques or tumors. Severe cases may be fatal by age 30. The gene for tuberous sclerosis can now be detected at an early stage of pregnancy.

See also TUBEROUS SCLEROSIS ASSOCIATION OF AMERICA; for address, see Appendix A.

Symptoms Symptoms include epilepsy and mental retardation, although intelligence may be normal in mild cases. Other problems include the development of nonmalignant TUMORS in the brain.

Treatment There is no cure; treatment is aimed at relieving symptoms, such a treating

EPILEPSY and removing tumors. Genetic counseling is recommended for affected families who are considering having children.

Tuberous Sclerosis Association of America   A group for persons with TUBEROUS SCLEROSIS, parents, physicians, and friends that provides patient service, public education, and physician awareness. The group is interested in finding cases of tuberous sclerosis and identifies the disease as soon as possible, expanding tuberous-sclerosis movement at local, state, and national levels. It also stimulates development, and improves the delivery of, services to patients. The group supports genetic research, offers counseling and contact service for patients and families, encourages the formation of parent support groups, and testifies before Congress. The association also maintains a speakers' bureau, conducts workshops, seminars, and lectures, and compiles statistics.

Founded in 1968, the group has 2,100 members and publishes the monthly newsletter *Tuberous Sclerosis Association of America*, brochures, flyers, fact sheets, and research bulletins. For address, see Appendix A.

tumors, brain   Abnormal growth in or near the brain which may or may not be malignant, these tumors are always serious because of the pressure they cause in the brain as they grow.

Abnormal growths in the brain may be primary (originating in brain tissue) such as GLIOMAS, MENINGIOMAS, ACOUSTIC NEUROMAS, and PITUITARY TUMORS, or secondary (arising from cancer cells which have spread to the brain from other parts of the body—usually the lungs or breast). Secondary brain tumors are always malignant.

Primary brain tumors are identified and classed according to their cell type, their location, and their degree of malignancy. A brain tumor's effect can be different depending on its location and its type.

While cancer in other parts of the body often spreads, primary brain tumors rarely do; if they do spread, it is usually to other parts of the CENTRAL NERVOUS SYSTEM (the brain and SPINAL CORD). Many brain tumors don't look like cancer cells under a microscope, and they are usually far more slow growing than other malignant tumors in other parts of the body. However, *any untreated brain tumor is malignant* because it has the potential to be fatal because of its location, if not its cell characteristics.

About 60 percent of brain tumors are gliomas, which are frequently malignant. Other primary tumors, usually benign, including meningiomas (arising from the meningeal membranes covering the brain); acoustic neuromas (on the acoustic nerve) and pituitary tumors (on the PITUITARY GLAND).

Children are prone to brain tumors located in the back of the brain, including two types of glioma: MEDULLOBLASTOMA and CEREBELLAR ASTROCYTOMA.

Incidence   In the United States, about 6 out of every 100,000 Americans will be diagnosed with a primary brain TUMOR every year; about 12,000 people will die. Tumors most often appear in people about 50 years old, but about one in every 3,000 children die from a primary brain tumor before the age of 10.

Alarmingly, the worldwide incidence of brain tumors has been increasing steadily for the past 20 years; in the United States, the incidence of brain cancer in those over age 75 has more than doubled since 1968, and in children, brain cancer has increased by 30 percent since 1973. Other statistics indicate that brain tumors are the fourth most-common cause of cancer-related death in women aged 15–34.

While some doctors believe that what has really increased is the rate of *diagnosis* because of more sophisticated brain scanners, others point out that the upward surge in tumors began *before* some of the more sensitive equipment was in use in the late 1970s. One Canadian study found that about a third of the increase in brain tumors could be attributed to improved diagnostic technology; this leaves two-thirds or more due to a true increase of incidence.

Causes A number of potential suspects have been identified, ranging from female hormones to chemical agents. Experts point out the increasing use of pesticides in this country parallel the rise in brain cancer. Other studies have implicated industrial and household chemicals, ionizing radiation (such as from X-RAYS), and electromagnetic fields (EMFs) caused by cellular telephone use, household appliances such as microwave ovens, and electric devices such as TVs and computers. The Environmental Protection Agency has labeled EMFs a Class B (or probable) carcinogen, which places them in a category with dioxin and DDT.

But while a Florida lawsuit raised questions in 1993 about whether certain types of cellular telephones (those with built-in antennas) cause brain cancer, there has been no proof that microwave radiation from these phones carries a health risk.

See CELLULAR PHONES AND BRAIN TUMORS.

Symptoms Compression of brain tissue by the tumor may cause weak muscles, sensory disturbances, speech problems, and epileptic SEIZURES. Pressure can also cause HEADACHES, especially in the morning, which may get worse during coughing or straining. Pressure may also cause vomiting, visual disturbances (blurred or double vision, partial visual loss), and impaired mental processes, and hearing problems (ringing or buzzing in the ears or partial hearing loss). Brain tumors may also cause behavior changes, such as problems with speaking, thinking or remembering, sluggishness, drowsiness, or changes in personality. There may also be problems in controlling muscles, paralysis, difficulty with balance, or trouble walking.

Diagnosis In order to locate the tumor and determine its extent, physicians use ANGIOGRAPHY together with various types of BRAINSCANS: CT SCANNING, MAGNETIC RESONANCE IMAGING (MRI), and X-ray studies.

Treatment Treatment of a brain tumor often depends on its classification and characteristics. For example, a medulloblastoma is usually treated with radiation of both the brian and spinal cord because this type of tumor has a tendency to spread throughout the entire central nervous system.

Tumors are often surgically removed when possible, but too often malignant tumors are inaccessible or too extensive to be removed. In this case, survival rates are not high; less than 20 percent of these patients survive one year.

When a tumor cannot be totally removed, as much of the growth as possible will be cut out to relieve pressure on the brain, followed by chemotherapy or radiation therapy. Corticosteroid drugs can be used to reduce tissue swelling around the tumor.

Radiation Radiation is the second most common treatment for brain tumors after surgery, usually administered soon after surgery. The cells of many malignant brain tumors are readily killed by radiation, which is why this type of treatment is almost always recommended. (One possible exception is the treatment of very young children, whose developing brains may be injured by the radiation.) Most tumors do shrink from the effects of radiation, although it may take some time for swelling and dead cells to diminish so that the true size of the growth can be seen.

A new type of radiation technique called STEREOTACTIC RADIOSURGERY, or *gamma knife*, is now being used for patients with inoperable brain tumors. In this technique, the surgeon uses a small directed beam of radiation to treat areas that may be inaccessible by conventional surgery or for patients who may not be able to withstand an operation. The one-time application is an outpatient procedure that may serve as a substitute for the 20 to 30 radiation treatments normally required. Using the precisely directed beams of radiation, surgeons can focus on and destroy the diseased tissue and spare nearly all of the surrounding healthy tissue.

The key is to locate the diseased tissue and program those coordinates into a linear accelerator—the unit that emits the radiation beam. The accelerator is rotated around the target area in the patient's brain, allowing high doses of radiation to be given directly to the designated site. The procedure usually takes an entire day and is performed with a local anesthetic. A CAT SCAN is used to determine the exact coordinates of the diseased tissue; with that information, doctors then affix a metal ring to the head, which helps the linear accelerator focus on the target area.

At present, this type of radiation is being used for patients with various types of brain tumors, as well as brain tumors that have not responded to conventional radiation therapy. It can also be used to treat malformed blood vessels in the brain that can cause seizures and are usually inoperable under normal situations.

Chemotherapy is also often used in the treatment of brain tumors, which work by interfering with various parts of the cell's cycle. Immunotherapy is also used with brain tumors.

tyrosine An AMINO ACID that plays a role in controlling blood pressure and is associated with alertness.

Scientists have found that tyrosine supplements may improve alertness during stress, lessening fatigue and boosting mental agility. Other studies found that giving tyrosine pills improved cognitive performance in the presence of loud, irritating noise.

However, some scientists caution that taking large doses of any amino acid may eventually disrupt the body's metabolic balance.

U

ultradian rhythms Rhythms that appear more than once per day (*ultra* for "beyond," or more than once a day). For example, the cycle of stages that occurs within the normal six-to-eight-hour period that humans sleep is one example of an ultradian rhythm. Several hormones (luteinizing hormone and follicle-stimulating hormone) are secreting into the bloodstream in an ultradian rhythm.

Some human ultradian rhythms occur without conscious knowledge—occurring about every hour-and-a-half during wakefulness and sleep, human adults experience a subtle cycle in brain activity. Verbal and spatial matching tasks also show that human alertness and cognitive performance also seem to run in 90-minute cycles. The nighttime portion of this ultradian rhythm—sleep—has been studied for many years. During sleep, the brain passes through several different states of activity in cycles of about 90 minutes.

See SLEEP AND THE BRAIN.

ultrasound scan Also known as *neurosonography*, this is a diagnostic technique utilizing a computer image produced by analysis of echoes of high-frequency sound generated by a device placed on the skin's surface, deflected from interfaces between structures of different density.

This technique is particularly useful in evaluating prenatal, neonatal, and infant-brain problems. Because the baby's skull before birth is poorly mineralized and not completely fused, sound waves can penetrate into the brain. Once the fontanelles close, the cranial bones disperse sound waves and make ultrasounds useless.

unconsciousness Loss of awareness of the self and one's surroundings caused by a drop in the activity of the reticular formation of the BRAINSTEM. Unconsciousness may either be brief (such as in FAINTING) or more profound (such as in a COMA). A CONCUSSION is a brief state of unconsciousness after a HEAD INJURY.

Sleep, on the other hand, is a normal form of *altered* consciousness.

Treatment To treat an unconscious person, first make sure the victim is breathing. Check airways and clear the mouth, if necessary. If the person is not breathing but the heart is beating, start artificial respiration. Loosen any tight clothing. Do not leave an unconscious person alone, and don't give anything to eat or drink to a person who is or has been unconscious.

United Cerebral Palsy Association A national voluntary federation of state and local affiliates aiding those with CEREBRAL PALSY and other disabilities and their families. The association hopes to prevent CP, minimize its effects, and improve the quality of life for those with the disorder. The association offers a wide range of services to those with CP and related handicaps, ranging from diagnosis and treatment to counseling and job retraining, residences, and sports activities. The group provides information and referrals, advocacy, and money for research. Founded in 1948, the association has 155 affiliates. For address, see Appendix A.

United Leukodystrophy Foundation This association for LEUKODYSTROPHY patients, their families, and medical-care professionals provides information on the disorder; assists in identifying sources of medical care, social services, and counseling; and coordinates a communication network among affected families. It also conducts educational and research programs and offers telephone referrals.

In addition, the group supports research into the causes, treatment, and prevention of leukodystrophies and coordinates cooperation between donor and government agencies, scientific programs, and the private sector.

Founded in 1982, the group has 2,500 members and sponsors an annual conference. Its publications include the quarterly newsletter *ULF News*. For address, see Appendix A.

United Parkinson Foundation This national support group for patients, family members, and medical personnel publishes reliable information about symptoms, medication, and therapy that is helpful to those with PARKINSON'S DISEASE and related disorders. The group also supports scientific research, helps patients, and family through medical referrals, education, and other means.

Founded in 1963, the group has 38,000 members and sponsors eight conferences a year. Its publications include the quarterly newsletter *United Parkinson Foundation Newsletter; Patient Experience, One Step at A Time,* and *Your Questions Answered*; the foundation also distributes an exercise tape and book. For address, see Appendix A.

United States Cerebral Palsy Athletic Association A support group for athletes with CEREBRAL PALSY, athletic officials, health-care professionals, and interested individuals to offer competitive athletic opportunities for athletes with CP and provides support and training assistance to athletes with varying degrees of disability. The group organizes multisport competitions at the local, regional, national, and international levels, and maintains an eight-level classification system to ensure that competition is based on the functional level of participants rather than their neurological capability.

The group also selects athletes to represent the United States in the Paralympic Games and other international competitions and provides referral services to assist members in obtaining support for local sports programs, develops fundraising programs, and operates a youth sports program which provides guidelines and help to young people with special needs who wish to learn a sport.

The group also conducts educational clinics and seminars, maintains a speakers' bureau and library and plans to make available to members liability insurance and reduced rates on special sports equipment.

Founded in 1986, the group has 3,000 members and publishes a quarterly newsletter. For address, see Appendix A.

V

vagus nerve Also known as the tenth cranial nerve, this nerve is the longest of all cranial nerves and is responsible for breathing, swallowing, taste, circulation, and digestion. It is a primary component of the parasympathetic nervous system, emerging from the MEDULLA OBLONGATA (part of the BRAINSTEM), through the neck and chest to the abdomen, with branches to most of the major organs of the body.

It affects other organs by releasing ACETYLCHOLINE, which is responsible for a wide range of bodily processes (narrows the bronchi, slows heart rate, boosts stomach acid and pancreatic juice production, stimulates gall bladder, and increases peristalsis). It is also involved in coughing, swallowing, sneezing, and speech.

If this nerve becomes too active, it can influence the development of a peptic ulcer by speeding up the production of stomach acid. It can also be damaged by infection, STROKE, or TUMORS. This type of damage could result in problems ranging with the gag reflex, swallowing, or hoarseness, to death.

See also CRANIAL NERVES.

Valium and the brain Valium (DIAZEPAM) is a BENZODIAZEPINE, one of the antianxiety drugs.

See TRANQUILIZERS AND THE BRAIN.

Varolio, Constanzo (1543–1575) The Italian surgeon and anatomist, who in 1573 illustrated the PONS, part of the BRAINSTEM overlooked earlier by the Belgian anatomist Andreas Vesalius (see VESALIUS, ANDREAS), who had produced the first anatomy book of the brain.

See also BRAIN IN HISTORY.

vasopressin Another name for ADH (antidiuretic hormone), this chemical functions as a NEUROTRANSMITTER in the brain—and it may also be part of the ink with which memories are written.

Vasopressin is released from the PITUITARY GLAND and acts on the kidneys to increase their reabsorption of water into the blood. It reduces the amount of water lost in the urine and helps control the body's overall water balance. Water is continually being taken into the body in food and beverages and is also produced by the chemical reactions in cells. At the same time, water is always being lost in urine, sweat, feces, and breath; vasopressin helps maintain the optimum amount of water in the body.

Its production is controlled by the HYPOTHALAMUS (located in the center of the brain), which detects changes in the concentration and volume of the blood. If the blood concentration loses water, the hypothalamus stimulates the pituitary gland to release more vasopressin, and vice versa.

External vasopressin is approved for treatment of diabetes as a way of preventing the frequent urination common in this disease. It is given via the nose or by injection, since high IV doses cause narrowing of blood vessels. Vasopressin has also been used to treat memory deficits of aging, senile DEMENTIA, ALZHEIMER'S DISEASE, KORSAKOFF'S SYNDROME, and AMNESIA.

Research has shown that when subjects are given vasopressin, they remember long lists of words better and seem to chunk and encode better. (Chunking, or grouping words together, is a trick that memory experts teach to improve memory). Vasopressin is also being studied as a possible memory enhancement drug.

Because cocaine, LSD, AMPHETAMINES, Ritalin, and Cylert (pemoline) cause the pituitary to step up the release of natural vasopressin, abuse of these drugs can result in a depleted pool of vasopressing and resulting mental slowness. On the other hand, alcohol and marijuana suppress the release of vasopressin.

Vasopressin is available by doctor's prescription in the United States. It is available in a nasal spray bottle and produces noticeable effect within seconds because it is absorbed by the nasal mucosa. However, it can produce a range of side effects from congestion to HEADACHE and increased bowel movements, abdominal cramps, nausea, drowsiness, and confusion. It has not been proved safe during pregnancy. Because it temporarily constricts small blood vessels, it should not be used by anyone with hypertension, angina, or ATHEROSCLEROSIS and should be used cautiously in the presence of EPILEPSY.

ventricle, brain One of four fluid-filled cavities of the brain. The lateral ventricles (paired first and second ventricles) are found one in each cerebral HEMISPHERE and communicate with the third ventricle in the center of the brain. The fourth ventricle is found between the BRAINSTEM and the CEREBELLUM. CEREBROSPINAL FLUID circulates within all the ventricles linked by special ducts and around the brain's outer rim before being reabsorbed by the blood. This fluid effectively reduces the weight of the brain, buffering the brain against trauma. The cerebrospinal fluid is secreted by tufted clusters of blood vessels called the *choroid plexus* that line the ventricles. As a person ages, the ventricles enlarge.

ventriculitis An inflammation of the VENTRICLES of the brain that is usually caused by an INFECTION. It may be caused by the rupture of a cerebral abscess into the cavity of the ventricle or from the spread of a severe form of MENINGITIS from the SUBARACHNOID SPACE.

ventriculoatriostomy A surgical procedure to relieve excess pressure due to the build-up of CEREBROSPINAL FLUID in HYDROCEPHALUS. The fluid is drained via a system of catheters into the jugular vein in the neck.

ventriculography An outdated type of procedure that illuminates the ventricular cavities within the brain to be seen on X-RAY film after air or a contrast medium has been introduced. This technique has largely been replaced by CAT SCANNING and MRI.

ventriculoscopy Examination of the VENTRICLES of the brain using a fiberoptic instrument.

ventriculostomy A surgical procedure to introduce a hollow needle into one of the lateral VENTRICLES of the brain to relieve elevated intracranial pressure, to obtain CEREBROSPINAL FLUID from a ventricle for testing, or to deliver antibiotics or contrast medium for X-RAY examination.

vertebrobasilar insufficiency Periods of dizziness, weakness, double vision, and speech problems that come and go because of the reduced flow of blood to the BRAINSTEM and CEREBELLUM. Usually, such a drop in blood flow is usually caused by fat deposits that narrow ardors (ATHEROSCLEROSIS) of arteries around the base of the brain.

vertigo A sensation of spinning (of either a person or the person's surroundings), this is a common complaint that is only rarely caused by disease. It is usually caused by a disturbance of the semicircular canals in the inner ear or the nerve tracts branching from the canals. Healthy people can experience vertigo on amusement-park rides, while sailing, or even while watching a movie.

On the other hand, *severe* vertigo (usually with other symptoms) is usually caused by disease, such as inflammation of the semicircular canals (labyrinthitis) or Minere's disease. Less commonly, it may be caused by a BRAIN TUMOR (on the BRAINSTEM) or by MULTIPLE SCLEROSIS. It may also be caused by psychological issues, when it may occur with agoraphobia.

Antihistamines may help prevent recurring attacks.

vestibular nerve Part of the VESTIBULO-COCHLEA NERVE, this nerve carries sensory impulse from the semicircular canals in the inner ear to the CEREBELLUM. Combined with information from the eyes and joints, this nerve controls balance.

vestibular system The system found in the inner ear that helps maintain balance and judge a person's position in space, even with the eyes shut. The three looped semicircular ducts of the system communicate with the saclike saccule and utricle. Hair cells on each structure are linked to nerve fibers; when a person moves his or her head, fluid flows through the ducts and sacs, moving hair cells that trigger signals from nerve fibers to the brain via the eighth cranial nerve (VESTIBULO-COCHLEAR NERVE).

Since different movements of the head can activate different sets of fibers, the semicircular ducts can register nodding, turning, or tilting of the head. The saccule and utricle relay to the brain the position of the head in relation to gravity. This is how a person is able to stand or walk in the dark.

vestibulocochlear nerve Another name for the eighth cranial nerve, this nerve is concerned with balance and hearing and carries sensory impulses from the inner ear to the brain. The nerve enters the brain between the PONS and the MEDULLA OBLONGATA (parts of the BRAINSTEM).

The vestibulocochlear nerve really has two parts, the VESTIBULAR NERVE and the ACOUSTIC NERVE (also called the *cochlear* or *auditory nerve*). Disorders of this nerve include TUMOR (ACOUSTIC NEUROMA) or INFECTION (such as MENINGITIS or ENCEPHALITIS).

See also CRANIAL NERVES.

vestibulo-ocular reflex This visual reflex located in the BRAINSTEM permits continued fixation of the eyes on an object while the head is in motion. With this sophisticated reflex, the neurons of the retina, the oculomotor system, and the vestibular system combine. It can best be understood by a simple test: A person who stares at an index finger while turning the head rapidly from side to side can easily retain focus on the finger; it is far more difficult to focus on the finger when the head is still and the finger is moved rapidly back and forth.

vincamine An extract of periwinkle, this drug is a vasodilator (widens blood vessels) and increases blood flow and oxygen use in the brain and has been used with some benefit for the treatment of memory defects.

In some studies, vincamine has shown some memory improvement in ALZHEIMER'S DISEASE patients and has normalized the brainwave patterns in elderly people with memory problems or with alcohol-induced ORGANIC BRAIN SYNDROME.

It has also been used to treat a variety of problems related to poor blood flow to the brain, including Meniere's syndrome, VERTIGO, sleep problems, mood changes, DEPRESSION, hearing problems, high blood pressure, etc.

However, there has been very little research on the drug and cognitive enhancement in normal subjects.

See also VINPOCETINE.

vinpocetine This derivative of VINCAMINE, a periwinkle extract, has fewer adverse effects and more benefits in memory enhancement, according to research. Marketed in Europe as Cavinton, the drug improves brain metabolism by improving blood flow and enhancing the use of GLUCOSE and oxygen.

It is often used to treat memory problems and other cerebral circulation disorders, such as STROKE, APHASIA, APRAXIA, HEADACHE, etc.

In one Hungarian study involving 882 patients with a range of neurological disorders, significant improvements were noted in 62 percent of the patients, including memorization of word lists.

In addition, at least one double-blind study of normal subjects indicated that the drug seemed to show significant short-term memory improvement within one hour after taking the drug.

vision The visual system is an extremely complex system in both organization and function. While vision occurs almost effortlessly for most people, it is far from a simple process.

The ability to see involves two main structures: the eye and the brain. When light reaches the eye, it passes into the retina, a thin web of nerve cells at the back of the eye. These cells respond to a wide range of information (such as color) in addition to filtering incoming information and sending it on to the optic nerves. At the back of the eyes, these optic nerves cross at the optic chiasma (or crossing). This means that the left optic tract carries information about objects in the right-hand field of vision, and vice versa.

Visual information is transmitted to a pair of nuclei on each side of the brain (the lateral geniculate nuclei) in an ordered pattern so that each half of the other visual field is precisely mapped onto the lateral geniculate on the opposite side of the brain. Scientists understand this map so well that in cases of STROKE or TUMOR, for example, they can pinpoint the exact location of BRAIN DAMAGE based on the type of visual deficit a person has. The lateral geniculate nuclei relay visual information to the primary VISUAL CORTEX, where it is again mapped in an extremely orderly fashion. From the visual cortex, the information is then transmitted to many other cortical areas involved in the higher aspects of visual processing, which is necessary in order to carry out activities associated with vision such as reading, writing, or recognizing objects. There are many regions of the cortex known

to be involved in visual processing, each serving a specific function and linked by many separate pathways. This division of labor could explain some of the more unusual aspects of some brain problems, such as why stroke patients can recognize some types of objects (like a book or chair) but not recognize their spouse's faces. Because these different objects have different features, damage to one area of the cortex may affect the perception of one type of feature but not others.

The brain must conduct extensive processing of visual information, allowing for pattern recognition and interpretation. These processes are based on work by the NEURONS, which are contained within an intricate pathway involving billions of individual NERVE CELLS. Scientists have discovered that many neurons are only involved with specific features of objects, such as the orientation of a bar, color, directional movement, or complex shapes. The retina also sends visual information to nuclei involved in controlling eye muscles responsible for turning the eyes to track objects and to coordinate movement of both eyes.

Proper functioning of the visual system depends on how well the neurons communicate in a coordinated fashion, using electrical and chemical signals generated by NEUROTRANSMITTERS, messengers, and other molecules.

Development The basic mechanism for vision is built into the brain at birth. Experiments with newborns reveal that they are already trying to find and fixate on objects within their surroundings. While babies can't see as well as adults, the basic reflexes important to vision are in place at birth, although the retinas are not well developed and the nerves from the eyes through the brain have not yet been covered with MYELIN. By two weeks of age, some babies' eye-brain development has progressed to the point where they can recognize patterns. Scientists reach this conclusion because babies who have reached this point spend more time looking at a pattern resembling a face than at patterns with random elements.

At birth, babies' eyes don't move as a unit and they find it difficult to look at an object. As the brain begins to improve its ability to control eye muscles, the ability to gaze at an object improves. By six weeks of age, infants can move their eyes to follow a ball through a 90-degree arc, and both eyes can focus on an object. Depth of field likewise develops during an infant's first months of life; experts estimate a six-month-old baby has visual acuity at about 20/120 (that is, objects can be clearly seen at 20 feet that a person with normal vision could see at 120 feet). By one year of age, an infant's vision (if developing normally) is 20/20.

Infant animal experiments have revealed that there appears to be a sensitive time for visual development. A two-month-old kitten deprived of visual stimuli for just four days may be permanently blind because the brain cells that register signals from the eyes stop working. Young infants, too, reach a critical stage when use of their eyes is essential for the development of the ability to see.

Because of the complicated interwoven pattern of physiological response, anatomic pathways, and neurochemical interactions, the function of the visual pathway is extremely difficult to understand. Despite many modern advances, neuroscientists still don't understand the fundamental nature of visual perception.

visual fields   The total area a person can see while looking straight ahead. Normally, the visual fields extend to about 90 degrees on either side of the middle of the face, but the field is narrower above and below (especially with deep-set eyes). Because the visual fields overlap in the middle ("binocular vision"), a defect in the field of one eye may not be apparent if both eyes are open.

While the total visual field is wide, visual acuity (sharpness) is not the same in all parts of the field. Objects on the periphery of the point at which a person focuses are far less sharp.

Similarly, partial loss of visual field is less noticeable than loss of central vision; even those who have had extensive damage to their visual field (such as from glaucoma or STROKE) may not be aware of it if their central visual acuity remains sharp.

visual occipital cortex   The area at the back of each cerebral HEMISPHERE, this is the part of the brain where we "see"—that is, where we register electrochemical impulses that arrive from the eyes. In the primary visual cortex, different columns of BRAIN CELLS register signals from different parts of the retina. From here, the signals are passed on to nearby visual areas for more refinement. In each visual area in the visual cortex, special cells react only to signals produced by special visual stimuli, such as movements in certain directions. Working together, these visual areas of the brain help us understand size, shape, and position of objects that we see.

See also VISION.

visual perception   See VISION.

vitamins and the brain   All communication in the brain depends on the function of NEUROTRANSMITTERS—chemicals that relay signals through the brain. To manufacture these important neurotransmitters, the brain needs adequate supplies of at least three B vitamins: FOLIC ACID, B_6 and B_{12}.

While the link between vitamins and cognition and memory is controversial, some studies have shown that better nutrition can lead to improved learning, IQ, and behavior, and several studies suggest that getting too little of these vitamins—especially folic acid and B_{12}—may interfere with mental or emotional well-being. Studies suggest that some people who are depressed or who show evidence of senile DEMENTIA may in fact have-deficiencies of folic acid or B_{12}; correcting these deficiencies improved the DEPRESSION or the memory problems. More important, studies suggest that even a slight lack of these B vitamins may slow down the thinking in otherwise healthy people. In one study, 250 apparently healthy older people revealed that those with the lowest blood levels of B_{12} and folic acid also scored lowest on memory and reasoning tests.

In a 1988 study, California researchers and a British research team found that vitamin and mineral supplementation boosted nonverbal IQ an average of six points among schoolchildren; in 1991 the team replicated their findings with an expanded study of 615 schoolchildren from six different schools and varied socioeconomic profiles. The children were randomly assigned to one of four different groups that received different vitamin-mineral supplements or placebo on a triple-blind basis (neither students, testers, nor scientists knew which child belonged to which group).

The group receiving the vitamins at 100 percent RDA scored a 3.7 point increase in the nonverbal IQ scores in three months; the 50 percent and 200 percent RDA groups experienced smaller but significant increases of 1.2 and 1.5 points, respectively. The results indicate that after a point, more is not necessarily better when it comes to vitamin supplementation. Not every child's IQ rose, but one-third experienced a dramatic 10-point jump, suggesting that some apparently normal children may in fact be subclinically nutritionally deficient.

The increase appeared in nonverbal scores, according to one of the researchers, because inadequate nutrition would be expected to show its earliest effects on the more biological intelligence measured by nonverbal tests. An increase in verbal intelligence might be expected only after some time, while the better-nourished brain had been stimulated by the environment.

See also VITAMINS, B-COMPLEX.

vitamins, B-complex The most important vitamins for top nervous system function. Vitamins B_1 (thiamine), B_6, and niacin must be obtained from the diet (especially organ meats, beans, and fresh vegetables) because they're not made by the body.

A lack of vitamin B_{12} may affect the healthy development of the NERVOUS SYSTEM (especially NERVE CELLS) because it synthesizes protein and fat. Without B_{12}, the MYELIN sheath (outer shell of the nerve cell) can't develop properly. Vegetarians are at high risk for B_{12} deficiency unless they consume alternate sources (including lentils, beans, sunflower seeds, peanuts, brown rice, asparagus, leafy greens, and broccoli).

A lack of vitamin B_1 causes peripheral nerve dysfunction and numbness in the hands and feet. Severe lack of this vitamin is often linked to alcoholism (because of poor diet) and can lead to the neurological disorder KORSAKOFF'S SYNDROME.

Excesses of these vitamins may also cause problems with the nervous system. Too much vitamin B_6 (doses exceeding 2 grams per day) can cause a severe neuropathy and impair senses of pain, touch, and temperature.

Voice of the Retarded This national organization of families and friends of mentally disabled people and mental health-care professionals advocates for the general welfare of mentally disabled individuals. The group works to improve services, monitors legislation, provides information, and provides resources to individuals, guardians, and families. The group also promotes freedom of choice and residential alternatives for mentally disabled persons and conducts research into the cause, prevention, and treatment of mental retardation. Founded in 1983, the group publishes a quarterly newsletter. For address, see Appendix A.

See also ASSOCIATION FOR CHILDREN WITH DOWN SYNDROME; ASSOCIATION FOR CHILDREN WITH RE-

TARDED MENTAL DEVELOPMENT; ASSOCIATION FOR RETARDED CITIZENS; CENTER FOR FAMILY SUPPORT; FEDERATION FOR CHILDREN WITH SPECIAL NEEDS; JARC; MENTAL RETARDATION ASSOCIATION OF AMERICA; NATIONAL ASSOCIATION OF DEVELOPMENTAL DISABIL-ITIES COUNCILS; NATIONAL DOWN SYNDROME CONGRESS; NATIONAL DOWN SYNDROME SOCIETY; PARENTS OF CHILDREN WITH DOWN SYNDROME; YOUNG ADULT INSTITUTE AND WORKSHOP.

W

WAIS-R See WECHSLER ADULT INTELLIGENCE SCALE REVISED.

Wechsler Adult Intelligence Scale Revised (WAIS-R) The best known and most common test used to assess general intellectual ability in people over age 16, providing a verbal, nonverbal, and overall intelligence quotient (IQ). It is also used to assess the cognitive ability of brain-damaged patients.

The WAIS consists of 11 subtests, including two verbal and performance scale subtests that assess several distinct cognitive functions. The verbal scale contains tests of common knowledge, vocabulary, comprehension of common situations, arithmetic, short-term memory, and abstract-thinking ability. The performance scale contains more timed tests, and high scores here depend less on previously established knowledge and problem-solving strategies.

Wechsler Intelligence Scale for Children Revised (WISC-R) A test designed for testing children between the ages of 6 and 16. It also yields verbal, nonverbal (performance), and full-scale IQ measurements. A discrepancy between verbal IQ and performance IQ often provides a clue to perception handicaps.

See also WECHSLER ADULT INTELLIGENCE SCALE REVISED (WAIS-R).

weight of the brain See BRAIN WEIGHT.

Wernicke, Carl (1848–1905) This nineteenth-century German neurologist who related nerve diseases to specific areas of the brain also investigated the localization of memory. He is best known for his descriptions of the APHASIAS (disorders interfering with the ability to communicate in speech or writing).

Wernicke studied at the University of Breslau before entering practice in Berlin, joining the faculty at Breslau where he remained until the year before his death.

In his book *Der aphasische Symptomenkomples* published in 1874, he tried to relate the various aphasias to impaired psychic processes in different parts of the brain and included the first accurate description of a sensory aphasia in the TEMPORAL LOBE. He showed that auditory word images appear to be located in a memory bank separate from that containing the images of the articulated words. Wernicke also noted a second language center farther back in the brain known today as WERNICKE'S AREA, which contains the records of individual words.

Wernicke went on to elaborate on different clinical syndromes in terms of damage to either the Wernicke area o r the area of the brain discovered by Paul Broca (see BROCA, PIERRE-PAUL).

He published *Textbook of Brain Disorders* (*Lehrbuch der Gehirnkrankheiten*) in 1891, trying to illustrate cerebral localization for all brain disease. Among the disorders he described in the book was WERNICKE'S ENCEPHALOPATHY, which is caused by a thiamine deficiency.

See also WERNICKE'S APHASIA; WERNICKE-KORSAKOFF SYNDROME.

Wernicke-Korsakoff syndrome This acute neurological condition is an uncommon brain disorder almost always due to the malnutrition that occurs in chronic alcohol dependence, although it can also occur in other conditions such as cancer with malnutrition. The disease consists of two stages: WERNICKE'S ENCEPHALOPATHY followed by Korsakoff's psychosis, each characterized by separate symptoms.

In the first stage (Wernicke's encephalopathy), the patient usually develops symptoms suddenly, including abnormal eye movements, problems in coordinating body movements, slowness, and confusion. There are also signs of NEUROPATHY, such as loss of sensation, pins and needles, or impaired reflexes. The level of consciousness progressively falls, and without treatment, this syndrome may lead to COMA and death.

The second stage (Korsakoff's psychosis, or KORSAKOFF'S SYNDROME) may follow if treatment is not instituted soon enough. In this stage, sufferers experience severe AMNESIA, apathy, and disorientation. Recent memories are affected more than distant memory; often, patients cannot remember what they did even a few moments ago, and they may make up stories to cover for their loss of memory.

See also WERNICKE, CARL; WERNICKE'S APHASIA.

Causes The disease is caused by a deficiency of thiamine (Vitamin B$_1$), which affects the brain and NERVOUS SYSTEM. This deficiency is probably caused by poor eating habits or an inherited effect in thiamine metabolism.

Treatment Wernicke's encephalopathy is a medical emergency requiring large doses of intravenous thiamine if the diagnosis is even suspected. Often, this treatment can reverse the symptoms within a few hours. In the absence of treatment, however, the disease will progress to Korsakoff's psychosis and at that stage is usually irreversible. The patient will experience permanent impairment of memory and is in need of constant supervision.

Wernicke's aphasia A disturbance of language characterized by poor comprehension but fluent production, albeit with many word and sound substitutions. It is caused by damage to WERNICKE'S AREA in the brain, a particular area in the dominant cerebral hemisphere.

Despite fluent speech, "internal speech" is impaired because of impaired comprehension, and speech content includes many errors in word selection and grammar. Writing is also impaired, and spoken or written commands are not understood. Wernicke's aphasia is associated with difficulty in accessing the meaning of words such as nouns.

See also WERNICKE, CARL; WERNICKE-KORSAKOFF SYNDROME.

Wernicke's area Language center responsible for the cognitive comprehension of speech.

See also WERNICKE, CARL; WERNICKE-KORSAKOFF'S SYNDROME; WERNICKE'S APHASIA.

Wernicke's encephalopathy See WERNICKE-KORSAKOFF SYNDROME.

whiplash-shaken-infant syndrome See SHAKEN-BABY SYNDROME.

white matter Name for white nerve fibers (as opposed to cell bodies, which appear gray). The white appearance comes from myelin, a fatty substance that surrounds axons, acting as an insulator to enhance electrical conduction of action potentials.

Willis, Thomas (1621–1675) The Oxford physician who studied cranial nerves, tracing blood flow to the brain. He believed that thought occurred in the CEREBRUM. He coauthored a book in 1664 in which he described the arterial system at the base of the brain (the Circle of Willis).

Wisconsin Card-Sorting Test A common way to assess FRONTAL-LOBE damage. The subject is given a deck of cards marked by a pattern with various symbol shapes, numbers, and colors. A card might have three blue stars or one red star or two green triangles.

The subject begins to sort cards and is given hints as to how they should be sorted by the tester's comments (such as placing all the cards with green triangles in one pile). A normal person quickly learns the proper sorting method; once the subject has learned to sort by the rule, the rule is changed and the subject must figure out what the new sorting rule is. Patients with frontal-lobe damage or KORSAKOFF'S SYNDROME tend to make a perseveration error at this point, continuing to sort the cards by the first rule. They have not lost the ability to understand that the rules have changed, but their understanding does not improve their behavior. They continue to sort by color, although each error brings the news that the action was wrong. Their mistake is not one of imagination or reasoning or any other type of intelligence but is an inflexibility in voluntary motor behavior. It is as if once they have decided to touch their fingers, it becomes impossible to touch their nose.

World Federation of Neurosurgical Societies   A group of national neurosurgical societies representing 12,000 NEUROSURGEONS that works for the advancement of neurological surgery. The federation sponsors a quadrennial congress and publishes *Federation News* and the quadrennial *Proceedings of International Congress.* For address, see Appendix B.

X

xanthinol nicotinate This form of niacin passes into cells much more easily than niacin itself; therein, it increases the rate of GLUCOSE metabolism and improves blood flow to the brain.

In recent studies, it was found to improve performance of healthy elderly subjects in a variety of short- and long-term memory tasks. Like niacin, however, excess doses can cause flushing and a variety of other mild symptoms.

X rays Invisible electromagnetic waves of very short wave length, some of which are absorbed and others of which pass through tissues; the shadow that is cast is projected onto a fluorescent screen or a film. X-rays are used to produce images of the brain and skill, in addition to other bones, organs, and internal tissues.

Discovered in 1895 by Wilhelm Conrad Roentgen, X rays can be used to penetrate all substances, but they have been used most often in medicine to diagnose and treat disease. While X-ray images of bone are quite distinct, pictures of soft tissues are less clear and are therefore of minimal benefit today in visualizing the brain. Still, they are used to evaluate skull fractures, cancer, and general alterations in the appearance of the skull (such as changes seen in PAGET'S DISEASE).

Since the 1920s, radiologists have used substances opaque to radiation as part of the X-ray technique. In ANGIOGRAPHY, contrast dye is injected into an artery or vein to provide images of blood vessels. Since the 1970s, many X-ray techniques have been surpassed by newer procedures that are both easier and safer to perform.

Instead, computer-aided X rays can show sections of the brain or scan its chemical activity. For example, in COMPUTERIZED AXIAL TOMOGRAPHY (CAT SCAN), an X-ray tube rotates around a patient's head, bombarding it with narrow X-ray beams. With computer help, the technique produces a brain cross-section projected on a TV screen that can be used to pinpoint blood clots, TUMORS, birth defects, or other damage.

Y

yoga This system of Hindu philosophy and physical discipline appears to have some affect on the /brain. The main form of yoga practiced in the West is hatha-yoga, in which the follower adopts a series of poses (or *asanas*) together with special breathing techniques. This maintains flexibility of the body, teaches physical and mental control, and is useful in relaxation.

Experiments in the 1960s showed that experts in yoga in fact were indeed capable of slowing normal body processes, such as the rate of oxygen consumption, heart rate, and breathing. Indian television cameras captured 46-year-old Ramanand Yogi sitting in a sealed box, in which he used little more than half the calculated minimum amount of oxygen required to maintain life. For one hour, he survived on a bare quarter of what his body should have needed.

In other tests, yogis produced sweat on the forehead only, while others slowed the heart rate while sitting still.

Young Adult Institute and Workshop A pioneer agency established to provide comprehensive programs that enable people with developmental disabilities, MENTAL RETARDATION, LEARNING DISABILITIES, emotional disturbances, or BRAIN DAMAGE to progress from dependency to a more self-sufficient role. The institute provides respite services to parents of mentally retarded and developmentally disabled people, conducts research, testifies before government hearings, sponsors conferences, and provides information. The institute produces weekly YAI *Children with Special Needs* and *On Our Own* TV programs

which provide counseling, training, referral, and other family support services.

The institute offers an alternative to institutionalization and focuses on developing supportive services to maintain individuals within the community. Programs also serve the multiply handicapped, including those who are deaf, blind, or have other physical disabilities. The group provides early intervention, residential, employment, socialization, recreational, parent-training, and clinical programs for those with various levels of retardation, as well as a variety of family support services.

In addition, the institute maintains day treatment programs in New York, in Manhattan and Brooklyn and Nassau and Westchester counties, evening adjustment centers in Manhattan and the Bronx, and community residential facilities throughout Brooklyn, the Bronx, Queens, Manhattan, and Nassau, Suffolk, and Westchester counties. Other programs include adjustment counseling, recreational activities, children's services, employment training and placement, remedial reading, money handling, budgeting, and sex education. For address, see Appendix A.

See also CENTER FOR FAMILY SUPPORT; FEDERATION FOR CHILDREN WITH SPECIAL NEEDS; JARC; MENTAL RETARDATION ASSOCIATION OF AMERICA; NATIONAL ASSOCIATION OF DEVELOPMENTAL DISABILITIES COUNCILS; NATIONAL DOWN SYNDROME CONGRESS; NATIONAL DOWN SYNDROME SOCIETY; PILOT PARENTS; VOICE OF THE RETARDED; ASSOCIATION FOR RETARDED CITIZENS; ASSOCIATION FOR CHILDREN WITH DOWN SYNDROME; ASSOCIATION FOR CHILDREN WITH RETARDED MENTAL DEVELOPMENT.

GLOSSARY

absolute refractory period The period after an impulse has been triggered during which a nerve fiber cannot carry a second impulse.

acetylcholine A neurotransmitter released at the synapses. After relaying a nerve impulse, acetylcholine is broken down by the enzyme cholinesterase. Physostigmine prolongs the activity of acetylcholine by blocking cholinesterase.

amino acid An organic compound that make up the primary components of proteins.

axon A long wirelike nerve fiber extending from the cell body of a neuron that sends nerve impulses (messages) to other neurons. In large nerves, the axon is covered with a sheath (neurilemma) made of myelin.

cell body The central part of a neuron that examines information received from other neurons.

cholinesterase Members of a class of enzymes that break down choline esters, such as acetylcholine.

cones Specialized light-sensitive cells in the retina that have a cone shape.

cytoplasm Cell material (including membranes, organelles, and fluid), not including the nucleus.

dendrite Branched ends of neurons that makes contact with other neurons at synapses and carries nerve impulses from them into the cell body.

differentiation Process of change during the development of a cell.

DNA The abbreviation for deoxyribonucleic acid, the genetic material of the cell located in the nucleus.

excitability The general capacity of cells to respond to irritation; this is highly enhanced in neurons and receptors.

extracellular spaces Fluid-filled areas between neighboring cells.

fibril A very tiny fiber or hairlike structure at the end of the axon.

ganglia Small groups of neurons in which nerve signals are processed.

glia A cell type that makes up the supportive tissue of the central nervous system. The brain is made up of glial cells and the much larger nerve cells.

habituate Gradual adaptation to an irritation (in nerve cells) that causes a decrease or halt to the generation of nerve impulses.

homeostasis The general capacity of a living organism to adjust to a chemical or physical stress so as to preserve a stable activity.

hyperpolarization An increase in the resting electrical potential across a nerve-cell membrane.

infarct A small area of dead brain tissue.

ions Charged particles generated from atoms or molecules by the loss or acquisition of electrons; this is important in neurons as a source of electrical potential.

lesions Tissue damage that may be caused by trauma or disease.

membrane Thin covering of a cell or tissue. Neurons are covered by a very thin membrane through which transmitter chemicals pass.

mitochondria Organelles found in all animal cells that is concerned with energy transformation.

motor end plate A flat disk at the end of a nerve. Motor end plates connect the nerve to the muscle.

myelin The fatty substance that surrounds axons and insulates the nerve.

nerve Bundle of axons through which signals pass to and from the brain.

nerve fiber Structures of a neuron, aside from the cell body; nerve fibers are such things as dendrites and axons.

nerve tracts Concentrations of parallel nerve axons running through the body.

neuroglial cells Special cells that are packed around and between the neurons that helps support the delicate nervous tissue.

neuromuscular junction The synapse where motor nerves contact a muscle.

neuron A nerve cell that passes signals to other neurons along the wirelike axon.

neurotransmitter A chemical the nervous system uses to carry messages from one neuron to another.

paresis Muscular weakness caused by disease of the nervous system that is usually considered to be lesser degree of weakness than full paralysis, although the two words may be used interchangeably.

peptide Short chain of amino acids.

permeability A measure of how porous a membrane is to molecules.

polarization The net difference in electrical charge generated across a membrane.

protein Long molecules consisting of chains of amino acids joined by peptide links.

receptor A sensor that is a special part of the dendrite that allows messages to be received and passed on to the nervous system. Typical receptors register touch (in the skin) and light (in the retina of the eye).

reflex An automatic response of the body that, at first, does not involve the brain, such as jerking away a hand from a flame.

refractory period The period of time necessary for the nerve-cell membrane to repolarize so that another impulse can pass.

resting membrane potential The electrical imbalance that exists across a normal, living cell membrane.

rods Light-sensitive cells in the retina in the shape of rods.

semipermeable membrane A type of membrane that only certain small molecules can penetrate.

skull The part of the skeleton which makes up the head, protecting the brain, eyes, and ears.

synapse The gap between neurons through which messages pass from one cell to another.

synaptic vesicle A capsule which contains sacs of neurotransmitters behind the presynaptic membrane.

threshold The level at which a depolarization is just enough to cause an action potential in an axon.

transmitter See *neurotransmitter*.

vesicle A small saclike structure that forms the brain during fetal development.

REFERENCES

"A window on the brain," *Discover*. 13(July 1992)16.

Adams, R.D., Victor, M., *Principles of Neurology*, (4th ed.). New York: McGraw-Hill, 1989.

Adler, Tina, "Infant C.P. protection," *Science News*. 147(Feb. 25, 1995)119.

———, "Slipping in new cells tricks Sly syndrome," *Science News*. 147(March 25, 1995)182.

———, "Single gene causes ataxia, cancer risk," *Science News*. 147(June 24, 1995)389.

Albright, A. Leland, Cervi, Alice and Singletary, Jane, "Intrathecal baclofen for spasticity in cerebral palsy," *JAMA*. 265(March 20, 1991)1418–22.

Aldrich, M.S., "Narcolepsy," *New England Journal of Medicine*. 323(1990)389.

Allison, Malorye, "Stopping the brain drain," *Harvard Health Letter*. 16(October 1991)6–8.

Alper, Joseph, "EEG + MRI: a sum greater than the parts," *Science*. 261(July 30, 1993)559.

ANA Committee on Ethical Affairs, "Persistent vegetative state: Report of the American Neurological Association Committee on Ethical Affairs," *Neurology*. 33(1993)386.

Annegers, J.F., "Seizures after head trauma," *Neurology*. 30(1980)683.

"Another round in the prion debate," *Science News*. 148(June 17, 1995)381.

Associated Press, "Alzheimer's has multiple causes, research shows," *Reading Eagle*. Aug. 1, 1995, p. A6.

August, Paul Nordstrom, *Brain Function*. New York: Chelsea House Publishers, 1988.

Aumick, Jane E., "Head trauma: guidelines for care," *RN*. 54(April 1991)26–32.

Baddeley, Alan, *The Psychology of Memory*. New York: Harper & Row, 1976.

Bagby, George, "Sensory sequelae: otologic and ophthalamologic interventions following minor neurologic injury," *Headlines*. 3:2(March/April 1992).

Baker, Sherry, "Palsy: trauma in the womb," *Health*. 23 (Feb. 1991)20.

Barinaga, Marcia, "Giving personal magnetism a whole new meaning," *Science*. 256(May 15, 1992)967.

———, "The brain reamps its own contours," *Science*. 258(Oct. 9, 1992)216–8.

———, "How scary things get that way," *Science*. 258(Nov. 6, 1992)887–8.

———, "Carbon monoxides: killer to brain messenger in one step," *Science*. 259(Jan. 15, 1993)309.

Becker, D.P., and Gudeman, S.K., *Textbook of Head Injury*. Philadelphia: Saunders, 1989.

Begley, Sharon, et al., "The human computer: how the brain works," *Newsweek*. (Feb. 7, 1983)40–7.

Begley, Sharon, "Graymatters," *Newsweek*. (CXXV/13(March 27, 1995)48–54.

Belliveau, J.W., Kennedy, D.N., et al., "Functional mapping of the human visual cortex by magnetic resonance imaging," *Science*. 254(Nov. 1, 1991)16–9.

Bennett, D.A., Gilley, D.W., Wilson, R.S., et al., "Chemical correlates of high signal lesions on magnetic resonance imaging in Alzheimer's disease," *Journal of Neurology*. 239(1992)186.

Benzel, E.C., et al., "Apnea testing for the determination of brain death," *Journal of Neurosurgery*. 76(1992)1029.

Black, P.M., "Brain tumors," *New England Journal of Medicine*. 324(1991)1471.

———, "Meningiomas," *Neurosurgery*. 32(1993)643.

Blakemore, Colin, *Mechanics of the Mind*. London: Cambridge University Press, 1977.

Blakeslee, Sandra, "How the brain might work: a new theory of consciousness," *The*

New York Times. 144(March 21, 1995)B7, C1.

_____ , "The mystery of music: how it works in the brain," *The New York Times.* 144(May 16, 1995)B5, C1.

Bloom, Floyd, Lazerson, Arlyne, and Hofstadter, Laura, *Brain, Mind and Behavior.* New York: W.H. Freeman and Co., 1985.

Bower, Bruce, "Brain study offers clues to hyperactivity," *Sciences News.* (Nov. 11, 1990)325.

_____ , "Clues emerge from vowels of the brain," *Science News.* 140(Sept. 21, 1991)180.

_____ , "Left brain may serve as language director," *Science News.* 141(March 7, 1992)149.

_____ , "Brain clues to energy-efficient learning," *Science News.* 141(April 4, 1992)215.

_____ , "Clues to the brain's knowledge systems," *Science News.* 142(9/5/92)148.

_____ , "Brain images show structure of depression," *Science News.* 142(Sept. 12, 1992)165.

_____ , "Baboons offer glimpses of left-brain brawn," *Science News.* 143(Jan. 23, 1993)54.

_____ , "The birth of schizophrenia: a debilitating mental disorder may take root in the fetal brain," *Science News,* 143(May 29, 1993)346-7.

_____ , "The social brain," *Science News.* 145(May 21, 1994)326-7.

_____ , "Images of intellect: brain scans may colorize intelligence," *Science News,* 146 (October 8, 1994)236-7.

_____ , "Brain faces up to fear, social signs," *Science News.* 146(Dec. 17, 1994)236-7.

_____ , "Brain scans tag sexes as world apart," *Science News.* 147(Feb. 18, 1995)101.

_____ , "Temperament, depression make volatile mix," *Science News.* 147(Feb. 25, 1995) 118.

_____ , "Brain activity calms down to expectations," *Science News.* 147(March 4, 1995) 38.

_____ , "Child sex abuse leaves mark on brain," *Science News.* 147(March 4, 1995) 340.

_____ , "Virus may trigger some mood disorders," *Science News.* 147(March 4, 1995)132.

_____ , "Schizophrenia drugs: A case for tapering," *Science News.* 147(March 25, 1995) 181.

_____ , "IQ's evolutionary breakdown: intelligence may have more facets than testers realize," *Science News.* 147(April 8, 1995) 220-2.

_____ , "Schizophrenia: fetal roots for GABA loss," *Science News.* 147(April 22, 1995)247.

_____ , "Map unfolds for brain's vision areas," *Science News.* 147(May 13, 1995)295.

_____ , "Brain changes linked to phantom-limb pain," *Science News.* 147(June 10, 1995)357.

_____ , "Understanding speech: I see what you mean," *Science News.* 147(June 17, 1995) 373.

_____ , "Brain data fuel alcoholism gene clash," *Science News.* 148(July 8, 1995)20.

Bracken, M.B., et al., "A randomized controlled trial of methylprednisolone or naloxone in the treatment of acute spinal cord injury," *New England Journal of Medicine.* 322(1990)1405.

"Brain gets thoughtful reappraisal," *Science News* 146(Oct. 29, 1994)284.

"Brain mapping offers clues," *USA Today* magazine. 119(April 1991)12.

Brandt, T., *Vertigo: Its Multisensory Syndromes.* London: Springer-Verlag, 1991.

Brash, Sarah, et al., *The Brain.* Alexandria, VA: Time-Life Books, 1990.

Broderick, Joseph, Brott, Thomas, et al., "The risk of subarachnoid and intracerebral hemorrhages in blacks as compared with whites," *The New England Journal of Medicine.* 326(March 12, 1992)733-6.

Brooks, A.C., "Low TSH: An early warning for stroke," *Science News.* 146(Nov. 11, 1994) 311.

Brown, Paul, and Chapman, Arthur, "EEG findings in Creutzfeldt-Jakob disease," *JAMA.* 269(June 23, 1993)3168.

Brownlee, Shannon, "Alzheimer's: is there hope?" *U.S. News & World Report.* 111(Aug. 12, 1991)40–7.

Brumback, Roger A., *Neurology and Clinical Neuroscience.* New York: Springer-Verlag, 1993.

Brust, J.C.M., *Neurological Aspects of Substance Abuse.* Boston: Butterworth-Heineman, 1993.

Buderi, Robert, "Can lab-grown cells thwart Parkinson's and Alzheimer's?" *Business Week* (March 25, 1991)89.

Burr, Chandler, "Homosexuality and biology," *The Atlantic.* 271(March 1993)47–61.

Byrne, T.N., "Spinal cord compression from epidural metastasis," *New England Journal of Medicine,* 327(1992)614.

Cady, R.K., et al., "Treatment of acute migraine with subcutaneous sumatriptan," *Journal of the American Medical Association,* 265:2831, 1991.

"Call of the left brain," *Science News.* 145(May 21, 1994)333.

Calvin, William H. and Ojemann, George A., *Conversations with Neil's Brain: The Neural Nature of Thought and Language.* N. Reading, Mass.: Addison-Wesley, 1995.

Camfield, C., et al., "Outcome of childhood epilepsy: A population-based study with a simply predictive scoring system for those treated with medication," *Journal of Pediatrics.* 122(1993)681.

Caplan, Louis R., "Diagnosis and treatment of ischemic stroke," *JAMA.* 266(Nov. 6, 1991)2413–8.

———, "Intracerebral haemorrhage," *The Lancet.* 339(March 14, 1992)656–8.

Carey, John, "Brain repair is possible," *Business Week.* (Nov. 18, 1991)62–3.

"Cellular damage: mobile telephones and cancer," *The Economist.* 326(Feb. 6, 1993) 88–89.

Chao, J., and Kikano, G.E., "Lead poisoning in children," *American Family Physician.* 47(1993):113.

Charness, M.E., Simon, R.P., and Greenberg, D.A., "Ethanol and the nervous system," *New England Journal of Medicine.* 321(1989)442.

Chase, Marilyn, "Inner music," *The Wall Street Journal.* (Oct. 13, 1993)A1(w).

Chiappa, K.H., "Pattern shift visual, brainstem auditory, and short-latency somatosensory-evoked potentials in multiple sclerosis," *Neurology.* 30(1980)110.

Clarke, Edwin, and Dewhurst, Kenneth, *An Illustrated History of Brain Function,* Los Angeles: University of California Press, 1972.

Clark, V.A., et al., "Factors associated with a malignant or benign course of multiple sclerosis," *Journal of the American Medical Association.* 248(1982)856.

Clouston, P.D., et al., "The spectrum of neurologic disease in patients with systemic cancer," *Annals of Neurology,* 31(1992)268.

Coffey, R.J., et al., "Intrathecal baclofen for intractable spasticity of spinal origin: results of a long-term multicenter study," *Journal of Neurosurgery.* 78:226, 1993.

Corina, David, Vaid, Jyotsna, and Bellugi, Ursula, "The linguistic basis of left hemisphere specialization," *Science.* 255(March 6, 1992)1258–60.

Corrick, James A., *The Human Brain: Mind and Matter.* New York: Arco Publishing, 1983.

Cotton, Paul, "Scientists chart course for brain map," *JAMA.* 269(March 17, 1993)1357.

Cowen, Ron, "In the valleys of thought," *Science News,* 146(Nov. 12, 1994)312.

Coyle, Joseph, and Puttfarcken, Pamela, "Oxidative stress, glutamate and neurodegenerative disorders," *Science.* 262(Oct. 29, 1993)689–95.

Craik, Fergus I.M., "Memory changes in

normal aging," *Current Directions in Psychological Science*, 3:5(October 1994)155-8.

Crease, Robert, "Images of conflict: magnetoencephalography vs. electroencephalograhy," *Science.* 253(July 26, 1991)374-5.

Cummings, J.L., and Benson, D.F., *"Dementia: A Clinical Approach"* (2nd ed.). Boston: Butterworth, 1992.

Curling, O.D., et al., "An analysis of the natural history of cavernous angiomas," *Journal of Neurosurgery*, 75(1991)702.

Dajar, Tony, "Monkeying with the brain," *Discover.* 13(Jan. 1992)70-1.

Dalessio, D.J., and Silberstein, S.D., *Wolff's Headache and Other Head Pain* (6th ed.). New York: Oxford University Press, 1993.

Daneshdoost, Leela, Gennarelli, Thomas, et al., "Recognition of gonadotroph adenomas in women," *The New England Journal of Medicine.* 324(Feb. 28, 1991) 589-94.

Davis, K.L., et al., "A double-blind placebo-controlled multicenter study of tacrine for Alzheimer's disease," *New England Journal of Medicine.* 327(1992)1253.

"Deciding to be born," *Discover.* 13(May 1992)10-1.

"DES sons show changes in brain function," *Science News.* 142(Nov. 7, 1992)318.

Diamond, Nina, "A brain is a terrible thing to waste," *Omni.* 15(August 1993)14.

"Don't take head bangs lightly," *Men's Health.* 6(Oct. 1991)11.

Drachman, D.A., et al., "Memory decline in the aged: Treatment with lecithin and physostigmine," *Neurology.* 32(1982)944.

Durand, M.L., et al., "Acute bacterial meningitis in adults," *New England Journal of Medicine.* 328(1993)21.

Dyck, P.J. et al., "Plasma exchange in polyneuropathy associated with monoclonal gammopathy of undetermined significance," *New England Journal of Medicine.* 325(21)(1991)1482.

Editorial, "Fetal-tissue transplants in Parkinson's disease," *New England Journal of Medicine.* 327(22)(1992)1589.

Ellis, Simon J., "Functional magnetic resonance: neurological enlightenment?" *Lancet.* 342(Oct. 9, 1993)882.

Elmer-Dewitt, Philip, "Dialing 'P' for panic," *Time.* 141(Feb. 8, 1993)56.

Evans, R.W., Baskin, D.S., Yatsu, F.M., *Prognosis of Neurological Disorders.* New York: Oxford University Press, 1992.

Ezzell, Carol, "Memories might be made of this," *Science News.* 139(May 25, 1991) 328-330.

_____ , "Receptor involved in brain injury found," *Science News.* 140(Nov. 23, 1991) 333.

_____ , "Watching the remembering brain at work," *Science News.* (Nov. 23, 1991).

_____ , "Monitoring memories moving in the brain,"*Science News.* 141(May 2, 1992)294.

_____ , "Gene therapy: brain cancer yes, AIDS no," *Science News.* 141(June 6, 1992) 372.

_____ , "A low-energy cause for Huntington's," *Science News.* 142(Oct. 31, 1992) 292.

Fackelmann, Kathy, "Natural sedatives linked to brain disorder," *Science News.* 138(July 21, 1990)38.

_____ , "Smoking silences critical pain messages," *Science News.* (Nov. 24, 1990)326.

_____ , "Fetus tells mother: it's time for labor," *Science News.* 140(Sept. 21, 1991) 182.

_____ , "Motherhood and cancer," *Science News.* 142(Oct. 31, 1992)298-300.

_____ , "Anti-inflammatories: New hope for Alzheimer's?" *Science News.* 145(Feb. 19, 1994)116.

_____ , "Artery surgery slashes risk of stroke," *Science News.* 146(October 8, 1994) 228.

_____ , "Brain changes may foretell Alzheimer's," *Science News.* 146(Dec. 17, 1994) 236-7.

Feniuk, W., et al., "Rationale for the use of 5HT-like agonists in the treatment of migraine," *Neurology*. 238:s57, 1991.

Foreman, Judy, "Estrogen may also help keep the brain working well," *Boston Globe*. (Jan. 10, 1994)42–3.

Franck, Irene, and Brownstone, David, *The Parent's Desk Reference*. New York: Prentice Hall, 1991.

Freundlich, Naomi, "Much Ado about NO," *Harvard Health Letter*. 18(Oct. 1993)6–8.

Friedman, Mel, and Weiss, Ellen, "What you should know about cerebral palsy," *Parents*. 66(May 1991)68–72.

Gibbons, Ann, "Databasing the brain," *Science*. 258(Dec. 18, 1992)1872–3.

Gilling, Dick, and Brightwell, Robin, *The Human Brain*. New York: Facts On File, 1982.

Ghikar, J., et al., "Idazoxan treatment in progressive supranuclear palsy," *Neurology*. 4(1991):986.

van Gijn, J., "Subarachnoid haemorrhage," *The Lancet*. 339(March 14, 1992)653–5.

Gladue, Brian, "The biopsychology of sexual orientation," *Current Directions in Psychological Science*, 3:5(October 1994)154–4.

Gleick, James, "Brain at work revealed through new imagery," *The New York Times* (Aug. 18, 1987)C12–14.

Goldberg, Jeff, "The empty mirror: a bizarre brain injury sheds light on the conscious mind," *Omni*. 14(May 1992)16.

Goldberg, Joan, "Peptide power," *American Health*. (June 1990)35–41.

Golden, David, "Building a better brain," *Life*. (July 1994)63–70.

Goleman, Dan, "The brain manages happiness and sadness in different centers," *The New York Times*. 144(March 28, 1995)B9, C1.

Grady, Denise, "The brains of gay men," *Discover*. 13(Jan. 1992)29.

Greenberg, David A., Aminoff, Michael J., and Simon, Roger P., *Clinical Neurology* (second edition). Norwalk, CT: Appleton & Lange, 1993.

Griffiths, Joan, "The mirthful brain," *Omni*. 14(August 1992)18.

Haggerty, Tim, "The humor in tumor," *Psychology Today*. 28/1(Jan./Feb. 1995)11.

Hall, S., and Bornstein, R.A., "The relationship between intelligence and memory following minor or mild closed-head injury: Greater impairment in memory than intelligence," *Journal of Neurosurgery*. 75(1991) 378.

Hambleton, P., "*Clostridium botulinum* toxins: A general review of involvement in disease, structure, mode of action and preparation for clinical use," *Journal of Neurology*. 239(1)(1992)16.

Heeger, David J., "The representation of visual stimuli in primary visual cortex," *Current Directions in Psychological Science*, 3:5(October 1994)159–63.

Heins, Henry C., "Simple tests—important answers about your newborn," *American Baby*. 54(Nov. 1992)16–7.

Hilts, Philip, "Photos show mind recalling a word," *The New York Times*. (Nov. 11, 1991)A10–11.

Hinton, Geoffrey, Plaut, David, and Shallice, Tim, "Simulating brain damage," *Scientific American*. 269(October 1993)76–82.

Hoehn, M.M., and Yahr, M.D., "Parkinsonism: Onset, progression and mortality," *Neurology*. 17(1967)427.

Hollander, H., McGuire, D., and Burack, J.H., "Diagnostic lumbar puncture in HIV-infected patients: Analysis of 138 cases," *American Journal of Medicine*, 96(1994)223.

Holloway, Marguerite, "Lethal cascade: a model for the neurologic damage found in AIDS," *Scientific American*. 268(March 1993)28–30.

Holzman, David, "Inflamed debate over neurotoxin," *Science*. 259(Jan. 1, 1993)25–6.

Hooper, Judith, "The brain's river of rewards," *American Health*. (Dec. 1987)36–41.

Hoppe, Kathryn, "GABA receptor linked to absence seizures," *Science News*. 142(July 25, 1992)54.

Hoppman, R.A., Peden, J.G., and Ober, S.K., "Central nervous system side effects of nonsteroidal anti-inflammatory drugs," *Archives of Internal Medicine*. 151(1991)1309.

"Hormone shows link to some obsessions," *Science News* 146(Oct. 29, 1994)277.

Howard, Rosanne, "Mild head injury: challenging emergency room decisions," *Headlines*. 3:2(March/April 1992)6–7.

Igarashi, Masanori, "Multiple brain abscesses," *The New England Journal of Medicine*. 329(Oct. 7, 1993)1083.

Ilano, A.L., and Raffin, T.A., "Management of carbon monoxide poisoning," *Chest*. 97(1990)165.

"Imaging clues to schizophrenia," *Science News*. 146(Oct. 29, 1994)284.

Jankovic, J., and Tolosa, E. (eds.), *Parkinson's Disease and Movement Disorders* (2nd ed.). Baltimore: Williams & Wilkins, 1993.

Kaiser, J., "Absent mouse gene leads to no-brainer," *Science News*. 147(April 1, 1995).

Katzman, R., and Jackson, J.E., "Alzheimer's disease: Basic and clinical advances," *Journal of American Geriatric Society*, 39(1991)516.

Kaufman, H.H., et al., "Delayed and recurrent intracranial hematomas related to disseminated intravascular clotting and fibrinolysis in head injury," *Neurosurgery*, 7(1980)445.

Kerr, Richard A., "Magnetism triggers a brain response," *Science*. 260(June 11, 1993)1590.

Kesselring, J., et al., "Acute disseminated encephalomyelitis: MRI findings and the distinction from multiple sclerosis," *Brain*, 113(1990)291.

Kim, S., Ashe, J., et al., "Functional magnetic resonance imaging of motor cortex: hemispheric asymmetry and handedness," *Science*. 261(July 30, 1993)615–7.

Kinoshita, June, "Severed from emotion," *Discover*. 13(July 1992)20.

_____ , "Mapping the mind," *The New York Times Magazine*. (Oct. 18, 1992)44.

Kirn, Tim, " 'Brain maps' may aid surgeons in not-too-distant future," *American Medical News*. 35(Sept. 14, 1992)17.

Klibanski, A., and Zervas, N.T., "Diagnosis and treatment of hormone-secreting pituitary tumors," *New England Journal of Medicine*. 324(1991)822.

Knudsen, Eric, and Brainard, Michael, "Visual instruction of the neural map of auditory space in the developing optic tectum," *Science*. 253(July 5, 1991)85–7.

Kolata, Gina, "Man's world, woman's world? Brain studies point to differences," *The New York Times*. 144(Feb. 28, 1995)B5, C1.

Kong, Dolores, "New MRI photographs brain in action," *The Boston Globe*. (Nov. 4, 1991)28–9.

Koopmans, R.A., et al., "Benign versus chronic progressive multiple sclerosis: Magnetic resonance imaging features," *Annals of Neurology*. 25(1989)74.

Kornblith, P.L., and Walker, M.C., "Chemotherapy for malignant gliomas," *Journal of Neurosurgery*, 68(1988)1.

Kosslyn, Stephen, and Koenig, Olivier, *Wet Mind: The New Cognitive Neuroscience*. New York: Macmillan, 1992.

Kroenki, K., et al., "Causes of persistent dizziness: a prospective study of 100 patients in ambulatory care," *Annals of Internal Medicine*. 117:898, 1992.

Lakie, M., Arblaster, L., et al., "Effect of stereotactic thalamac lesion on essential tremor," *The Lancet*. 340(July 25, 1992)206–7.

Lance, J.W., *The Mechanism and Management of Headache* (5th ed.). London: Butterworth, 1993.

Laurence, Leslie, "Don't have a stroke!" *Ladies' Home Journal* (Nov. 1993)112–8.

"Less-invasive brain imaging in humans," *Science News.* 145(Jan. 15, 1994).

Levine, David, "A Compass in the Brain?" *American Health*, (Jan./Feb. 1994)30.

Lipkin, Richard, "Protecting nerve cells after injury," *Science News.* (Sept. 3,1994)157.

Lipman, Marvin, "Is it senility?" *Consumer Reports on health.* (Dec. 1993)139.

Llinas, Rodolfo, R., *The Biology of the Brain: From Neurons to Networks.* New York: W.H. Freeman and Co., 1988.

Luckasson, R. (ed.), *Mental Retardation: Classification and Systems of Support* (9th ed.). Washington, DC: American Association on Mental Retardation, 1992.

"Magnetic resonance imaging in epilepsy," (editorial), *The Lancet.* 340(Aug. 8, 1992)343-5.

Maguire, Jack, *Care and Feeding of the Brain: A Guide to Your Gray Matter.* New York: Doubleday, 1990.

Marchal, Gilles, Serrati, Carlo, et al., "PET imaging of cerebral persusion and oxygen consumption in acute ischemic stroke," *The Lancet.* 341(April 10, 1993)925-7.

Martin, Joseph, "Molecular genetics of neurological diseases," *Science.* 262(Oct. 29, 1993)674-6.

Masand, P., Murray, G.B., and Pickett, P., "Psychostimulants in post-stroke depression," *Journal of Neuropsychiatry.* 3(1991)23.

McGuire, D., and So, Y.T., "Neurologic Dysfunction in HIV: Intracranial Disorders, in P.T. Cohen, M. Sande, and P. Volberding (eds.) *AIDS Knowledge Base.* Boston: Little, Brown, 1994.

McGuire, P.K., Shah, G., and Murray, R., "Increased blood flow in Broca's area during auditory hallucinations in schizophrenia," *The Lancet.* 342(Sept. 18, 1993)703-7.

Miller, D.H., Morrissey, S.B., and McDonald, W.I., "The prognostic significance of brain MRI at presentation with a single episode of suspected demyelination: A five-year follow-up study," *Neurology.* 42(1992)427.

Mitiguy, Judith, "New applications of diagnostic techniques," *Headlines.* (March/April 1992)2-5, 8-10.

Mishkin, Mort, and Appenzeller, Tim, "The anatomy of memory," *Scientific American.* 256:6(June 1987)80-89.

Mohr, J.P. (ed.), *Manual of Clinical Problems in Neurology* (2nd edition). Boston: Little, Brown and Co., 1989.

Moir, Anne, and Jessel, David, *Brain Sex.* New York: Dell, 1989.

Molitch, Mark E., "Gonadotrop-cell pituitary adenomas," *The New England Journal of Medicine,*" 324(Feb. 28, 1991)626-7.

Mortensen, M.E., and Walson, P.D., "Chelation therapy for childhood lead poisoning: The changing scene in the 1990s," *Clinical Pediatrics.* 32(1993)284.

Muller, T., Moller, T., Berger, T., Schnitzer, J., and Kettenmann, H., "Calcium entry through kainate receptors and resulting potassium-channel blockade in Bergmann glial cells," *Science.* 256(June 12, 1992) 1563-5.

Munoz, Douglas, Pelisson, Denis, and Guitton, Daniel, "Movement of neural activity on the superior colliculus motor map during gaze shifts," *Science.* 251(March 15, 1991)1358-60.

Nadis, Steve, "The energy-efficient brain," *Omni.* 14(Feb. 1992)16.

National Institute of Medicine press release, "New Findings Suggest Possible Link Between DPT Vaccine and Certain Forms of Brain Dysfunction in Rare Cases," (March 2, 1994).

Nelson, L.M., et al., "Risk of multiple sclerosis exacerbation during pregnancy and breast-feeding," *JAMA,* 259(1988)3441.

Ohman, J., Servo, A., Heiskanen, D., "Risk factors for cerebral infarction in good-grade patients after neurysmal subarachnoid hemorrhage and surgery: A prospective study," *Journal of Neurosurgery.* 74(1991)14.

Ornstein, Robert, and Thompson, Richard F., *The Amazing Brain.* Boston: Houghton Mifflin, 1984.

Ornstein, Robert, and Sobel, David, *The Healing Brain.* New York: Simon & Schuster, 1987.

Patchell, R.A., et al., "A randomized trial of surgery in the treatment of single metastasis to the brain," *New England Journal of Medicine,* 332(1990)494.

Paty, D.W., et al., "MRI in diagnosis of MS: A prospective study with comparison of clinical evaluation, evoked potentials, oligoclonal banding and CT," *Neurology,* 38(1988)180.

Peitersen, E., "The natural history of Bell's palsy," *American Journal of Otology.* 4(1982)107.

Pennisi, Elizabeth, "Memory loss tied to stress . . . and to shrinking brains" *Science News.* 144(Oct. 10, 1993)332.

_____ , "Food cravings tied to brain chemicals," *Science News.* 144(Nov. 13, 1993)310.

_____ , "Color-By-Number neurons," *Science News.* 144(Nov. 20, 1993),332.

_____ , "Microglial madness: When the brain's immune system turns from friend to foe," *Science News.* 144(Dec. 4, 1993)378–9.

_____ , "A molecular whodunit: new twists in the Alzheimer's mystery," *Science News.* 145(Jan. 1, 1994)8–11.

_____ , "Seeing synapses: New ways to study nerves," *Science News.* (Jan. 26, 1994)135.

_____ , "Is this the way Bobby Fisher does it?" *Science News.* 145(May 21, 1994)327.

_____ , "Fragile X repeats clog protein synthesis," *Science News.* (Sept. 3, 1994)157.

_____ , "Mice, flies share memory molecule," *Science News* 146(Oct. 15, 1994)244.

_____ , "One team, two clues in Alzheimer's puzzle," *Science News.* 146(Nov. 11, 1994)308–9.

Pfister, H.W., Feiden, W., and Einhaupl, K.M., "Spectrum of complications during bacterial meningitis in adults: Results of a prospective clinical trial," *Archives of Neurology,* 50(1993)575.

Pipitone, Paul, "Flawed Neurotrauma treatment," *Headlines.* 3:2(March/April 1992)26.

_____ , "Medication to cross the blood-brain barrier," *Headlines.* 3:2(March/April 1992)26.

_____ , "Chemical block to nerve cell regeneration discovered," *Headlines.* 3:2(March/April 1992)27.

_____ , "Study on substance abuse and brain injury," *Headlines.* 3:2(March/April 1992)27.

_____ , "Brain reorganization explored in stroke recovery," *Headlines.* 3:2(March/April 1992)27.

Polich, John, "Cognitive Brain Potentials," *Current Directions in Psychological Science,* 2/6(Dec. 1993)175–9.

Porter, S.B., and Sande, M., "Toxoplasmosis of the central nervous system in the acquired immunodeficiency syndrome," *New England Journal of Medicine,* 327(1992):1643.

Raloff, Janet, "Brain Warping," *Science News.* 144(Dec. 11, 1993)392–4.

_____ , "Brain warping: will electronic idiot savants become a doctor's best friends?" *Science News.* 144(Dec. 11, 1993)392–4.

_____ "Lead may foster immune attack on brain," *Science News.* 147(Jan. 14, 1995)23.

_____ , "Drug of darkness: can a pineal hormone head off everything from breast cancer to aging?" *Science News.* 147(May 13, 1995)300–1.

" 'Reading minds' the autistic way," *Science News.* 148(June 17, 1995)381.

Rennie, John, "Kitty, we shrunk your brain," *Scientific American.* 268(April 1993)29.

Restak, Richard M., *Receptors.* New York: Bantam, 1995.

Richardson, J.P., and Knight, A.L., "The

prevention of tetanus in the elderly," *Archives of Internal Medicine*. 151(9)(1991)1712.

Robb-Nicholson, Celeste (ed.), "Migraine," *Harvard Women's Health Watch*. July 1995, pp. 2–3.

Rose, Steven, *The Conscious Brain*. New York: Alfred A. Knopf, 1973.

Rosebush, P., and Stewart, T.A., "Prospective analysis of 24 episodes of neuroleptic malignant syndrome," *American Journal of Psychiatry*. 146(1989)717.

Rosenberg, R. (ed), *Comprehensive Neurology*. New York: Raven Press, 1991.

Rosenthal, Elizabeth, "Dead complicated," *Discover*. 13(October 1992)28–30.

Samuels, Martin A. (ed.), *Manual of Neurologic Therapeutics* (5th ed.). Boston: Little, Brown and Co., 1995.

Sande, M.A., and Volberding, P.A. (eds.), *The Medical Management of AIDS* (2nd ed). Philadelphia: W.B. Saunders, 1990.

Sanders, Kenton, "Nitric oxide and the nervous system," *The Lancet*. 339(Jan. 4, 1992)50–1.

Schieber, Marc, and Hibbard, Lyndon, "How somatotopic is the motor cortex hand area?" *Science*. 261(July 23, 1993)489–92.

Schlaggar, Bradley, and O'Leary, Dennis, "Potential of visual cortex to develop an array of functional units unique to somatosensory cortex," *Science*. 252(June 14, 1991)1556–60.

Schmeck, Harold, "Study identifies part of brain as important site of anxiety," *The New York Times*. (Feb. 24, 1989)A13.

Schmoker, J.D., et al., "An analysis of the relationship between fluid and sodium administration and intracranial pressure after head injury," *Head Trauma*, 33(1992)476.

Schneider, L.S., Pollock, V.E., and Lyness, S.A., "A meta-analysis of controlled trials of neuroleptic treatment in dementia," *Journal of the American Geriatric Society*. 38(1990)553.

Science News editors, "Making cerebral sense of words," *Science News*. 147(March 11, 1995)157.

_____ , "Brain's singular way with language," *Science News*. 147(April 1, 1995)202.

_____ , "EMFs on the brain?" *Science News*. 147(April 1, 1995)44.

_____ , "Molecular clue to schizophrenia," *Science News*. 147(April 1, 1995)202.

_____ , "Genetic hint to schizophrenia," *Science News*. 147(May 13, 1995)297.

_____ , "Lucky catch: Reeling in the reeler gene," *Science News*. 147(May 13, 1995)297.

_____ , "Unexpected role for skin gene in brain," *Science News*. 147(May 13, 1995)297.

_____ , "Another round in the prion debate," *Science News*. 147(June 17, 1995)383.

_____ , " 'Reading minds' the autistic way," *Science News*. 147(June 17, 1995)381.

_____ , "Chlordane's lingering neurotoxicity," *Science News*. 148(July 15, 1995)47.

_____ , "Do songbirds sing of Alzheimer's?" *Science News*. 148(Aug. 26, 1995)139.

_____ , "Stealth surgery on brain tissue," *Science News*. 148(Aug. 26, 1995)137.

Scriver, Charles R., "Phenylketonuria—genotypes and phenotypes," *The New England Journal of Medicine*. 324(May 2, 1991) 1280–1.

Seachrist, Lisa, "Gene for early, aggressive Alzheimer's," *Science News*. 148(July 8, 1995)23.

_____ , "Mimicking the brain: using computers to investigate neurological disorders," *Science News*. 148(July 22, 1995)62–3.

Selkoe, Dennis, "Amyloid protein and Alzheimer's disease," *Scientific American*. 265(Nov. 1991)68–76.

_____ , "Aging brain, aging mind," *Scientific American*. 267(Sept. 1992)134–42.

Seligman, Martin, and Yellen, Amy, "What is a dream?" *Behavioral Research Therapy*. 25:1(1987)1–24.

Service, Robert, "Making modular memories," *Science*. 260(June 25, 1993)1876.

Shah, A., and Lisak, R.P., "Immunopharma-cologic therapy in myasthenia gravis," *Clinical Neuropharmacology.* 16(2)1993,97.

Shreeve, James, and Crabb, Charlene, "Touching the phantom," *Discover.* 14 (June 1993)34–42.

Siegel, Jerome, Nienhuis, Robert, et al., "Neuronal activity in narcolepsy: identifi-cation of cataplexy-related cells in the me-dial medulla," *Science.* 252(May 31, 1991)1315–8.

Simon, R.H., and Syre, J.T., *Strategy in Head Injury Management.* Norwalk, CT: Ap-pleton & Lange, 1987.

Simpson, D.M., and Wolfe, D.E., "Neuro-muscular complications of HIV infection and its treatment," *AIDS.* 5(1991)917.

Skinner, Karen, "The chemistry of learning and memory," *Chemical and Engineering News,* 69(Oct. 7, 1991)24–42.

Skolnick, Andrew, "New ultrasound evi-dence appears to link prenatal brain dam-age, cerebral palsy," *JAMA.* 265(Feb. 28, 1991)948–9.

———, "Magnetic resonance spectroscopy may offer early look at HIV disease-mediated changes in brain," *JAMA.* 269(March 3, 1993)1084.

"Sleep no more: role of the superchiasmatic nuclei in the sleep-wake cycle," *Discover.* 14(July 1993)14–5.

Snell, Richard S., *Neuroanatomy.* Boston: Lit-tle, Brown and Co., 1992.

Squire, Larry, and Zola-Morgan, Stuart, "The medial temporal lobe memory sys-tem," *Science.* 253(Sept. 20, 1991)1380–6.

Starkstein, S.E., et al., "Mania after brain injury: Neurological and metabolic find-ings," *Annals of Neurology,* 27(1990)652.

Steen, Edwin B., and Montagu, Ashley, *Anatomy and Physiology.* New York: Harper & Row, 1985.

Steering Committee of the Physicians' health study Research Group, "Final report on the aspirin component of the ongoing phy-sicians' health study," *New England Journal of Medicine.* 321(1989)129.

Stein, Douglas, "Compulsive eating, ritual, and addiction: Outside suggestions may trigger 'pig-out' brain programs," *Omni.* 16(November 1993)14.

Steriade, Mircea, McCormick, David, and Sejnowski, Terrence, "Thalamocortical os-cillations in the sleeping and aroused brain," *Science.* 262(Oct. 29, 1993)679–85.

Stipp, David, "Partial recall: amnesia studies show brain can be taught at subconscious level," *The Wall Street Journal* (Oct. 5, 1993)A1(E).

Stroebel, G., "Tracing Earliest Neurons' Mi-gration," *Science News.* 144(11/13/93)308.

Suplee, Curt, "Physiology: Art of motor neuron maintenance," *The Washington Post.* 118(June 12, 1995)A2.

Sussman, Vic, "The art of staying alive: resus-citation attempts usually fail," *U.S. News & World Report.* 115(Oct. 18, 1993)70–1.

Tarleton, J.C., and Saul, R.A., "Molecular genetic advances in fragile-X syndrome," *Journal of Pediatrics,* 122(1993)169.

Temkin, N.R., et al., "A randomized, double blind study of phenytoin for the pre-vention of post-traumatic seizures," *New England Journal of Medicine,* 323(1990)497.

"Thalamic lesions in infancy," (editorial) *The Lancet.* 339(May 9, 1992)1143–5.

"This is your brain on alcohol," *Consumer Reports on Health.* (March 1994)34.

Thompson, Larry, "Healy approves an un-proven treatment," *Science.* 259(Jan. 8, 1993)172.

Tomlinson, Elaine, *Children with Cerebral Palsy: A Parent's Guide.* Kensington, MD: Woodbine, 1990.

"Tracking the brain's language streams," *Sci-ence News.* 143(June 19, 1993)399.

Travis, J., "Alzheimer's mice betray cognitive drop," *Science News.* 147(June 10, 1995)358.

———, "Brain scans hint why elderly forget faces," *Science News.* 148(July 15, 1995)36.

_____ , "One Alzheimer's gene leads to another," *Science News*. ;148(Aug. 19, 1995)118.

"Triple Tourette's," *Science News*. (Feb. 24, 1990).

Troost, B.T., and Patton, J.M., "Exercise therapy for positional vertigo," *Neurology*. 42:1441, 1992.

Trotter, Bob, "Better memory through chemistry," *American Health*. 10(April 1991)12.

UC Berkeley Wellness Letter editors, "A lousy story," *UC Berkeley Wellness Letter*. May 1995, p. 6.

Van der Meche, F.G.A., Schmitz, P.I.M., and the Dutch-Guillain-Barre Study Group, "A randomized trial comparing intravenous immune globulin and plasma exchange in Guillain-Barre syndrome," *New England Journal of Medicine*. 326(17)(1992)1123.

Vecht, C.J., et al., "Treatment of single brain metastasis: Radiotherapy alone or combined with surgery?" *Annals of Neurology*, 33(1993)583.

Victor, M., Adams, R.D., and Collins, G.H., *The Wernicke-Korsakoff Syndrome and Related Neurological Disorders* (2nd ed.). Philadelphia: Davis, 1989.

Victor, Susanne, and Lausberg, Gerhard, "Malignant glioma of the brain: a study of 100 operated patients," *JAMA*. 267(Feb. 5, 1992)642.

Wappner, R.S., "Biochemical diagnosis of genetic diseases," *Pediatric Annals*. 22(1993)282.

Watson, Ronald R., "Caffeine: Is it dangerous to health?" *American Journal of Health Promotion*. 2:4(Spring 1988)13–21.

Weiner, William J., and Goetz, Christopher G., *Neurology for the Non-Neurologist* (3rd ed.). Philadelphia: J.B. Lippincott Co., 1994.

Weiner, William J., and Singer, C., "Parkinson's disease and nonpharmacologic treatment programs," *Journal of the American Geriatric Society*. 37(1989)359.

_____ , *Emergency and Urgent Neurology*. Philadelphia: J.B. Lippincott, 1992.

Weiss, Rick, "Human brain neurons grown in culture," *Science News*. 137(May 5, 1990)276.

_____ , "Brain chemical offers hope for treating nerve disorders," *The Washington Post*. 118(Jan. 26, 1995).

Welch, K.M.A., "The therapeutics of migraine," *Current Opinions in Neurological Neurosurgery*. 6:264, 1993.

"What has four legs . . ." *Time*. 140(Sept. 14, 1992)20.

Whitley, R.J., "Viral encephalitis," *New England Journal of Medicine*, 323(1990)242.

Wilkins, R. H., and Rengachary, S.S. (eds.), *Neurosurgery*. New York: McGraw-Hill, 1985.

Williams, R.L., and Karacan, I., *Sleep Disorders: Diagnosis and Treatment*. New York: John Wiley, 1978.

Wilson, F., Scalaidhe, S., and Goldman-Rakic, P., "Dissociation of object and spatial processing domains in primate prefrontal cortex," *Science*. 260(June 25, 1993)1955–8.

Winckelgren, Ingrid, "How the brain 'sees' borders where there are none," *Science*. 256(June 12, 1992)1520–1.

Wolpow, Edward R., "After the fall: Mild head injury," *Harvard Health Letter*. 16(April 1991)1–3.

Wright, James E., "Exercise and your brain: Can you prepare for a peak performance?" *Shape*. 12(April 1993)54–5.

Wu, C., "Sometimes a bigger brain isn't better," *Science News*. 148(Aug. 19, 1995) 116.

Youmans, J.R. (ed.), *Neurological Surgery*. Philadelphia: Saunders, 1982.

Yu, R.K., et al., "Autoimmune mechanism in peripheral neuropathies, *Annals of Neurology*. 27(Suppl.)(1990)S30.

APPENDIX A: SELF-HELP ORGANIZATIONS (PARTIAL LIST)

ACOUSTIC NEUROMA

Acoustic Neuroma Association
PO Box 398
Carlisle, PA 17013
(803) 280-5715

ALZHEIMER'S DISEASE

Alzheimer's Association
919 N. Michigan Ave., Ste. 1000
Chicago, IL 60611
(312) 335-8700

Alzheimer's Disease and Related Disorders Assoc.
70 East Lake St.
Chicago, IL 60601
(800) 621-0379; (312) 496-9265

Alzheimer's Disease International
919 N. Michigan Ave., No. 1000
Chicago, IL 60611
(312) 335-5777

Alzheimer's Foundation, The
8177 South Harvard
M/C 114
Tulsa, OK 74137
(918) 631-3665

AMYOTROPHIC LATERAL SCLEROSIS

Amyotrophic Lateral Sclerosis Association
21021 Ventura Blvd. #321
Woodland Hills, CA 91364
(818) 340-7500; (800) 782-4747

ALS Research Foundation
Pacific Medical Center
PO Box 7999
San Francisco, CA 94120
(415) 923-3604

ATAXIA

National Ataxia Foundation
600 Twelve Oaks Center
15500 Wayzata Boulevard
Wayzata, MN 55391
(612) 473-7666

Friedreich's Ataxia Group in America
PO Box 116
Oakland, CA 94611
(415) 655-0833

ATTENTION DEFICIT DISORDER/HYPERACTIVITY
(see also Learning Disabilities)

Center for Hyperactive Child Information
PO Box 66272
Washington, DC 20035
(703) 920-7495

Children and Adults with Attention Deficit
Disorder
499 NW 70th Ave., Ste. 308
Plantation, FL 33317

Coalition for the Education and Support of
Attention Deficit Disorder
PO Box 242
Osseo, MI 55369
(612) 425-0423

Council for the Education and Support of
Attention Deficit Disorder
PO Box 242
Osseo, MI 55369
(612) 425-0423

Council for Learning Disabilities
PO Box 40303
Overland Park, KS 66204
(913) 492-8755

Learning Disabilities Association of America
4516 Library Rd.
Pittsburgh, PA 15234
(412) 341-1515

National Attention-Deficit Disorder Association
PO Box 488
West Newbury, MA 01985
(508) 462-0495; (800) 487-2282

National Center for Learning Disabilities
381 Park Ave. S., Ste. 1420
New York, NY 10016
(212) 545-7510

National Networker
PO Box 32611
Phoenix, AZ 85064
(602) 941-5112

Time Out to Enjoy (TOTE)
c/o CDR
208 S. La Salle, No. 1330
Chicago, IL 60604
(312) 444-9484

AUTISM

Autism Network International
PO Box 1545
Lawrence, KS 66044

Autism Services Center
605 9th St.
PO Box 507
Huntington, WVA 25710
(304) 525-8014

Autism Society of America
1234 Massachusetts Ave. NW
Suite 1017
Washington, DC 20005
(301) 657-0881; (800) 3-AUTISM

BATTEN'S DISEASE

Batten's Disease Support and Research
    Association
2600 Parsons Ave.
Columbus, OH 43207
(800) 448-4570

BIRTH DEFECTS

March of Dimes Birth Defects Foundation
1275 Mamaroneck Ave.
White Plains, NY 10605
(914) 428-7100

BRAIN DAMAGE

The Family Survival Project for Brain-Damaged
    Adults
(415) 921-5400

National Brain Injury Research Foundation
1612 K St. NW, Ste. 204
Washington, DC 20006
(202) 331-8445

National Head Injury Foundation
333 Turnpike Road
Southboro, MA 01772
(617) 485-9950

BRAIN RESEARCH

Division of Basic Brain and Behavioral Sciences
National Institute of Mental Health

National Institute of Neurological Disorders and
    Stroke
9000 Rockville Pike
Building 31, Room 8A06
Bethesda, MD 20892
(301) 496-5751

Brain Information Service
43-367 CHS/UCLA School of Medicine
Los Angeles, CA 90024
(310) 825-3417

National Brain Injury Research Foundation
1612 K St. NW, Ste. 204
Washington, DC 20006
(202) 331-8445

National Foundation for Brain Research
1250 24th St. NW, Ste. 300
Washington, DC 20037
(202) 293-5453

BRAIN TUMORS

Acoustic Neuroma Association
PO Box 398
Carlisle, PA 17013
(717) 249-4783

American Brain Tumor Association
2720 River Road
Des Plaines, IL 60018
(800) 886-2282

Association for Brain Tumor Research
2910 West Montrose Ave.
Chicago, IL 60618
(312) 286-5571

Brain Tumor Foundation for Children
751 DeKalb Industrial Way
Decatur, GA 30033
(414) 292-3536

Brain Tumor Society
60 Birmingham Parkway
Boston, MA 02135
(617) 783-0340

Elekta
8 Executive Park West
Atlanta, GA 30329
(800) 535-7355

Friends of Brain Tumor Research
2169 Union St.
San Francisco, CA 94123
(415) 563-0466

National Brain Tumor Foundation
323 Geary St.
Suite 510
San Francisco, CA 94102
(800) 934-CURE

National Cancer Institute
(800) 4-CANCER

NIH Neurology Institute/Brain Tumor
Box 5801
Bethesda, MD 20824
(800) 352-9424

CEREBRAL PALSY

National Association of Sports for Cerebral Palsy
66 E. 34th St.
New York, NY 10016
(212) 481-6300

United Cerebral Palsy Association
7 Penn Plaza, Suite 804
New York, NY 10010
(212) 268-6655; (800) USA-SUCP; (717) 396-7965
    (for publication list)

United States Cerebral Palsy Athletic Association
34518 Warren Rd., Ste. 264
Westland, MI 48185
(313) 425-8961

CRANIOSYNOSTOSIS

Society for Children with Craniosynostosis
PO Box 1522
Denver, CO 80201
(303) 722-9992

CRI DU CHAT SYNDROME

5p- Society
11609 Oakmont
Overland Park, KS 66210
(913) 469-8900

DEVELOPMENTAL DISABILITIES
(see Down Syndrome; Mental Retardation)

DOWN SYNDROME

Association for Children with Down Syndrome
2616 Martin Ave.
Bellmore, Long Island, NY 11710
(516) 221-4700

Down's Syndrome International
11 N. 73rd Terrace, Rm. K
Kansas City, KS 66111
(913) 299-0815

National Association for Down Syndrome
PO Box 4542
Oakbrook, IL 60521
(312) 325-9112

National Down's Syndrome Adoption Exchange
(914) 428-1236

National Down Syndrome Congress
1605 Chantilly Dr., Suite 250
Atlanta, GA 30324
(800) 232-6372; (404) 633-1555

National Down Syndrome Society
666 Broadway
New York, NY 10012
(212) 460-9330; (800) 221-4602 (except New York);
    (800) 460-9330 in New York

Parents of Children with Down Syndrome
c/o Association for Retarded Citizens
11600 Nebel St.
Rockville, MD 20852
(301) 984-5792

DYSAUTONOMIA

Dysautonomia Foundation
20 E. 46th St., 3rd fl.
New York, NY 10017
(212) 949-6644

EPILEPSY

Epilepsy Concern Service Group
1282 Wynnewood Dr.
West Palm Beach, FL 33417
(407) 683-0044

Epilepsy Foundation of America
4351 Garden City Dr., Suite 406
Landover, MD 20785
(301) 459-3700; (800) EFA-1000

GUILLAIN-BARRE SYNDROME

Guillain-Barre Syndrome Foundation
International
PO Box 262
Wynnewood, PA 19096
(215) 667-0131

HEADACHE

National Headache Foundation
5252 N. Western Ave.
Chicago, IL 60625
(800) 843-2256; (800) 523-8858 in IL

American Council for Headache Education
(ACHE)
Suite 200
875 Kings Highway
Woodbury, NJ 08096
(800) 255-ACHE

HEAD INJURY

National Head Injury Foundation
333 Turnpike Rd.
Southboro, MA 01772
(617) 485-9950

HUNTINGTON'S DISEASE

Hereditary Disease Foundation
606 Wilshire Blvd., Suite 504
Beverly Hills, CA 90401
(213) 458-4183

Huntington's Disease Society of America
140 West 22nd St.
New York, NY 10011
(800) 345-4372; (212) 242-1968 in NY

Huntington Society of Canada
Box 333
Cambridge, Ontario
CANADA N1R 5T8

HYDROCEPHALUS

Guardians of Hydrocephalus Research
Foundation
2618 Avenue Z
Brooklyn, NY 11235
(718) 743-GHRF; (800) 458-8655

National Hydrocephalus Foundation
Rte. 1, River Road
Box 210A
Joliet, IL 60436
(815) 467-6548

JOSEPH DISEASE

International Joseph Disease Foundation
PO Box 2550
Livermore, CA 94551
(510) 443-4600

LEARNING DISORDERS

Association for Children and Adults with
Learning Disabilities
4156 Library Rd.
Pittsburgh, PA 15234
(412) 341-1515

AVKO Educational Research Foundation
3084 W. Willard Rd.
Birch Run, MI 48415
(313) 686-9283

Council for Learning Disabilities
9013 West Brooke Drive
Overland Park, KS 66212
(913) 492-3840

National Center for Learning Disabilities
99 Park Ave., 6th Flr.
New York, NY 10016
(212) 687-7211

Orton Dyslexia Society, The
724 York Rd.
Baltimore, MD 21204
(800) ABCD-123; (301) 296-0232

SAT Admissions Testing Program for
Handicapped Students
CN 6603
Princeton, NJ 08541
(609) 734-5068

LEUKODYSTROPHY

United Leukodystrophy Foundation
2304 Highland Dr. Sycamore, IL 60178
(815) 895-3211

MENTAL HEALTH/MENTAL ILLNESS

American Mental Health Association
1021 Prince St.
Alexandria, VA 22314
(703) 684-7722; (800) 433-5959

National Alliance for the Mentally Ill
2101 Wilson Blvd., Ste. 302
Arlington, VA 22201
(703) 524-7600

Mental Illness Foundation
370 7th Ave., Ste. 222
New York, NY 10024
(212) 629-0755

MENTAL RETARDATION
(See also DOWN SYNDROME)

American Network of Community Options
and Resources
4200 Evergreen Ln, Ste. 315
Annandale, VA 22003
(703) 642-6614

Association for Retarded Citizens
500 E. Border St.
Ste. 300
Arlington, TX 76010
(817) 261-6003

Association for Children with Retarded
Mental Development
162 5th Ave., 11th Flr.
New York, NY 10010
(212) 741-0100; (800) WOW-ACRM

Fragile X Foundation
PO Box 30023
Denver, CO 80203
(800) 835-2246, x. 58

Fragile X Support
1380 Huntington Dr.
Mundelein, IL 60060
(312) 680-3317

People First International
PO Box 12642
Salem, OR 97309
(503) 362-0336

Pilot Parents
3610 Dodge St., Ste. 101
Omaha, NE 68131

Special Olympics
1350 New York Ave., NW, Ste. 500
Washington, DC 20005
(202) 628-3630

MIGRAINE

National Migraine Foundation
5252 North Western Ave.
Chicago, IL 60625
(312) 878-7715

MULTIPLE SCLEROSIS

National Multiple Sclerosis Society
205 East 42nd St.
New York, NY 10017
(212) 986-3240; (800) 624-8236

Multiple Sclerosis Foundation
6350 N. Andrews Ave.
Fort Lauderdale, FL 33309
(305) 776-6805; (800) 441-7055

MUSCULAR DYSTROPHY

MD Association
810 Seventh Ave.
New York, NY 10019
(212) 586-0808

NARCOLEPSY
(see SLEEP DISORDERS)

NEUROFIBROMATOSIS

National Neurofibromatosis Foundation
141 5th Ave.
Suite 7-S
New York, NY 10010
(212) 460-8980

PAIN

Chronic Pain Outreach
822 Wycliff Ct.
Manassas, VA 22110
(703) 368-7357

National Chronic Pain Outreach
    Association, Inc.
4922 Hampden Lane
Bethesda, MD 20814
(301) 652-4948

PARKINSON'S DISEASE

American Parkinson Disease Association
116 John St.
Suite 417
New York, NY 10038
(718) 981-8001; (800) 223-APDA

National Parkinson Foundation
1501 NW Ninth Ave.
Miami, FL 33136
(800) 327-4545; (800) 433-7022 in FL;
    (305) 547-6666 in Miami

Parkinson Disease Foundation
Wm. Black Medical Bldg.
640 West 168th St.
New York, NY 10032
(212) 923-4700; (800) 457-6676

Parkinson's Educational Program
1800 Park Newport #302
Newport Beach, CA 92660
(800) 344-7872; (714) 640-0218 in CA

Parkinson Support Groups of America
11376 Cherry Hill Rd., #204
Beltsville, MD 20705
(301) 937-1545

United Parkinson Foundation
360 W. Superior St.
Chicago, IL 60610
(312) 664-2344

PHENYLKETONURIA (PKU)

PKU Parents
8 Myrtle Lane
San Anselmo, CA 94960
(415) 457-4632

RETT SYNDROME

International Rett Syndrome Association
8511 Rose Marie Dr.
Ft. Washington, MD 20744
(301) 856-3334

REYE'S SYNDROME

National Reye's Syndrome Foundation
426 North Lewis
Byran, OH 43506
(419) 636-2679; (800) 233-7393;
    (800) 231-7393 in OH

SCHIZOPHRENIA

American Schizophrenia Association
900 North Federal Highway, #330
Boca Raton, FL 33432
(407) 393-6167

National Alliance for Research on Schizophrenia
    and Depression
60 Cutter Mill Rd., Ste. 200
Great Neck, NY 11021
(516) 829-0091

SLEEP DISORDERS/NARCOLEPSY

American Narcolepsy Assn.
425 California St., #201
San Francisco, CA 94104
(415) 788-4793; (800) 222-6085

American Sleep Apnea Association
2700 E. Main St., Ste. 206
Columbus, OH 43209
(614) 239-4200

Association of Sleep Disorders Centers
604 2nd St., SW
Rochester, NY 55902
(507) 287-6006

Brain Information Service
43-367 CHS/UCLA School of Medicine
Los Angeles, CA 90024
(310) 825-3417

Narcolepsy and Cataplexy Foundation of
    America
1410 York Ave., Ste. 2D
Mail Box #22
New York, NY 10021
(212) 628-6315

SPINA BIFIDA

Spina Bifida Association of America
1700 Rockville Pike, Suite 250
Rockville, MD 20852
(301) 770-SBBA; (800) 621-3141

Spina Bifida Adoption Referral Program
1955 Florida Dr.
Xenia, OH 45385
(513) 372-2040

SPINAL INJURIES

American Paralysis Association
500 Morris Ave.
Springfield, NJ 07081
(800) 225-0292; (201) 379-2690 in NJ

American Spinal Injury Association
250 E. Superior, Rm. 619
Chicago, IL 60611
(312) 908-3425

National Spinal Cord Injury Hotline
c/o American Paralysis Association
PO Box 187
Short Hills, NJ 07078
(800) 526-3456

National Spinal Cord Injury Association
600 West Cummings Park
Suite 2000
Woburn, MA 01801
(617) 964-0521; (800) 962-9629

Paralyzed Veterans of America
801 18th St., NW
Washington, DC 20006
(202) 872-1300

Spinal Cord Society
Wendell Rd.
Fergus Falls, MN 56537
(218) 739-5252

STROKE

American Heart Association
7272 Greenville Ave.
Dallas, TX 75231
(800) 242-8721; (214) 750-5300

National Stroke Association
300 East Hampden Ave., Suite 240
Englewood, CO 80110
(800)-STROKES; (303) 771-1700

National Institute of Neurological Disorders
and Stroke
Building 31
Room 8A-06
9000 Rockville Pike
Bethesda, MD 20892
(800) 352-9424

Stroke Clubs International
805 12th St.
Galveston, TX 77550
(409) 762-1022

STURGE-WEBER SYNDROME

Sturge-Weber Foundation
PO Box 460931
Aurora, CO 80015
(800) 627-5482; (303) 369-7290

TARDIVE DYSKINESIA/DYSTONIA

Tardive Dyskinesia/Tardive Dystonia National
Association
4244 University Way, Northeast
PO Box 45732
Seattle, WA 98145
(206) 522-3166

TAY-SACHS

National Tay-Sachs and Allied Diseases
Association, Inc.
2001 Beacon St.
Brookline, MA 02146
(617) 277-4463

TOURETTE SYNDROME

Tourette Syndrome Association
42-40 Bell Blvd.
Bayside, NY 11361
(718) 224-2999; (800) 237-0717

Tourette Syndrome Foundation of Canada
173 Owen Boulevard
Willowdale, Ontario
CANADA M2P 1GB

TREMOR

International Tremor Foundation
360 West Superior St.
Chicago, IL 60610
(312) 664-2344

TRIGEMINAL NEURALGIA ASSOCIATION

PO Box 785
Barnegat Light, NJ 08006
(609) 361-1014

TUBEROUS SCLEROSIS

National Tuberous Sclerosis Association
8000 Corporate Dr., Ste. 120
Landover, MD 20785
(800) 225-6872; (301) 459-9888

APPENDIX B. PROFESSIONAL ORGANIZATIONS

American Academy of Cerebral Palsy and
   Developmental Medicine
1910 Byrd Ave., Suite 118, PO Box 11086
Richmond, VA 23230
(804) 282-0036

American Academy of Neurological and
   Orthopaedic Surgeons
2320 Rancho Dr., Ste. 108
Las Vegas, NV 89102
(702) 385-6886

American Academy of Neurological Surgery
Dept. of Neurosurgery
Temple University Hospital
3401 N. Broad St.
Philadelphia, PA 19140
(215) 221-4068

American Academy of Somnology
PO Box 29124
Las Vegas, NV 89126
(702) 594-5746

American Association of Neurological Surgeons
22 S. Washington St., Ste. 100
Park Ridge, IL 60068
(708) 692-9500

American Board of Neurological Microsurgery
2320 Rancho Dr., Ste. 108
Las Vegas, NV 89102
(702) 385-6886

American Board of Neurological and Orthopedic
   Medicine and Surgery
2320 Rancho Dr., Ste. 108
Las Vegas, NV 89102
(702) 385-6886

American Board of Orthopaedic
   Microneurosurgery
2320 Rancho Dr., Ste. 108
Las Vegas, NV 89102
(702) 385-6886

American Epilepsy Society
638 Prospect Ave.
Hartford, CT 06105
(203) 232-4825

American Neurological Association
2221 University Ave. SE, Ste. 350
Minneapolis, MN 55414
(612) 378-3290

American Pain Society
5700 Old Orchard Rd., first floor
Skokie, IL 60077
(708) 966-5595

American Society for Clinical Evoked Potentials
14 Soundview Ave., No. 51
White Plains, NY 10606
(914) 761-4713

American Society for Stereotactic and Functional
   Neurosurgery
6550 Fannin St., No. 2139
Houston, TX 77030
(713) 790-6015

Association of Sleep Disorders Centers
604 2nd St., SW
Rochester, MN 55902
(507) 287-6006

AVKO Education Research Foundation
3084 West Willard Rd.
Birch Run, MI 48415
(313) 686-9283

Cajal Club
c/o Dr. David Whitlock
Univ. of Colorado Health Sciences Center
Dept. of Cellular & Structural Biology, B-111
4200 E. 9th Ave.
Denver, CO 80262
(303) 270-8201

Child Neurology Society
475 Cleveland Ave. N., Ste. 220
St. Paul, MN 55104
(612) 641-1584

Congress of Neurological Surgeons
506 Oak St.
Cincinnati, OH 45219
(513) 872-2657

Council for Learning Disabilities
9013 West Brooke Dr.
Overland Park, KS 66212
(913) 492-3840

Hereditary Disease Foundation
1427 7th St., Ste. 2
Santa Monica, CA 90401
(213) 458-4183

International Academy for Child Brain
 Development
8801 Stenton Ave.
Philadelphia, PA 19118
(215) 233-2050

International Association for the Study of Pain
909 NE 43rd St., Ste. 306
Seattle, WA 98105
(206) 547-6409

International Federation of Clinical
 Neurophysiology
6550 Fannin St., No. 2139
Houston, TX 77030
(713) 790-6015

International Neural Network Society
1250 24th St., Ste. 300
Washington, DC 20037
(202) 466-4667

International Pain Foundation
909 NE 43rd St., Ste. 306
Seattle, WA 98105
(206) 547-2157

National Coalition for Research in Neurological
 Disorders
1250 24th St., NW, Ste. 600

Washington, DC 20037
(202) 293-5453

National Committee on the Treatment of
 Intractable Pain
1333 New Hampshire Ave., NW
Washington, DC 20036
(202) 452-4836

Neurodevelopmental Treatment Association
PO Box 70
Oak Park, IL 60303
(708) 386-2454

Neurosurgical Society of America
2074 Abington Rd.
Cleveland, OH 44106
(216) 844-5949

Society of Neurological Surgeons
750 Washington St.
Box 178
Boston, MA 02111
(617) 956-5858

Society of Neurosurgical Anesthesia and Critical
 Care (SNACC)
11512 Allecingie Pky.
Richmond, VA 23235
(804) 379-5513

World Federation of Neurosurgical Societies
5841 S. Maryland Ave.
Chicago, IL 60637
(312) 702-6158

APPENDIX C. GOVERNMENTAL ORGANIZATIONS

National Institute on Aging
9000 Rockville Pike
Bethesda, MD 20205
(301) 496-9265

National Institute of Neurological Disorders and
    Stroke
National Institutes of Health
9000 Rockville Pike
Building 31, Room 8A-16
Bethesda, MD 20205
(301) 496-5751

INDEX

This index is designed to be used in conjunction with the many cross-references within the A-to-Z entries. The main A-to-Z entries are indicated by **boldface** page references. The general subjects are subdivided by the A-to-Z entries. Tables are indicated by "t" following the page locator and glossary items by "g".

A

AAMI *see* age-associated memory impairment
abducent nerve **1**
abortive poliomyelitis 206
ABR test *see* auditory brainstem response (ABR) test
abscess, brain **1**
absolute refractory period 274g
Academy of Aphasia **1**
acalculia **1**
acetaminophen 114
acetylcholine **1–2**, 274g *see also* anticholinergics; cholinergic
  aging 5
  Alzheimer's disease 14
  basal forebrain 40
  learning 141
  neurotransmitter actions 188t
  nimodipine 189
  nucleus basalis of Meynert 191
  parasympathetic nervous system 197
  scopolamine 220
  tetrahydroaminoacridine 249
  vagus nerve 262
acetylcholinesterase 2, 16, 17
acetyl coenzyme A 66
ACHE *see* American Council for Headache Education
acoustic nerve 2, **2**, 117
acoustic neuroma **2–3**, 287
Acoustic Neuroma Association 3, 287, 288
acoustic reflex 3
acromegaly 111, 205
ACTH *see* adrenocorticotropic hormone
acute idiopathic polyneuritis *see* Guillain-Barre syndrome
acyclovir 90
ADC *see* AIDS dementia complex
ADD *see* Children and Adults with Attention Deficit Disorder
addiction **3–4**, 166 *see also specific drug*; substance abuse
adenosine triphosphate (ATP) **4**, 107, 127
Ader, Robert 127
ADH *see* vasopressin
ADHD *see* attention deficit hyperactivity disorder

adrenal glands 94, 179
adrenaline *see* epinephrine
adrenergic hormones 238
adrenocorticotropic hormone (ACTH) **4**, 73, 101
AEP *see* auditory-evoked potentials
aerobic exercise 96
Africa 230
African Americans
  meningioma 157
  multiple sclerosis 168
  phenylketonuria 202
  stroke 240
age-associated memory impairment (AAMI) 15
aggression *see* fear and aggression
aging and the brain **5–6**, 12, 187
agnosia **6–7**
agraphia **7**, 32
AIDS and the brain **7**, 7t, 75
AIDS dementia complex (ADC) **7–8**, 7t
alcohol and the brain **8–11**, 9t
  addiction 3, 4
  appetite suppressants 31
  caffeine 54
  central nervous system depressants 59
  delirium tremens 78
  fetal alcohol syndrome 99–100
  Korsakoff's syndrome 135
  tremor 254
  vasopressin 263
  Wernicke-Korsakoff syndrome 269
alexia **11**
alkaloids *see* cocaine and the brain
alpha antagonists 246
alpha-fetoprotein 25
alpha waves **11**, 150
ALS *see* amyotrophic lateral sclerosis
ALS Forbes Norris Research Center **11**
ALS Research Foundation 287
aluminum 14
Alzheimer, Alois 12, 180
Alzheimer's Association **11–12**, 287
Alzheimer's disease **12–17**
  aging 5, 6
  amnesia in 22
  areas affected by
    basal forebrain 40
    nucleus basalis of Meynert 191

  biochemistry of
    acetylcholine 2
    calcium 55
    cholinergic hypothesis of Alzheimer's disease 66
    protein kinase C 211
  memory disorders in 156
  neurofibrillary tangles and 180
  self-help organizations 287
  treatment of
    choline 66
    Cognex 69
    dehydroepiandrosterone 77
    deprenyl 79
    estrogen 95
    ginkgo biloba 107
    Hydergine 123
    hyperzine A 124, 125
    indomethacin 127
    lecithin 142–143
    nerve-growth factor 178
    oxiracetam 194
    phosphatidylserine 202
    physostigmine 202
    pramiracetam 209
    pregnenolone 210
    tetrahydroaminoacridine 249
    vasopressin 262
    vincamine 264
Alzheimer's Disease and Related Disorders Association 287
Alzheimer's Disease International 17, 287
Alzheimer's Foundation, The 287
amantadine 60, 198, 246
ambenonium chloride (Mytelase) 170
amblyopia **17–18**
American Academy for Cerebral Palsy and Developmental Medicine 18, 295
American Academy of Neurological and Orthopaedic Surgeons 18, 295
American Academy of Neurological Surgery 18, 295
American Academy of Neurology 18
American Academy of Somnology **18–19**, 295
American Association of Neurological Surgeons 19, 295
American Bar Association 47